METHODS IN MOLECULAR BIOLOGY

Series Editor
John M. Walker
School of Life and Medical Sciences
University of Hertfordshire
Hatfield, Hertfordshire, UK

For further volumes:
http://www.springer.com/series/7651

For over 35 years, biological scientists have come to rely on the research protocols and methodologies in the critically acclaimed *Methods in Molecular Biology* series. The series was the first to introduce the step-by-step protocols approach that has become the standard in all biomedical protocol publishing. Each protocol is provided in readily-reproducible step-by-step fashion, opening with an introductory overview, a list of the materials and reagents needed to complete the experiment, and followed by a detailed procedure that is supported with a helpful notes section offering tips and tricks of the trade as well as troubleshooting advice. These hallmark features were introduced by series editor Dr. John Walker and constitute the key ingredient in each and every volume of the *Methods in Molecular Biology* series. Tested and trusted, comprehensive and reliable, all protocols from the series are indexed in PubMed.

Malaria Control and Elimination

Edited by

Frédéric Ariey

INSERM 1016 Institut Cochin, Service de Parasitologie-Mycologie, Université Paris Descartes, Hôpital Cochin, Paris, France

Frédérick Gay

Faculté de Médecine, AP-HP, Sorbonne Université, Groupe Hospitalier Pitié-Salpêtrière, Paris, France

Robert Ménard

Malaria Infection and Immunity Unit, Institut Pasteur, Paris, France

Humana Press

Editors
Frédéric Ariey
INSERM 1016 Institut Cochin
Service de Parasitologie-Mycologie
Université Paris Descartes
Hôpital Cochin
Paris, France

Frédérick Gay
Faculté de Médecine
AP-HP, Sorbonne Université
Groupe Hospitalier Pitié-Salpêtrière
Paris, France

Robert Ménard
Malaria Infection and Immunity Unit
Institut Pasteur
Paris, France

ISSN 1064-3745 ISSN 1940-6029 (electronic)
Methods in Molecular Biology
ISBN 978-1-4939-9549-3 ISBN 978-1-4939-9550-9 (eBook)
https://doi.org/10.1007/978-1-4939-9550-9

This Humana imprint is published by the registered company Springer Science+Business Media, LLC part of Springer Nature.
The registered company address is: 233 Spring Street, New York, NY 10013, U.S.A.

Preface

Great strides have been made in the last two decades in our capacity to fight malaria. At the fundamental level, the turn of the twenty-first century has witnessed many technical breakthroughs: the sequencing of the genomes of the three organisms (i.e., parasite, mosquito, and human) involved in the disease, molecular genetic tools to modify the parasite genome, and cell biological methods to characterize phenotypes. Together, these technological achievements have allowed for tremendous progress in our understanding of the infectious process and the host-parasite interactions involved. They have been the topic of a recent Springer book published in 2013, which was mainly aimed at laboratories working on basic malaria research.

At an applied level, controlling malaria worldwide has dramatically ameliorated since the early 2000s. The demonstration of the efficacy and large-scale use of insecticide-treated bed nets, the first-line use of artemisinin-based combination therapies, and the scale-up of effective intervention methods have all contributed to an important lessoning of the malaria burden during the first decade of this century. In just a few years, between 2010 and 2017, malaria morbidity decreased by 10% and mortality by 30% worldwide, despite an African population increase of about 20%. Excitingly, the momentum built around these successes has ushered in higher goals. In October 2007 at the Malaria Forum in Seattle, Bill and Melinda Gates called for the global eradication of malaria, which was instantaneously endorsed by the World Health Organization Director-General Margaret Chan.

Unfortunately, during the last few years, the news from the field revealed a halt in progress toward elimination. In the 2017 World Malaria Report, the WHO highlights the remarkable progress achieved in tackling one of humanity's oldest diseases, while also pointing out worrying trends. The global response to control malaria is at a crossroad, and there is an urgent need for remobilization; a second breath must be found. The gain in expertise accumulated so far, and especially during the last decades, must be the basis of a new era of malaria control and elimination.

The goal of this book is to provide a global overview of the goals, rationale, and scientific basis for malaria control and elimination, as well as tools, methods, and strategies to that end. Clearly, the issues relevant to such a vast topic are so numerous that their exhaustive presentation would exceed the size of a typical *Springer Protocols* book. Therefore, priority has been given to some of the most important and promising methods. With a few exceptions, most chapters of the book are in a discursive form rather than in the protocol format of the typical Methods in Molecular Biology books.

The book contains 20 chapters divided into six parts. Part 1 concentrates on malaria epidemiology. An opening chapter by the WHO recounts the history of major malaria elimination efforts and focuses on the current status of country-led and country-driven malaria elimination programs. The subsequent chapters in this section overview the current malaria situation in Africa, Asia-Oceania, and Latin America, addressing in each case the specific issues that need to be resolved to near or complete elimination regionally.

Part 2 focuses on some of the tools that are critical to malaria management: conventional and unconventional diagnostic methods, ELISA protocols to monitor antibodies to malarial antigens, and controlled human malaria infections (CHMI), a major recent technical advance that should greatly accelerate the validation of new malaria therapeutics and vaccines in humans.

Part 3 deals with antimalarial drugs and resistance to these drugs. It includes chapters on clinical trials for assessing the therapeutic efficacy of antimalarial drugs, the site-directed gene editing methods for dissecting antimalarial drug resistance, and the current understanding of the molecular basis of resistance to artemisinin. The section ends with a chapter summarizing the currently available antimalarial drugs for elimination programs and their implementation strategies.

Part 4 examines vaccination approaches against malaria. The section starts with a chapter on the preclinical and phase 1 and 2 clinical trials of vaccine development in general. The remaining chapters of the section present the current developmental status of RTS,S/AS01, the most advanced malaria vaccine, as well as the live preerythrocytic vaccines and blood-stage vaccines.

Part 5 centers on vector control and includes an overview of the use of insecticide-treated nets, a description of the methods for sampling *Anopheles* populations using traps, and an update on resistance to various insecticides.

Part 6 ends the book by presenting two personal perspectives, one on the hopes and disillusions of using herbal remedies against malaria in Madagascar and another on the currents that shaped past control strategies and the prospects for current ones.

Finally, we wish to sincerely thank the authors for their valuable contributions. We hope that this book will be useful to all those involved in malaria control and elimination worldwide, from students to health practitioners and field researchers, and that it will help them make malaria elimination a reality wherever possible.

Paris, France

Frédéric Ariey
Frédérick Gay
Robert Ménard

Contents

Contributors

PEDRO L. ALONSO • *Global Malaria Programme, World Health Organization, Geneva, Switzerland*

RAKOTONDRAFARA ANDRIAMALALA • *Institut Pasteur de Madagascar, Antananarivo, Madagascar; Centre National d'Application de Recherche Pharmaceutique, Antananarivo, Madagascar*

FRÉDÉRIC ARIEY • *INSERM 1016, Institut Cochin, Université Paris Descartes, Paris, France; Service de Parasitologie-Mycologie, Hôpital Cochin, Paris, France*

CÉCILE ARTAUD • *Centre de Recherche Translationnel, Institut Pasteur, Paris, France*

LAWRENCE AYONG • *Malaria Research Unit, Centre Pasteur du Cameroun, Yaoundé, Cameroon*

STEFFEN BORRMANN • *Institute for Tropical Medicine, Eberhard Karls University of Tübingen, Tübingen, Germany*

PAUL T. BREY • *Medical Entomology and Vector-Borne Disease Laboratory, Institut Pasteur du Laos, Vientiane, Laos*

PIERRE CARNEVALE • *Institut de Recherche pour le Développement (IRD), Portiragnes, France*

MARCIA C. CASTRO • *Department of Global Health and Population, Harvard T.H. Chan School of Public Health, Boston, MA, USA*

CHETAN E. CHITNIS • *Malaria Parasite Biology and Vaccines Unit, Department of Parasites and Insect Vectors, Institut Pasteur, Paris, France*

JEROME CLAIN • *UMR 261, IRD, Université Paris Descartes, Paris, France*

MEHUL J. DHORDA • *Mahidol-Oxford Tropical Medicine Research Unit, Faculty of Tropical Medicine, Mahidol University, Bangkok, Thailand; WorldWide Antimalarial Resistance Network–Asia Regional Centre, Bangkok, Thailand; Nuffield Department of Medicine, Centre for Tropical Medicine and Global Health, University of Oxford, Oxford, UK*

ARJEN M. DONDORP • *Mahidol-Oxford Tropical Medicine Research Unit, Faculty of Tropical Medicine, Mahidol University, Bangkok, Thailand; Nuffield Department of Medicine, Centre for Tropical Medicine and Global Health, University of Oxford, Oxford, UK*

CAROLE ELSE EBOUMBOU MOUKOKO • *Faculty of Medicine and Pharmaceutical Science, University of Douala, Douala, Cameroon*

MARCELO U. FERREIRA • *Department of Parasitology, Institute of Biomedical Sciences, University of São Paulo, São Paulo, SP, Brazil*

DAVID A. FIDOCK • *Department of Microbiology and Immunology, Columbia University Irving Medical Center, New York, NY, USA; Division of Infectious Diseases, Department of Medicine, Columbia University Irving Medical Center, New York, NY, USA*

GAWRIE LOKU GALAPPATHTHY • *Global Malaria Programme, World Health Organization, Geneva, Switzerland*

FRÉDÉRICK GAY • *UMR S 1136 équipe SUMO, Institut National de la Santé et de la Recherche Médicale (INSERM), Institut Pierre Louis d'Epidémiologie et de Santé Publique (iPLESP), Sorbonne Université, Paris, France; Assistance Publique Hôpitaux de Paris (AP-HP), Hôpital Pitié–Salpêtrière, Paris, France*

MAGELLAN GUEWO-FOKENG • *Department of Biochemistry, Faculty of Science, University of Yaoundé 1, Yaoundé, Cameroon*

ABDERAOUF HAMZA • *Université Paris Sud, Orsay, France; Service de Génétique Moléculaire, Hôpital Universitaire Necker-Enfants Malades, Paris, France*

ALEXANDRA HISCOX • *Laboratory of Entomology, Wageningen University and Research, Wageningen, Netherlands; International Centre of Insect Physiology and Ecology, Nairobi, Kenya*

XIAO HONG LI • *Global Malaria Programme, World Health Organization, Geneva, Switzerland*

ARSÈNE INDRIAMBELO • *Faculté des Sciences, Université de Toliara, Toliara, Madagascar; Institut Pasteur de Madagascar, Antananarivo, Madagascar*

GATHONI KAMUYU • *Centre for Infectious Diseases, Heidelberg University Hospital, Heidelberg, Germany*

LEILA KARA • *Université Paris-Descartes, Paris, France; INSERM CIC 1417, F-CRIN I-REIVAC, Paris, France; Assistance Publique Hôpitaux de Paris, Hôpital Cochin, Paris, France*

RINTER K. KIMATHI • *KEMRI Wellcome Trust Research Programme, Centre for Geographic Medicine Research-Coast, Kilifi, Kenya*

ASTRID KNOBLAUCH • *Faculté des Sciences, Université de Toliara, Toliara, Madagascar; Global Health Institute, Stony Brook University, Stony Brook, NY, USA*

JAN KOLACZINSKI • *Global Malaria Programme, World Health Organization, Geneva, Switzerland*

ROSSITZA KURDOVA-MINTCHEVA • *Independent Scholar, Sofia, Bulgaria*

ODILE LAUNAY • *Université Paris-Descartes, Paris, France; INSERM CIC 1417, F-CRIN I-REIVAC, Paris, France; Assistance Publique Hôpitaux de Paris, Hôpital Cochin, Paris, France*

KIM A. LINDBLADE • *Global Malaria Programme, World Health Organization, Geneva, Switzerland*

LAURA MAC-DANIEL • *Health Sciences Division, Burn and Shock Trauma Research Institute, Loyola University Chicago, Maywood, IL, USA*

VALERIE MAKOGE • *Institute of Medical Research and Medicinal Plants Studies (IMPM), Ministry of Scientific Research and Innovation, Yaoundé, Cameroon*

KAI MATUSCHEWSKI • *Department of Molecular Parasitology, Institute of Biology, Humboldt University, Berlin, Germany*

WILFRED FON MBACHAM • *Faculty of Science, University of Yaoundé 1, Yaoundé, Cameroon*

DIDIER MÉNARD • *Biology of Host-Parasite Interactions Unit, Malaria Genetic and Resistance Group, Pasteur Institute, Paris, France*

ROBERT MÉNARD • *Malaria Infection and Immunity Unit, Institut Pasteur, Paris Cedex 15, France*

LINDA M. MURUNGI • *KEMRI Wellcome Trust Research Programme, Centre for Geographic Medicine Research-Coast, Kilifi, Kenya*

MAMADOU OUSMANE NDIATH • *G4 Malaria Group, Institut Pasteur de Madagascar, Antananarivo, Madagascar; MRC Unit The Gambia at the London School of Hygiene and Tropical Medicine, Banjul, The Gambia*

CAROLINE L. NG • *Department of Pathology and Microbiology, University of Nebraska Medical Center, Omaha, NE, USA*

ABDISALAN NOOR • *Global Malaria Programme, World Health Organization, Geneva, Switzerland*

Faith H. A. Osier • *KEMRI Wellcome Trust Research Programme, Centre for Geographic Medicine Research-Coast, Kilifi, Kenya; Centre for Infectious Diseases, Heidelberg University Hospital, Heidelberg, Germany*
Kevin Palmer • *Department of Tropical Medicine and Pharmacology, John A. Burns School of Medicine, Honolulu, HI, USA*
Harison Rabarison • *Faculté des Sciences, Université d'Antananarivo, Antananarivo, Madagascar*
Mamy Arilandy Rakotomamonjy • *Ecole Doctorale Génie du Vivant et Modélisation, Faculté des Sciences, Université de Mahajanga, Madagascar*
Milijaona Randrianarivelojosia • *Faculté des Sciences, Université de Toliara, Toliara, Madagascar; Institut Pasteur de Madagascar, Antananarivo, Madagascar*
Michel Ratsimbason • *Centre National d'Application de Recherche Pharmaceutique, Antananarivo, Madagascar*
Georges Snounou • *IDMIT Department, IBFJ, DRF, CEA-Université Paris Sud 11-INSERM U1184, Immunology of Viral Infections and Autoimmune Diseases (IMVA), Fontenay-aux-Roses, France*
Julie-Anne A. Tangena • *Medical Entomology and Vector-Borne Disease Laboratory, Institut Pasteur du Laos, Vientiane, Laos*
James Tuju • *KEMRI Wellcome Trust Research Programme, Centre for Geographic Medicine Research-Coast, Kilifi, Kenya; Department of Biochemistry, Pwani University, Kilifi, Kenya*
Aneesh Vijayan • *Malaria Parasite Biology and Vaccines Unit, Institut Pasteur, Paris, France; Centre for Infection and Immunity, Institut Pasteur de Lille, Lille, France*
Lorenz von Seidlein • *Mahidol-Oxford Research Unit, Faculty of Tropical Medicine, Mahidol University, Bangkok, Thailand*
Chansuda Wongsrichanalai • *Independent Scholar, Bangkok, Thailand*

Part I

Epidemiology

Chapter 1

Country-Owned, Country-Driven: Perspectives from the World Health Organization on Malaria Elimination

Kim A. Lindblade, Xiao Hong Li, Gawrie Loku Galappaththy, Abdisalan Noor, Jan Kolaczinski, and Pedro L. Alonso

Abstract

Malaria has infected and killed humans since long before history began recording evidence of the parasite's pernicious influence. The extraordinary discoveries of the *Plasmodium* parasite by Charles Louis Alphonse Laveran in 1880, and the role of the *Anopheles* mosquito in transmission of the parasite to humans by Sir Ronald Ross in 1897, led to an understanding of the parasite life cycle and ultimately to the development of interventions that would interrupt disease transmission. Almost as soon as the insecticidal properties of dichlorodiphenyltrichloroethane (DDT) were discovered in 1939, the public health profession began battling to achieve a world free of malaria. That vision persists as the aim of all malariologists and, increasingly, the goal of all nations that remain endemic for malaria. This chapter recounts the history of malaria eradication and elimination efforts throughout the world and focuses on the current status of country-led and country-driven malaria elimination programs, along with the technical strategies recommended by the World Health Organization (WHO) for achievement of malaria elimination.

Key words Malaria, Control, Elimination, Eradication, Transmission, Surveillance, Countries

1 The Origins, Successes, and Failures of the Global Malaria Eradication Program

The discovery of the insecticidal properties of DDT in 1939 brought about a radical change in malaria control strategies. Experiences from national control programs that adopted DDT as part of indoor residual spraying (IRS) during the late 1940s and early 1950s showed that transmission could be interrupted and that malaria did not necessarily return if spraying stopped [1]. Apart from some disappointing results from Africa and the Philippines, DDT appeared to be effective everywhere, leading malaria experts to believe that the eradication (*see* **Note 1**) of malaria was achievable.

Encouraged by the early successes of using DDT against malaria, and the discovery of chloroquine (and the class of 8-aminoquinolines drugs), WHO embarked on the Global Malaria

Frédéric Ariey et al. (eds.), *Malaria Control and Elimination*, Methods in Molecular Biology, vol. 2013,
https://doi.org/10.1007/978-1-4939-9550-9_1, © Springer Science+Business Media, LLC, part of Springer Nature 2019

Eradication Program (GMEP) in 1955. As expressed during the first meeting of the Expert Committee on Malaria, "never before has an international body faced such great opportunities over wide areas for the practical control of one of the world's greatest afflictions" [2]. The global public health community believed that in the long term, eradication was financially more attractive than control. The emergence of vector resistance to DDT, first reported in Greece in 1951, was also a stimulus for the launch of the GMEP as experts feared the loss of a potent intervention. However, there were criticism and doubts, mainly on the feasibility of eradication in vast areas with poor communication, adverse environments, poor or nonexistent public health systems, and limited understanding of the implications of undertaking a malaria eradication campaign [3]. Importantly, the GMEP decided that sub-Saharan Africa was not ready for elimination because of the long transmission seasons, the high degree of endemicity, and the weak infrastructure [4].

Soon after launching the GMEP, the WHO Expert Committee on Malaria was called to design the eradication campaign [5]. Eradication was defined as "ending of the transmission of malaria and the elimination of the reservoir of infective cases in a campaign limited in time and carried out to such a degree of perfection that when it comes to an end, there is no resumption of transmission" [5]. The campaign eventually included five phases: pre-eradication, preparatory, attack, consolidation, and maintenance (*see* **Note 2**). The predominant intervention was IRS with DDT or another approved insecticide. The Expert Committee developed standardized and rigid guidelines for action on the basis of vertical, time-limited interventions. Implementation of eradication campaigns puts great emphasis on the need for exceptionally good organization and planning outside the routine activities of the health departments. The feasibility of eradication was seen as dependent on good management, methods, and money.

Success, although slower than anticipated, was at first remarkable outside of sub-Saharan Africa [6]. Nevertheless, as areas advanced into the consolidation phase of the program, full implementation of the strict requirements of the campaign was hardly possible anywhere. Resurgences of transmission began occurring in areas that had entered the consolidation and maintenance phases, necessitating reversion to the attack phase in those locations. At the same time, reports of insecticide resistance increased between 1955 and the early 1960s, followed by the emergence of chloroquine resistance between 1958 and 1959. Increasingly, WHO recognized that, even outside tropical Africa, not all endemic areas responded to the prescribed attack measures despite being correctly implemented.

Progress slowed after 1966 [6]. The GMEP faced financial constraints during these years. Undoubtedly, the 1968–1969 resurgence of malaria in Sri Lanka (then Ceylon), a country that had been considered a model for the training of malariologists, shook the confidence of the eradication program. In 1969, 14 years after the launch of the GMEP, the 22nd World Health Assembly had to recognize that there were countries where eradication was not feasible in the short term and that a strategy of control was an appropriate step toward future eradication in those areas: "In the regions where eradication does not yet seem feasible, control of malaria with the means available should be encouraged and may be regarded as a necessary and valid step towards the ultimate goal of eradication" [7].

Although the GMEP was widely perceived as a failure, in relation to the stated objectives and planned time frame (10 years), its impact was, nevertheless, tremendous. The GMEP drastically altered the global distribution of malaria, which in the 1950s was widely prevalent in Asia and the Americas [6] and succeeded in eliminating malaria from most of Europe, North America, the Caribbean, and parts of Asia and Venezuela. The GMEP made important contributions beyond its specific impact on malaria. These included indirect effects on the general improvement of health, contributions to the understanding of malaria epidemiology worldwide, the planning, implementation and management of health programs, and the development of peripheral health services.

2 Changing Course

Although malaria eradication remained the ultimate, overarching objective of global malaria activities after the 1969 resolution ending the GMEP, WHO changed tactics in the early 1970s to malaria control, defined as implementation of measures of indefinite duration aimed at reducing the incidence of malaria. In spite of WHO's efforts at regional and country level to develop a viable malaria control strategy, the 1970s witnessed a decline of financial support leading to a general weakening of antimalarial programs throughout the world. Countries had great difficulties transforming eradication to control programs [6]. The capabilities of malaria-endemic countries to continue their antimalarial operations were further reduced by the world economic crisis in the early 1970s. These factors, combined with changes in land use in some countries, led to massive malaria epidemics. Resistance of malaria parasites to the primary antimalarial, chloroquine, became widespread during this period [8].

The rapidly deteriorating malaria situation during the 1970s became a serious concern for the WHO. This concern was particularly provoked by massive epidemics in the Indian subcontinent between 1973 and 1976 and in Turkey in 1977. In 1985, the World Health Assembly urged a review of the malaria situation and current control activities [9]. By the beginning of the 1990s,

WHO estimated that there were 300–500 million cases of malaria and 1.5–2.7 million deaths from the disease, with 90% of the cases occurring in sub-Saharan Africa.

Continued monitoring of the implementation of control strategies and concerns regarding the progress that was being achieved led WHO to call for a Ministerial Conference on Malaria Control in Amsterdam in October 1992. The revised global malaria control strategy adopted by the Ministers of Health in Amsterdam was endorsed by the World Health Assembly (WHA) in 1993 [10]. The global strategy called for rational use of existing and future tools to control malaria. Implementation of the strategy depended on a change of emphasis from highly prescriptive, centralized control programs to flexible, cost-effective, and sustainable programs adapted to local conditions and responding to local needs.

3 Malaria Control Scaled Up for Impact

Several important events occurred early in the first decade of the twenty-first century that would have profound impacts on malaria elimination. First, a series of randomized controlled trials of insecticide-treated bednets (ITNs) confirmed the efficacy of ITNs in reducing the incidence of malaria and all-cause child mortality in endemic areas of Africa, including those with the highest levels of transmission [11], and long-lasting insecticide formulations were developed that made widespread scale-up of ITNs feasible [12]. The impact of ITNs and their successors, the long-lasting insecticidal nets (LLINs), transformed vector control around the world. Second, in 1998 the Roll Back Malaria (RBM) initiative was launched to halve the malaria mortality in Africa by 2010 through scale-up of effective intervention methods [4]. The RBM initiative placed significant emphasis on the reduction of disease burden in the most endemic countries in Africa. Third, in 2001, WHO first recommended the use of artemisinin-based combination therapies (ACTs) for countries where *Plasmodium falciparum* malaria was resistant to standard antimalarial therapies [13]. ACTs replaced failing drugs and were highly effective at reducing morbidity and mortality, although they were not widely used within Africa until after 2009 [4]. Fourth, in 2002 the Global Fund for AIDS, Tuberculosis and Malaria was formed to end the epidemics of the three diseases. Since its inception, the Global Fund has raised more than US$ 9 billion for malaria and provides approximately 50% of all global funding for malaria efforts. Finally, in 2005, the US government launched the President's Malaria Initiative, providing more than US$ 5.6 billion for malaria in Africa and the Greater Mekong Subregion to date. Donor funding for malaria rose from <US$

200 million per year in the early 2000s to more than US$ 1.8 billion by 2010 [14].

Increased funding for malaria led to widespread scale-up of control interventions, and by 2010 the cumulative impact around the world, and particularly in sub-Saharan Africa, was becoming measureable. The World Malaria Report 2011 reported a decrease in malaria incidence by 17% and malaria mortality rates by 25% between 2000 and 2010, with significantly greater reductions in Europe (99.5%), the Americas (60%), and the Western Pacific (38%). In Africa, eight countries and one subnational region reported >50% reductions in either confirmed malaria cases or malaria admissions and deaths. These reductions were associated with intense coverage of malaria control interventions [14].

4 Current Elimination Efforts: Bottom-Up, Country-Driven

Beginning in the 1990s, multiple countries and regions declared national or subnational malaria elimination goals, despite the global focus having switched from eradication to control of malaria after the perceived failure of the GMEP. In 1991, after achieving substantial reductions in malaria incidence in certain regions of the country, Oman initiated a pilot malaria elimination program that was expanded to the entire country after transmission was successfully interrupted in the initial target district [15]. In 1997, five North African countries (Algeria, Egypt, Libya, Morocco, and Tunisia) adopted a regional elimination initiative that helped Morocco eliminate residual foci and contributed to the renewal of WHO interest in elimination [16]. Haiti and the Dominican Republic developed a joint proposal in 2000 to eliminate malaria as a public health problem from the island of Hispaniola [17]. Several countries of the Eastern Mediterranean Region decided to target malaria elimination in the early part of the 2000s: Yemen planned to eliminate malaria from a subnational region in 2002 and was followed by national elimination goals from Saudi Arabia (2004), Iraq (2005), and the Islamic Republic of Iran (2005). In 2005, the countries of the European Region signed the Tashkent Declaration, recognizing the need to move from malaria control to elimination at the national level [18]. Argentina, Paraguay, and Malaysia had also notified WHO of their intent to pursue malaria elimination by 2006 [13].

WHO convened an informal consultation on elimination and prevention of reintroduction of malaria in Morocco in 2002 to review experiences from the Eastern Mediterranean and European regions [19]. In May 2007, WHO elaborated guiding principles for assessing the feasibility of malaria elimination [20]. At the time, 7 of 107 malaria-endemic countries were reporting no locally acquired infections, and the United Arab Emirates (UAE) had just been certified malaria-free, the first country since the 1980s to receive WHO certification.

Building on the momentum toward national and regional elimination of malaria generated by WHO and many national governments, Melinda Gates and her husband, Microsoft chairman Bill Gates, called for the global eradication of malaria at the Malaria Forum in Seattle in October 2007. Although there was not universal agreement that a global eradication effort could succeed, the proposal of such an ambitious and inspiring goal by a well-respected, innovative, and wealthy donor challenged international organizations, development agencies, nongovernmental institutions, as well as national governments of malaria-endemic countries to accelerate their malaria agendas. At the Malaria Forum, WHO Director-General Margaret Chan embraced the goal of eradicating malaria, stating, "We have to make it work in the interest of humanity. I, for one, pledge WHO's commitment to move forward with all of you" [21].

Following quickly on the heels of the Malaria Forum, WHO convened a panel of experts in Geneva in January 2008 to examine the technical issues facing malaria control and the feasibility of eradicating malaria [22, 23]. The expert group concluded that areas with low and unstable transmission should be encouraged to proceed to elimination because existing tools had the potential to interrupt local transmission. However, the committee cautioned that eliminating transmission from areas with stable high transmission was extremely unlikely with current tools, although significant reductions in morbidity and mortality could be achieved in those areas.

The successful certification of the UAE as malaria-free in 2007 was followed by Morocco (2010), Turkmenistan (2010), and Armenia (2011) [24]. The achievement of malaria-free status by Kazakhstan in 2001 and the Maldives in the 1980s was recognized by WHO in 2012 and 2016, respectively. However, it was the certification of malaria elimination in Sri Lanka in 2016 that was hailed as a remarkable public health achievement, buoying hopes around the world for a future free of malaria.

The achievement of malaria elimination in Sri Lanka has been viewed as a watershed moment for malaria in large part because the country had been held up as the prime example of the failed potential of the GMEP. Sri Lanka joined the GMEP in 1958 although by that point it had already significantly reduced malaria transmission from between 2 and 3 million cases annually in the 1940s to fewer than 100,000 cases. By 1963, Sri Lanka reported just 17 indigenous cases [25], but the success was short-lived. Between 1967 and 1968, the country experienced a significant resurgence in malaria after vector control activities and surveillance were scaled back due to the low number of cases. Sri Lanka suffered large epidemics in the 1980s and early 1990s, but soon thereafter, malaria control strategies successfully reduced transmission to the point that the country could again consider elimination. Enhanced surveillance systems to detect and treat malaria infections in mobile and displaced populations were established, while both IRS and ITNs were deployed to reduce receptivity in key areas. By 2008, with fewer than 1000 infections per year, the country declared a goal of achieving malaria pre-elimination by 2012 [26]. Despite the extreme challenges posed by a 30-year civil war, Sri Lanka actually achieved complete interruption of transmission by 2012. The last indigenous case in Sri Lanka was reported in October 2012 [27]. Certification of malaria elimination in Sri Lanka was awarded by WHO in September 2016 to great international acclaim.

Beginning in 2013, WHO recognized the need for a new global strategy for malaria and embarked on a series of consultations and meetings to shape the strategy. Endorsed by the WHA in 2015, the *Global Technical Strategy for Malaria 2016–2030* (GTS) lays out three pillars and two supporting elements for malaria [28] (Fig. 1). One of the central pillars is "Accelerate efforts towards elimination and attainment of malaria-free status." All countries are urged to intensify efforts to reduce transmission of malaria, particularly in geographical areas where transmission is already low, through deployment of core interventions as well as intensified attention to transmission foci and use of population-based medicine strategies to clear the parasite reservoir.

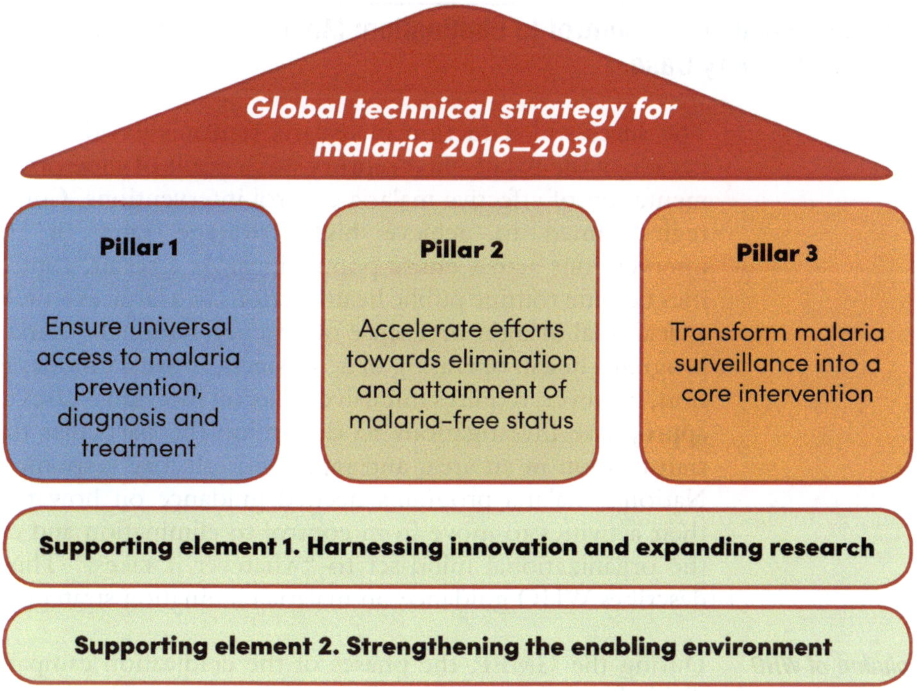

Fig. 1 Pillars and supporting elements of the *Global Technical Strategy for Malaria 2016–2030*

The massive scale-up and effective use of core malaria control tools since 2000 led to a significant decline in the global malaria burden, and more countries moved toward elimination. In 2010, 37 countries reported fewer than 10,000 indigenous malaria cases; by 2016, this number had increased to 44 [29]. In April 2016, WHO published an analysis of countries with the potential to eliminate indigenous transmission of malaria by 2020. This assessment was based on annual trends in the total number of indigenous cases, the country own declared elimination objective, and the judgments of WHO and other experts. A total of 21 countries were identified: Algeria, Botswana, Cabo Verde, Comoros, South Africa, and Swaziland (African region); Iran and Saudi Arabia (Eastern Mediterranean region); Belize, Costa Rica, Ecuador, El Salvador, Mexico, Paraguay, and Suriname (region of the Americas); Bhutan, Nepal, and Timor-Leste (South-East Asia region); and China, Malaysia, and the Republic of Korea (Western Pacific region) [30]. WHO launched an initiative to support the 21 countries to reach zero malaria cases by 2020 (referred to as the Elimination 2020, or E-2020 countries). The inaugural Global Forum of Malaria-Eliminating Countries was held in Geneva in March 2017 [31]. The main objectives of the E-2020 initiative are to monitor individual country progress, share lessons learned, identify operational research needs to accelerate progress, and advocate for resource needs.

5 Reorienting Focus from Control to Elimination: Moving from Business as Usual to Responding to Every Case

The successful reduction in malaria transmission during the first decade of the twenty-first century was a result of widespread implementation of effective malaria control interventions. Control strategies aimed to achieve high coverage rates of the core interventions across entire populations. As a result, control activities became routine public health actions to a large extent. Without a clear goal in sight or a sense of urgency, national malaria control programs began operating in a "business as usual" mode. Elimination, however, requires intensive focus on individual cases and foci, appropriate investigations to determine the particular drivers of transmission in an area, and rapid and effective response actions. National malaria programs needed guidance on how to refocus their activities to move from control to elimination and changing the organizational mind-set to "whatever it takes." This section describes WHO guidance on malaria elimination strategies.

5.1 Evolution of WHO Malaria Elimination Guidance

During the GMEP, the phases of the eradication campaign were divided into pre-eradication, preparatory, attack, consolidation, and maintenance [32]. Specific activities were linked to each phase along with parasitologic criteria for when countries could move from one stage to the next. In 2007, WHO published *Malaria Elimination: A Field Manual for Low and Moderate Endemic Countries*, the first global guidance for malaria elimination since the end of the GMEP [20]. Based on this manual, countries were recommended to transition between stages of control, pre-elimination, elimination, and prevention of reintroduction. The transition from control to pre-elimination could occur when slide positivity rates among fever cases was less than 5%. While these criteria were only meant to be indicative, the practical result was that high-burden countries felt relegated to remaining perpetually in control status.

In 2017, WHO published the *Framework for Malaria Elimination* as an update to the 2007 manual [33]. One of the innovations in the 2017 document was recognition that all countries, no matter where they are found on the malaria transmission continuum, can take specific actions to accelerate toward elimination. In high-burden countries, these actions should take the form of improving quality and coverage of vector control, strengthening passive surveillance, and improving access to diagnostic and treatment services. Rather than specific parasitologic criteria, countries are encouraged to focus and sharpen activities when they have the capacity to do so, which is determined both by the strength and flexibility of their health-care system and the level of malaria transmission. "Accelerating" toward elimination is an appropriate metaphor capturing this change in guidance, as it suggests constant forward progress with gradual but continual improvements providing positive feedback to the process and thereby increasing momentum.

The WHO *Framework* provides descriptions of four essential components to a malaria elimination strategy: (a) universal access to malaria prevention, diagnosis, and treatment; (b) surveillance as an intervention; (c) population-wide medicine strategies; and (d) case and focus investigations. Figure 2 from the *Framework* provides an illustration of where along the transmission continuum these different components might be initiated and subsequently strengthened by certain time-limited efforts. Components (b) and (d) are both related to surveillance but reflect different levels of intensity and focus on individual cases and transmission foci. Components (a) and (c) both include malaria treatment, but component A focuses on symptomatic individuals who seek treatment, whereas (c) emphasizes population-based strategies that target an asymptomatic reservoir or populations that don't seek care from traditional health facilities.

No single intervention or package of interventions will achieve malaria elimination in all settings; rather, interventions should be tailored and focused as appropriate for the setting and level of transmission. Subnational stratification of elimination interventions recognizes that the transmission continuum operates within as well

Illustrative intervention package

This package of intervention strategies can be adapted for different geographical areas in a country. The choice of interventions should be based on transmission intensity (from "high" to "very low" to zero and maintaining zero) and also on operational capacity and system readiness. The diagram should be seen as illustrative rather than prescriptive, as the onset and duration of interventions will depend on local circumstances. The shading in the boxes showing components indicates the enhancements and quality required as programmes progress towards elimination, with darker colours indicating more intense actions and shading from light to dark indicating enhancement of the quality and scale or focus of the work.

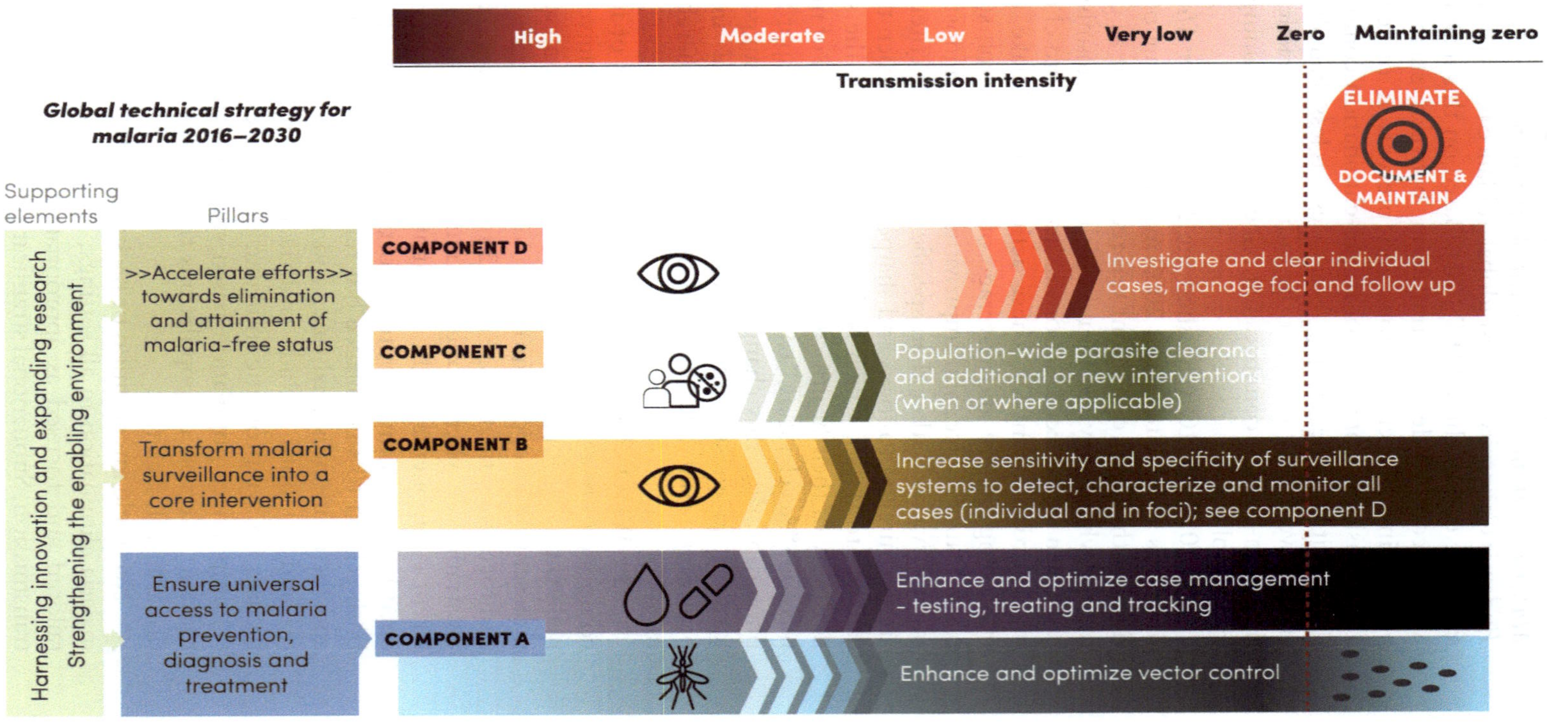

Acceleration – as represented by arrow bars (>>>>>) here – relates to time-limited efforts made across all components in order to (1) achieve universal/optimal coverage in malaria prevention and case management (Component A**), and increase sensitivity and specificity of surveillance systems so they are able to detect, characterize and monitor all malaria cases and foci (**Component B**); and (2) bring malaria transmission to sufficiently low levels (with or without population-wide parasite clearance and other strategies, **Component C as an option**) where remaining cases can be investigated/cleared and foci can be managed and followed up (**Component D**).*

Fig. 2 Illustrative malaria elimination intervention packages (from the *Framework for Malaria Elimination*) as between countries. Because of variation in the effectiveness of interventions by place and time, the impact of strategies should be evaluated regularly to guide the country malaria elimination program.

5.2 Surveillance

Malaria elimination efforts differ from control programs in the degree of emphasis that is placed on surveillance. When the national goal is reduction in the burden of malaria, the role of surveillance is to allocate resources appropriately, monitor disease trends in terms of person, place and time, and measure the impact of malaria control interventions broadly. In contrast, as countries or regions progress toward elimination, surveillance must become a key intervention in itself to identify individual cases, limit onward transmission, and prove that elimination has been achieved.

Recognition of the importance of surveillance in elimination and eradication goes back to the global eradication efforts. The GMEP specifically recognized the importance of surveillance to detect and treat all infections at the later stages of eradication campaigns, thereby interrupting transmission, particularly when afebrile infections were numerous [34]. The concept of surveillance "as an intervention" was explicitly defined in a series of papers laying out a research agenda for malaria eradication in 2011 [35]. In elimination programs, emphasis is placed on detection and treatment of all infections likely to result in secondary cases. By identifying and appropriately treating these infections, onward transmission is interrupted, while the surveillance data can be used to identify areas of continuing transmission to appropriately target effective interventions.

The reclassification and reorientation of surveillance from a routine, supportive activity to one that is used proactively to reduce transmission has been an essential element of malaria elimination. Surveillance is classically divided into two types of case detection: passive, in which infections are identified in symptomatic individuals who seek care from health facilities or community health volunteers, and active, in which health-care workers detect infections proactively through community screening or testing. While much of the elimination guidance has focused on the role of active surveillance in elimination, passive surveillance is, in fact, of equal or greater importance to achievement of elimination. In most settings, passive surveillance, based on parasitologic malaria diagnosis conducted either in primary health-care facilities or by community health volunteers, will cover a much larger proportion of the population at risk of malaria transmission than could be achieved with active surveillance, assuming that the majority of the population has access to health facilities or community health volunteers. Passive surveillance in health facilities has the potential to be more effective at identifying, diagnosing, and treating malaria infections and more sustainable over the long-term than active surveillance given the health facility infrastructure, trained health personnel, supervision by district and provincial health teams, and logistics systems.

Proactive case detection is necessary when traditional health facilities are not accessed, as may be the case for marginalized or undocumented populations, or when the population is located in remote or hard-to-reach areas that are not covered by traditional health facilities. Proactive surveillance may also be useful to identify foci of relatively high transmission. Proactive surveillance can be established through mobile clinics, community health workers, or periodic surveys. Countries approaching elimination must systematically review their data to identify populations at risk who might not be adequately covered by passive surveillance systems and extend surveillance activities to them proactively.

Reactive case detection has a different goal and scientific underpinning than proactive case detection. Malaria cases tend to cluster at very low transmission levels, and a symptomatic case identified, usually through passive surveillance at a health facility, may lead back to a cluster of cases in and around the location where the index case was infected. It is hypothesized that by treating and thereby clearing infections around the index case, transmission in the focus may be eliminated or reduced. In practice, reactive case detection strategies have not proven to be highly effective on their own [36], but when reactive case detection is integrated within a thorough investigation of the drivers of transmission in an area and an appropriate response plan including vector control is implemented, transmission can be interrupted. Reactive case detection may also serve a useful purpose during the last stages of an elimination effort by demonstrating an *absence* of additional cases to support certification of elimination of malaria transmission.

Strong passive surveillance is also key to the success of active surveillance strategies. Whether proactive case detection occurs through prospective surveys in areas or populations identified through surveillance as having ongoing malaria transmission, or reactive case detection is implemented around a symptomatic index case, active case detection strategies rely on quality data obtained through passive surveillance systems.

Good passive surveillance is also a key element of plans to prevent re-establishment. Once elimination has been achieved, continued vigilance is required to identify and test suspected malaria patients, provide them with appropriate antimalarial treatment, and ensure complete clearance of their infection to minimize the chances they generate local transmission. Because imported cases can occur anywhere within a malaria-free country, the passive surveillance system across the country has to be primed to test all patients meeting the suspected case definition to ensure good case management, with extra efforts to reduce the risk of onward transmission in areas with moderate to high degrees of receptivity for transmission.

When countries are close to achieving malaria elimination, and the number of cases is very few, focus investigations become a key activity. Foci are considered defined and circumscribed areas that contain the epidemiological and ecological factors necessary for malaria transmission. In elimination settings, they are the small geographical areas that have the last few remaining cases. The purpose of focus investigations is to rapidly and thoroughly identify the determinants of malaria transmission in the area to develop an effective response plan to eliminate transmission and prevent re-establishment. Focus investigations can also be thought of as "focused" investigations because they target a small area and identify the essential elements contributing to continued or resurgent malaria transmission.

Focus investigations should start from a standard set of hypotheses as to the reasons for continued or resurgent malaria transmission and then use appropriate epidemiological and entomological methods to uncover the factors responsible. An initial set of hypotheses (loosely in order of likelihood) should include (1) suboptimal quality or coverage of vector control interventions, (2) ineffective case management, (3) increased receptivity, (4) increased rate of parasite importation, (5) increased susceptibility of the human population, (6) change in vector behavior, (7) reduced efficacy of vector control (e.g., insecticide resistance), and (8) reduced efficacy of antimalarials.

5.3 Vector Control

The purpose of vector control is both to decrease the size of the vector population and to prevent transmission by reducing human-vector contact. The principal eradication strategy employed during the GMEP was IRS with DDT, and surveillance was only considered important during the end-stage. In contrast, surveillance is now understood to be a critical and early elimination strategy. The current emphasis on surveillance as an intervention has occasionally been interpreted to mean that vector control is a less important strategy, but that is not the case. Vector control, principally LLINs and IRS, is an essential component of an effective elimination strategy and may be required in some areas even after elimination to prevent re-establishment. Resurgences of malaria have been linked to withdrawal of vector control. WHO recommends that vector control not be withdrawn while transmission continues, and after interruption, scale-back of vector control should only be undertaken after a careful review of malariogenic potential and consideration of the surveillance, case management, and response capacity [37].

Entomological surveillance is an important activity to guide the selection of vector control interventions. Entomological surveillance monitors key information on vector behavior, likely breeding sites and insecticide susceptibility that might lead to modifications of the elimination strategy over time. Entomological surveillance also contributes to characterizing the level of receptivity of an area. Receptivity is a measure of the capacity of the local vector population to transmit malaria parasites and is determined by how frequently, when and where *Anopheles* sp. bite the human population, and how rapidly and efficiently parasites undergo sexual reproduction and produce infective stages in the vector. Several methods can be used to measure receptivity, and WHO is developing guidance on how best to measure and classify receptivity to inform elimination and prevention of re-establishment strategies.

The malariogenic potential of an area is determined by the levels of receptivity of the vector population and the vulnerability of the human population to parasite importation. Vulnerability reflects the frequency of importation of malaria parasites, as well as the intrinsic capacity of the human population to be infected and develop gametocytes. Vulnerability is generally thought of in terms of the movement of human populations, but along international borders, it is also possible that infective mosquitoes can be responsible for importing parasites. In highly receptive areas, even low levels of vulnerability can result in significant onward transmission, and vector control must be applied with high degrees of coverage and quality; surveillance as an intervention will not be sufficient on its own to eliminate transmission in highly receptive areas [38]. In areas with low receptivity, however, imported parasites can be diagnosed and treated with good surveillance and case management. Subnational regions that have interrupted malaria transmission, and countries that have been certified as malaria-free, need to monitor the receptivity of their malaria-free areas and institute appropriate vector control to limit the potential for onward transmission of imported parasites [37].

5.4 Population-Wide Medicine Strategies

Once all core malaria interventions have been implemented fully and at high quality, additional, time-limited activities to accelerate malaria elimination can be deployed. Currently, only mass drug administration (MDA) is recommended by the WHO as a population-wide medicine strategy. MDA consists of administering a full therapeutic course of antimalarial medicine (irrespective of the presence of symptoms or infection) to a defined population living in a defined geographical area (except for those for whom the medicine is contraindicated) at approximately the same time and often at repeated intervals [39]. MDA to accelerate malaria elimination should be considered under specific conditions: (1) High coverage of the entire population at risk should be achievable, and the campaign should be time-limited with a clear exit strategy. (2) The drug used should have a very high safety profile. The drug(s) chosen may be directed against asexual stages (e.g., ACT) or may also target the sexual stages (e.g., low-dose primaquine). And (3) there should be limited risk of reintroduction of parasites into the area where MDA is applied.

MDA often has to be repeated over multiple rounds to have a significant impact [40]. Mathematical modeling suggests that the key factor influencing the effectiveness of MDA is the percentage of the total population that participates in MDA at least once during the year [41]. High coverage can be achieved during a single round of MDA or through multiple rounds that specifically target the population that was not covered in previous rounds. However, areas with highly mobile populations may not be good candidates for MDA or will require innovative solutions to achieving higher coverage and targeting imported infections.

5.5 Putting It All Together

The illustration from Fig. 1 found in the *Framework for Malaria Elimination* suggests how countries can tailor appropriate packages of interventions based on their location along the malaria continuum. As malaria at subnational level within countries may be as heterogeneous as between countries, the continuum concept also applies within countries. Taking advantage of within-country heterogeneity in malaria transmission is one of the strategies by which countries can begin accelerating toward elimination through targeting areas of lower transmission and lower malariogenic potential to achieve subnational elimination.

Subnational stratification of malaria transmission is the process of dividing the country into small regions according to their level of malaria transmission, degree of receptivity, population vulnerability, and other factors that affect both the technical and operational aspects of malaria programs. In settings with high transmission, the malaria program typically stratifies subnational areas such as districts or provinces, sometimes using data from household surveys. As countries progress toward elimination, finer-scale mapping is required, and stratification should be more specific, ideally at the level of localities or health facility catchment areas [42]. As countries near elimination, strata give way to foci as transmission remains only in small, discrete areas.

On the basis of the results of stratification exercises and understanding of the epidemiological, ecological, and social features of each area, national malaria programs can determine the appropriate package of interventions. If stratification exercises are conducted appropriately, subnational regions can move toward elimination at their own pace, thus accelerating the process of elimination nationwide. While the WHO does not officially certify subnational areas as free of elimination, countries can use subnational verification of malaria-free status as stepping-stones along their roadmap to national elimination.

6 National and Global Oversight of Malaria Elimination

6.1 Independent National Malaria Advisory Committees

The WHO recommends that countries embarking on elimination programs establish an independent national malaria advisory committee. The purpose of such a committee is to provide an external view of progress and gaps in malaria elimination programs, assist in adapting WHO guidance to the national context, and review malaria trends and progress toward elimination.

The committee should be independent from the national malaria program to provide a frank and open review of the program activities, strengths, and weaknesses. Several countries that have established similar committees have benefitted from retired academic or government malaria experts as committee chairpersons. The terms of reference for the committee include:

1. Advise the national malaria program on the implementation of the National Strategic Plan for malaria elimination.
2. Monitor progress toward elimination.
3. Provide assistance in adapting WHO guidelines and policies.
4. Identify bottlenecks toward elimination, develop potential responses to address these issues, and evaluate bottleneck resolution.
5. Support the national malaria program in the preparation of the national elimination report to be submitted to the WHO Malaria Elimination Certification Panel (MECP).
6. Advise the national program on the plan to prevent re-establishment of malaria transmission.
7. Form ad hoc thematic working groups, e.g., surveillance, case management, and vector control (depending on country needs).

6.2 Malaria Elimination Oversight Committee

In 2017, WHO established the Malaria Elimination Oversight Committee (MEOC) [43]. The purpose of the MEOC is to monitor and guide global malaria elimination activities as part of a transparent, responsive, and effective approach to malaria elimination in countries and regions actively pursuing or close to that goal. The MEOC reviews progress toward elimination and the quality and coverage of malaria elimination strategies in order to provide recommendations on how to accelerate elimination and prevent re-establishment of transmission. The MEOC is constituted by and reports to WHO/GMP.

The terms of reference for the MEOC are to:

1. Evaluate national and regional progress toward malaria elimination according to established milestones and timelines.

2. Determine the need for corrective actions to address programmatic or operational bottlenecks, and evaluate plans developed to address such issues.
3. Identify any risks to malaria elimination that need to be addressed by the WHO, regional initiatives, or national programs.
4. Provide observations and/or draft recommendations to the WHO/GMP with respect to policies or guidance related to malaria elimination, for MPAC consideration.
5. Question the status quo and confront difficult issues.

The MEOC will have up to ten full and two adjunct members. Full members are malaria and public health senior experts, while adjunct members are representatives from eliminating countries. The committee met for the first time in 2018 to review progress of the E-2020 countries toward elimination.

7 WHO Certification of Malaria Elimination and Prevention of Re-establishment to Maintain Gains

The 13th World Health Assembly requested the WHO "to establish an official register listing areas where malaria eradication has been achieved, after inspection and certification by a WHO evaluation team" [44]. The criteria by which malaria could be confirmed to be eliminated were discussed and debated over multiple meetings of the WHO Expert Committee on Malaria during the GMEP. Several basic principles were acknowledged: (1) malaria eradication does not necessitate the elimination of anopheline mosquitoes; (2) after elimination has been achieved, it is expected that imported cases may lead to a few secondary cases, but the finding of introduced cases does not necessarily mean that malaria transmission has been re-established; and (3) *P. vivax* infections were assumed to not "die out" in less than 2 and a half to 3 years after transmission has ended, therefore requiring a period of post-elimination surveillance of 3 years [5]. The Expert Committee on Malaria determined that an adequate surveillance system would need to operate for at least 3 years without finding any indigenous cases, but the Committee also required that vector control measures be discontinued during the last two of those years to prove that transmission had been interrupted and could be sustained without further need for vector control.

Since the GMEP, the criteria by which certification of malaria-free status is awarded have evolved only slightly (*see* Appendix). The use of the past 3 consecutive years as the period of post-elimination surveillance has been maintained. However, due to resurgence of transmission in several countries as a result of the scale-back of vector control, the post-elimination surveillance period is no longer required to pass 2 years without vector control. One important change made by the 16th meeting of the WHO Expert Committee on Malaria in 1974 was the addition of a national plan to maintain malaria-free status by preventing re-establishment of transmission. The current *Framework for Malaria Elimination* recognizes two main categories of criteria: the first is related to proof beyond a reasonable doubt that the country has been free of indigenous transmission for at least the past 3 consecutive years and the existence of an appropriate program to prevent re-establishment.

A methodology for the inspection of countries to determine whether certification criteria had been met was first provided in at the eighth meeting of the Expert Committee on Malaria [45] and further deliberated in the tenth meeting [46]. Certification procedures were to begin when a country made an official request to the WHO. As no evaluation team could be expected to establish proof that elimination has been achieved by direct assessment, such as blood survey, within the comparatively short period of its visit, the burden of proof of achievement of malaria-fee status fell on the country requesting certification. An independent team visits the country to verify the data provided by the country to prove its claim and develops an evaluation report. The Expert Committee on Malaria was to review the report and provide a recommendation to the WHO on whether or not a concerned country should be granted malaria-free status.

The Expert Committee of Malaria did not meet after 2000. As a result, the WHO established a Malaria Elimination Certification Panel (MECP) in 2017 to advise WHO on whether certification can be granted to applicant countries [43]. This panel is entrusted to review the national elimination report, make field visits to verify the data provided by the country, develop an evaluation report, and reach a consensus on whether the malaria-free status should be granted to the applicant countries or not. The latest update of procedure of certification of malaria elimination was laid out in the *Framework for Malaria Elimination* [33].

The first list of certified countries in the official register was published in December 1963 [47]. Two countries (St. Lucia and Grenada) and one subnational region (northern Venezuela) that had been officially certified by WHO were included on the list. In the same publication, a supplemental list of countries where malaria never existed or disappeared spontaneously was included. Between 1955 and 2010, 32 countries and territories were officially certified and entered in the WHO official register [24]. The malaria-free status of Armenia, Maldives, Sri Lanka, and Kyrgyzstan were published in 2017 [48].

The criteria and procedures used to certify countries were considered sound as the majority of countries that have entered into the official register have maintained their malaria-free status. Nevertheless, some certified countries and territories have experienced indigenous malaria outbreaks but ultimately managed to interrupt transmission. Singapore experienced an outbreak in April–May 1993, but transmission was interrupted within 3 weeks of the start of the outbreak [49]. In 2006, 44 years after malaria was eliminated, Jamaica had an outbreak of *P. falciparum* but managed to interrupt transmission by 2009. Mauritius also suffered malaria epidemics in the 1980s and 1990s after being declared malaria-free in 1973. It took the country nearly 30 years to eliminate malaria again [50]. The *Framework for Malaria Elimination* now includes criteria for re-establishment of malaria transmission (*see* **Note 3**) after certification that could result in a country losing its certification status [33]. The MECP will advise the WHO on whether countries have met criteria for re-establishment through standardized and transparent procedures similar to those used for certification.

The 16th meeting of the Expert Committee on Malaria clearly pointed out, "[certification] should be considered as an operational accomplishment, rather than as a guarantee of a permanent epidemiological situation" [51]. Countries must continue to prevent re-establishment of transmission until malaria is eradicated from the world. Preventing re-establishment of malaria transmission requires vigilance and proper management of areas that are receptive to transmission and vulnerable to the importation of parasites. A high-performing health system, as well as strong leadership and sustainable funding, is critical to preventing the re-establishment of malaria once a country has achieved certification [50].

8 Conclusions

The goal to eradicate malaria dates back to the GMEP and remains the vision of the WHO and the global malaria community. While the vision of a world free of malaria has remained constant, crucial experience has been gained that has informed the evolution of strategies and approaches over time, from a rigid, top-down GMEP to the current flexible, adaptive, bottom-up, country-led elimination efforts. As political will is one of the principal components of an effective elimination strategy, the increasing numbers of countries that are choosing elimination as their strategic goal is an important signal that the current elimination efforts have a significant chance for success.

However, 2016 saw the first evidence that progress toward a world free of malaria had been stalled when 5 million more malaria cases were reported than in the previous year [29]. This reversal can be partially attributed to stagnation in funding. The annual investment required by 2020 to meet the 2030 targets of the global malaria strategy has been estimated at US$ 6.5 billion; in 2016, only US$ 2.7 billion were invested in malaria control and elimination efforts globally.

At the same time, more countries than ever before are closing in on malaria elimination, with 44 countries achieving fewer than 10,000 malaria cases, up from 37 in 2010. With renewed attention to certification of malaria-free status, WHO expects 4–6 countries to be certified by 2019. Achievements of malaria elimination serve as important beacons of hope to countries that are still facing enormous challenges from malaria. These achievements must be accelerated and protected, while efforts to reduce the continuing high burden of malaria in the rest of the world are also enhanced.

9 Notes

1. While the term "eradication" was used during the WHO-led Global Malaria Eradication Program to refer to individual countries, we now define eradication as the permanent reduction to zero of the worldwide incidence of all human malaria infections [52]. In contrast, malaria elimination is the achievement of zero incidence of indigenous malaria cases in a defined geographical area, with the need to continue control measures to prevent re-establishment of transmission. Elimination does not require the extermination of disease vectors or a complete absence of reported malaria cases in the country: imported malaria cases will continue to be detected due to international travel and may on occasion lead to the occurrence of second generation infections.
2. The phase of "pre-eradication" was added later when it became clear that many countries required significant health systems strengthening before embarking on eradication.
3. A minimum indication for re-establishment of malaria transmission after certification would be the occurrence of three or more indigenous cases of the same species per year in the same focus for 3 consecutive years.

Appendix: Changes in Criteria for WHO Certification of Malaria-Free Status Over Time

Source document	Criteria	Reasons for changes
Expert Committee on Malaria, 6th report [52]	1. Proof that an adequate surveillance system has operated in the area for at least 3 years, in at least 2 of which no specific anopheline control measures have been carried out 2. Evidence that no indigenous cases were discovered 3. All cases detected are either imported, relapsed, induced, or introduced	
Expert Committee on Malaria, 8th report [45]	Further elaborate the proof of adequate surveillance, role of passive detection system, active detection, annual blood examination rate >10%, quality of laboratory service	Definition of what constituted "adequate surveillance" and its relation to the discontinuation of vector control led to difficulties in applying the criteria
Expert Committee on Malaria, 10th report [46]	Annual blood examination rate can be less than 10%, adequacy of general health service and of the system of notification, and epidemiological follow-up should be taken into account	Recognition that general health services will be responsible for the implementation of vigilance activities
Expert Committee on Malaria, 12th report [53]	Recommended that a system of vigilance should be in place	Recognition that the risk of imported malaria always exists until the global eradication goal has been achieved

(continued)

Expert Committee on Malaria, 16th report [51]	A detailed plan for vigilance activities to maintain the achieved malaria eradication that tailors to the local context should be in place and should be updated regularly to adapt to changes in receptivity and vulnerability	Recognition that the resurgence of malaria in some areas resulted largely from faulty forecasting of the general health service's ability to maintain eradication
Malaria elimination: a field manual for low and moderate Endemic countries [20]	1. A good surveillance mechanism with full coverage of all geographical areas 2. A national malaria case register, notification, and full immediate reporting by public and private health services 3. Adequate health services for early detection and effective treatment and follow-up of imported malaria cases 4. High-quality laboratory services to diagnose malaria, based on microscopy 5. Epidemiological investigation of every malaria case 6. A national, comprehensive plan of action with continued political and financial support to carry out activities needed to prevent re-establishment of transmission 7. A system for awareness, prevention of mosquito bites, and chemoprophylaxis for travelers to prevent imported malaria	The criteria related to surveillance after the withdrawal of vector control was deleted due to recognition that premature withdrawal of vector control would likely result in a resurgence of transmission More guidance on what constituted proof of adequate surveillance was added Emphasized a high quality of entomological surveillance as a prerequisite of certification

(continued)

	8. A central computerized geo-referenced database of cases and latest foci 9. Entomological surveillance and monitoring of insecticide resistance in areas with high receptivity 10. A functional border coordination system, wherever relevant 11. Capacity for early detection of and rapid response to epidemics 12. Sero-epidemiological surveys can support validation of the interruption of local transmission	
A Framework for Malaria Elimination [33]	1. Local malaria transmission by *Anopheles* mosquitoes has been fully interrupted, resulting in zero incidence of indigenous cases for at least the three past consecutive years 2. An adequate surveillance and response system for preventing re-establishment of indigenous transmission is fully functional (in particular the curative and preventive services and the epidemiological service) throughout the territory of the country	Criteria were grouped into two major categories, with additional details on the type of proof that would be required to establish each criterion. Sero-epidemiological data was not included as laboratory procedures have yet to be validated and standardized

References

1. Livadas G (1952) Is it necessary to continue indefinitely DDT residual spraying programmes? Relevant observations made in Greece. WHO, Geneva
2. World Health Organization (1947) Expert committee on malaria: 1st report. World Health Organization, Geneva
3. World Health Organization (1955) Eighth World Health Assembly. Official records of the World Health Organization. World Health Organization, Geneva
4. Snow R, Amratia P, Kabaria C et al (2012) The changing limits and incidence of malaria in Africa: 1939-2009. Adv Parasitol 78:169–262
5. World Health Organization (1957) Expert committee on malaria: 6th report. World Health Organization, Geneva
6. Nájera JA (1999) Malaria control. Achievements, problems and strategies. Roll back malaria communicable diseases. World Health Organization, Geneva
7. World Health Organization (1973) Malaria. In: Handbook of resolutions and decisions of the World Health Assembly and the Executive Board. World Health Organization, Geneva
8. Packard R (2014) The origins of antimalarial-drug resistance. N Engl J Med 371:397–399
9. World Health Organization (1986) Expert committee on malaria: 18th report. World Health Organization, Geneva
10. World Health Organization (1993) A global strategy for malaria control. World Health Organization, Geneva
11. Philips-Howard P, Nahlen B, Kolczak M et al (2003) Efficacy of permethrin-treated bed nets in the prevention of mortality in young children in an area of high perennial malaria transmission in western Kenya. Am J Trop Med Hyg 68(4 Suppl):23–29
12. Ordonez Gonzalez J, Kroeger A, Avina A et al (2002) Wash resistance of insecticide-treated materials. Trans R Soc Trop Med Hyg 96:370–375
13. World Health Organization (2006) WHO briefing on malaria treatment guidelines and artemisinin monotherapies. World Health Organization, Geneva
14. World Health Organization (2011) World Malaria Report 2011. World Health Organization, Geneva
15. Hassan KS (2017) World malaria day: our story with malaria in Oman. Sultan Qaboos Univ Med J 17:133–134
16. World Health Organization (2006) Informal consultation on malaria elimination: setting up the WHO agenda. World Healh Organization, Geneva
17. Pan American Health Organization (2000) Roll Back Malaria in Meso America: Report of the meeting held in the Dominican Republic with the participation of Central American countries, Mexico, Haiti and the Dominican Republic. Pan American Health Organization, Washington, DC
18. World Health Organization (2006) From malaria control to elimination in the WHO European region 2006–2015. World Health Organization Regional Office for Europe, Copenhagen
19. World Health Organization (2002) Informal consultation on the elimination of residual malaria foci and prevention of re-introduction of malaria. World Health Organization, Cairo
20. World Health Organization (2007) Malaria elimination: A field manual for low and moderate endemic countries. World Health Organization, Geneva
21. Bill & Melinda Gates Foundation (2007) Malaria Forum: collaboration, innovation, impact. Bill & Melinda Gates Foundation, Seattle WA
22. Mendis K, Rietveld A, Warsame M et al (2009) From malaria control to eradication: The WHO perspective. Tropical Med Int Health 14:802–809
23. World Health Organization (2008) Global malaria control and elimination: report of a technical review. World Health Organization, Geneva
24. World Health Organization (2012) World Malaria Report 2012. World Health Organization, Geneva
25. Abeyasinghe R, Galappaththy G, Gueye C et al (2012) Malaria control and elimination in Sri Lanka: Documenting progress and success factors in a conflict setting. PLoS One 7:e43162
26. Sri Lanka Ministry of Health Anti-Malaria Campaign (2008) Strategic Plan for Phased Elimination of Malaria from Sri Lanka. Sri Lanka Ministry of Health, Colombo
27. Sri Lanka Ministry of Health Anti-Malaria Campaign (2014) National malaria strategic plan for elimination and prevention of re-introduction—Sri Lanka. Sri Lanka Ministry of Health, Colombo
28. World Health Organization (2015) Global technical strategy for malaria 2016–2030. World Health Organization, Geneva

29. World Health Organization (2017) World malaria report 2017. World Health Organization, Geneva
30. World Health Organization (2016) Eliminating malaria. World Health Organization, Geneva
31. World Health Organization (2017) Malaria elimination: report from the inaugural global forum of countries with potential to eliminate malaria by 2020. Wkly Epidemiol Rec 92:578–585
32. Nájera J, González-Silva M, Alonso P (2011) Some lessons for the future from the Global Malaria Eradication Programme (1955–1969). PLoS Med 8:e1000412
33. World Health Organization (2017) A framework for malaria elimination. World Health Organization, Geneva
34. Yekutiel P (1960) Problems of epidemiology in malaria eradication. Bull World Health Organ 22:669–683
35. malERA Consultative Group on Monitoring, Evaluation and Surveillance (2011) A research agenda for malaria eradication: Monitoring, evaluation, and surveillance. PLoS Med 8: e1000400
36. van Eijk A, Ramanathapuram L, Sutton P et al (2016) What is the value of reactive case detection in malaria control? A case-study in India and a systematic review. Malar J 15:67
37. Global Malaria Programme (2015) Risks associated with scale-back of vector control after malaria transmission has been reduced. World Health Organization, Geneva
38. Gerardin J, Bever C, Bridenbecker D et al (2017) Effectiveness of reactive case detection for malaria elimination in three archetypical transmission settings: a modelling study. Malar J 16:248
39. World Health Organization (2017) Mass drug administration for falciparum malaria. World Health Organization, Geneva
40. Eisele T, Bennett A, Silumbe K et al (2016) Short-term impact of mass drug administration with dihydroartemisinin plus piperaquine on malaria in Southern Province Zambia: A cluster-randomized controlled trial. J Infect Dis 214:1831–1839
41. Brady O, Slater H, Pemberton-Ross P et al (2017) Role of mass drug administration in elimination of *Plasmodium falciparum* malaria: a consensus modelling study. Lancet 5: e680–e687
42. Cox J, Sovannaroth S, Soley L et al (2014) Novel approaches to risk stratification to support malaria elimination: an example from Cambodia. Malar J 13:1
43. Global Malaria Programme (2017) WHO malaria policy advisory committee (MPAC) meeting. World Health Organization, Geneva
44. World Health Organization (1960) Thirteenth World Health Assembly Resolution WHA 13.55. World Health Organization, Geneva
45. World Health Organization (1961) Expert committee on malaria: 8th report. World Health Organization, Geneva
46. World Health Organization (1964) Expert Committee on Malaria: 10th report. World Health Organization, Geneva
47. (1963) Status of malaria eradication during first semester 1963. Wkly Epidemiol Rec 38:612–617
48. (2017) Armenia, Maldives, Sri Lanka and Kyrgyzstan certified malaria-free. Wkly Epidemiol Rec 92:573–577
49. (1993) Malaria. Localized outbreak. Wkly Epidemiol Rec 68:285–286
50. Tatarsky A, Aboobakar S, Cohen J et al (2011) Preventing the reintroduction of malaria in Mauritius: a programmatic and financial assessment. PLoS One 6:e23832
51. World Health Organization (1974) Expert committee on malaria: 16th report. World Health Organization, Geneva
52. World Health Organization (2017) WHO malaria terminology. World Health Organization, Geneva
53. World Health Organization (1966) Expert committee on malaria: 12th report. World Health Organization, Geneva

Chapter 2

Current Situation of Malaria in Africa

Wilfred Fon Mbacham, Lawrence Ayong, Magellan Guewo-Fokeng, and Valerie Makoge

Abstract

Malaria infection is one of the major causes of deaths in the African continent. The high burden of malaria in Africa is due to *P. falciparum*, which adapts and cospecializes with *Anopheles gambiae*, the most effective and widespread malaria vector. Since 2000, the incidence of malaria has been reduced by 17% and malaria mortality rates by 26%. However, the rate of decline has stalled and even reversed in some regions since 2014. In 2017 as described by the latest World malaria report, 219 million malaria cases were reported, up from 2017 million cases reported in 2016 in 91 countries, and the global tally of malaria deaths reached 435,000 deaths, compared with 451,000 estimated deaths in 2016. Despite these achievements, the African region continues to account for about 92% of malaria cases and deaths worldwide. Therefore, it is important to master the current situation of malaria in Africa to see how to better plan its elimination. In this chapter, we present the current situation and prospective means to improve it, including a salutogenesis approach.

Key words Malaria, Burden, Salutogenesis, Africa

1 Introduction

Based on the data provided by the world malaria report 2018, worldwide, there is a noticeable decrease in the number of malaria cases. In 2017, an estimated 219 million cases of malaria occurred worldwide (95% CI: 203–263 million), compared with 239 million cases in 2010 (95% CI: 219–285 million) and 217 million cases in 2016 (95% CI: 200–259 million). Compared with 2013 and 2014, nine million more malaria cases were estimated to have occurred globally in 2017. Of an estimated 219 million cases in 2017, 92% were in the WHO African Region (Fig. 1). About 3.4% of estimated cases globally were caused by *P. vivax*, but outside the African continent this proportion was more than 50%.

In 2017, the African continent alone accounted for 80% of all malaria cases globally, with the highest proportion in Nigeria (25%); followed by the Democratic Republic of the Congo (11%); Mozambique (5%); Ghana, Burkina Faso, Niger, and Uganda (4%); Mali,

Frédéric Ariey et al. (eds.), *Malaria Control and Elimination*, Methods in Molecular Biology, vol. 2013,
https://doi.org/10.1007/978-1-4939-9550-9_2,

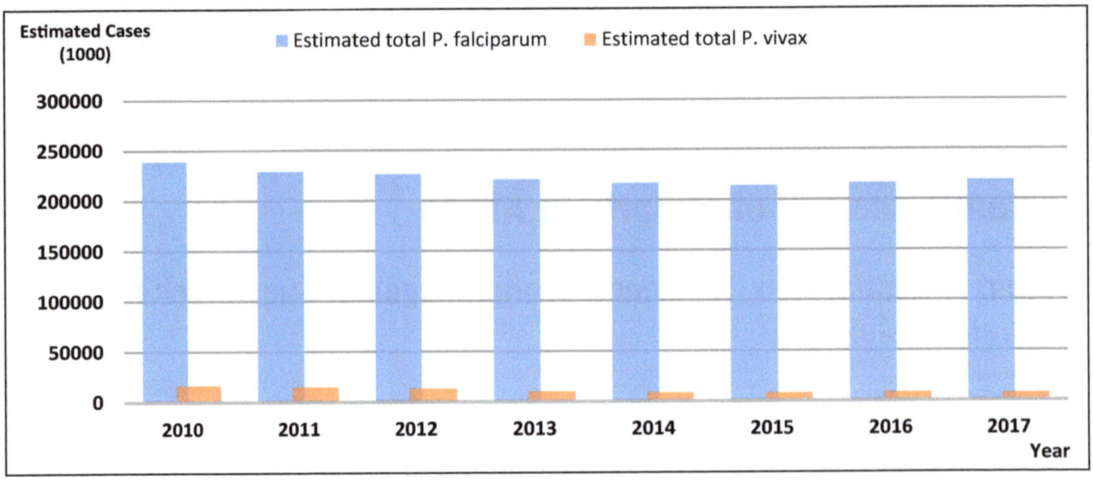

Fig. 1 Estimated malaria cases, 2010–2017

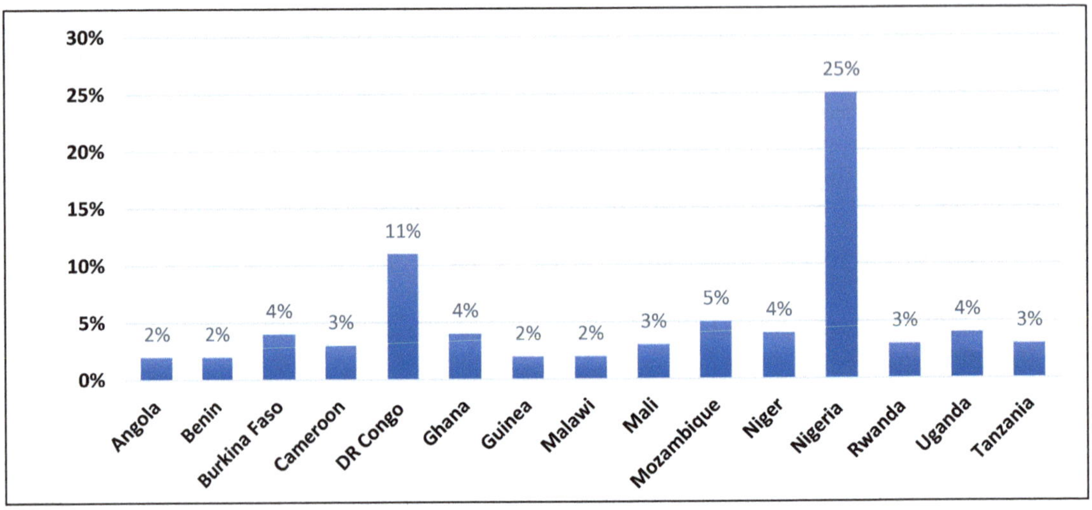

Fig. 2 Estimated total malaria cases in Africa, 2017

United Republic of Tanzania, Cameroon, and Rwanda (3%); and 2% for Guinea, Angola, Benin, and Malawi (Fig. 2). In the same year, 82% of estimated vivax malaria cases occurred in Afghanistan (09%), Ethiopia (09%), India (48%), Indonesia (08%), and Pakistan (10%).

Malaria-related mortality data showed that globally around 435,000 deaths were caused by malaria in 2017. More than 90% of these were from the African continent. This represents broadly similar levels of deaths to 2015, when 469,000 deaths were estimated to have occurred globally. Approximately 80% of all deaths in 2017 occurred in 17 countries, all of which are in the WHO African Region, except for India. Nigeria, Democratic Republic of the Congo, Burkina Faso, and India accounted for 58% of all malaria deaths globally. From 2010 to 2017, there is a nonnegligible decrease in the number of deaths associated with malaria in Africa (Fig. 3).

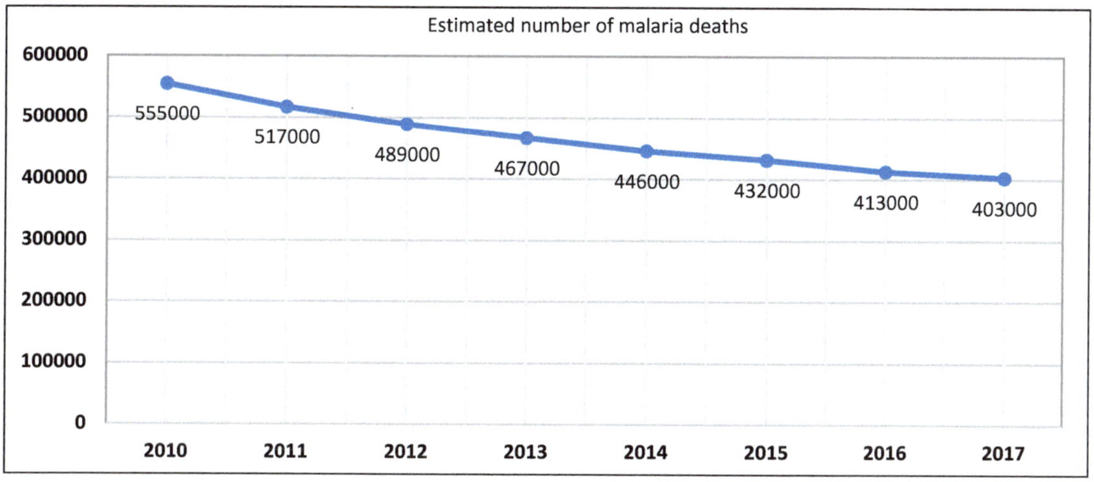

Fig. 3 Estimated number of malaria deaths in Africa, 2010–2017

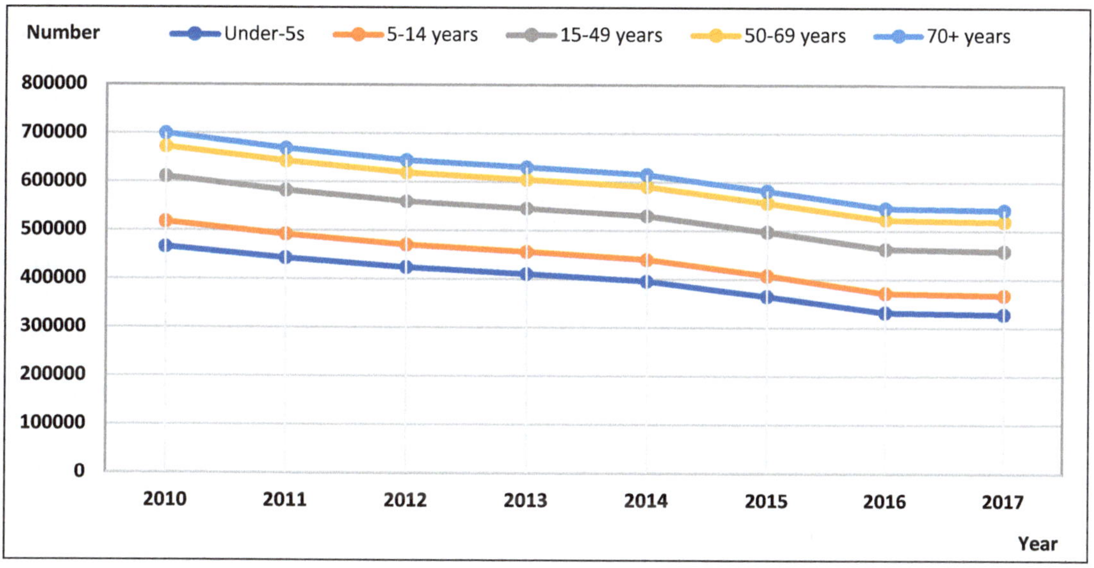

Fig. 4 Estimated number of malaria deaths by age in sub-Saharan Africa, 2010–2017

Age-specific categorization shows that the highest mortality rates are recorded from 2010 to 2017 in children under 5, followed by people over 70 in sub-Saharan Africa (Fig. 4).

2 Bed Net, Drug Coverage, and Mortality of Malaria: Projection for 2030

Huge efforts have been done globally to control malaria with the objective to ultimately eradicate malaria [1]. The use of insecticide-treated mosquito nets is one of the most important tools in malaria control and elimination strategies. This reduces more than 50% of malaria cases and 17% of deaths in children under 5 [2]. In sub-Saharan Africa, 16 countries accounted for more than 80% of deliveries of insecticide-treated mosquito nets in the period 2014–2016. These countries were Nigeria (78.0 million), Democratic Republic of the Congo (61.2 million), Uganda (35.6 million), Ethiopia (33.0 million), United Republic of Tanzania (29.2 million), Ghana (19.6 million), Mozambique (17.6 million), Côte d'Ivoire (16.9 million), Kenya (16.9 million), Senegal (15.1 million), Burkina Faso (14.6 million), Mali (14.1 million), Sudan (13.6 million), Cameroon (13.6 million), Madagascar (12.7 million), and Malawi (12.4 million). In this geographic area, several studies have also demonstrated and confirmed the beneficial effects at the individual and community level of insecticide-treated mosquito nets on malaria-related morbidity and mortality [3, 4]. Despite all this, the use of insecticide-treated mosquito nets remains below universal coverage; this may be due to the fact that malaria knowledge, which is an important factor in the design and implementation of malaria control programs, continued to be very inadequate and mostly false regarding the etiology and prevention of the disease [5–12]. A recent study [13] demonstrated that in 5 years (2012–2017), with a sample of 7535 residents recruited from 2066 households in Mutasa District, Zimbabwe (seasonal malaria transmission), Choma District, Zambia (low transmission), and Nchelenge District, Zambia (high transmission), most of the 3836 adult participants correctly linked mosquito bites to malaria (85.0%), mentioned at least one malaria symptom (95.5%), and knew of the benefit of sleeping under an insecticide-treated mosquito net. In these localities, factors as age, household size, and socioeconomic status were also associated with the bed net use. The study finally concluded that the implementation and delivery of malaria control and elimination tools need to consider socioeconomic equity gaps and to target school-age children to ensure access to, and improve the utilization of, insecticide-treated mosquito nets. Added to this, a considerable drop was observed in the number of artemisinin-based combination therapies (ACTs) purchased by countries, mainly for the public sector of around 70% and above, from 393 million in 2013 to 337 million in 2014 and 311 million in 2015, followed by a sharp increase to 409 million in 2016. The number of ACT treatments distributed by national malaria control programs to the public sector increased from 192 million in 2013 to 198 million in 2016. These malaria treatments were distributed for the most part (99%) in 2016 and the same percentage was observed in 2017 (206 million ACTs) in the WHO African region [14, 15].

By 2030, as postulated by the WHO and according to existing theories on health behavior change, high levels of knowledge about causality, transmission, and prevention through the use of insecticide-treated mosquito nets as well as other means and treatment by ACTs may facilitate attitudinal changes, leading to the adoption of positive preventive practices that reduce the risk of exposure to *Plasmodium* and reduce the risk of malaria transmission [16], thus facilitating malaria elimination.

3 Malaria Transmission

There are more than 400 different species of *Anopheles* mosquito, with around 30 that are malaria vectors of major importance. All of the important vector species bite between dusk and dawn. The intensity of transmission depends on factors related to the parasite, the vector, the human host, and the environment. Transmission is stronger in areas where the mosquito life span is longer, allowing the parasite to complete its development in the mosquito, and especially where human density is high, giving more probability to bite humans rather than animals. More than 90% of global malaria cases are in Africa because of the longer life span and the human biting capacity of vector species found in the African continent. Transmission also depends on climatic conditions that may affect the number and survival of mosquitoes, such as rainfall patterns, temperature, humidity ecological zones and even among areas in close proximity [17–24]. In many areas, transmission is seasonal, with the peak during and just after the rainy season.

In large parts of Sahelian and sub-Sahelian Africa, the highest rate of transmission occurs only for a few months during the year, although few observational studies have recorded in detail the incidence of malaria per month over a period of several years. In tropical Africa, where most of the year is favorable for malaria transmission, it is largely determined by seasonal changes in rainfall. By comparing the incidence of malaria each month with the monthly rainfall in areas where both were determined, it has been possible to estimate from rainfall patterns, the areas of Africa where malaria is likely to be concentrated during 3 or 4 months of the year and where malaria incidence is estimated to exceed 100 cases per 1000 children per year [25]. These areas lie predominantly in the Sahelian and sub-Sahelian regions of Africa, where the burden of malaria continues to be very high.

Forest ecosystems contribute significantly to increase malaria transmission because of its influence on temperature buffering, rainfall, humidity, tree canopy [26], flora, fauna [27], high organic content in breeding pools [28], and lack of infrastructure. A global assessment indicates that "closed forests in areas at risk of malaria cover about 4.8 million km^2" [29]. The living populations in these forest areas are therefore at a very high risk of infection and malaria development, that is, about 1.4 billion, representing 11.7 million population for 1.5 million km^2 in the Amazon, 18.7 million population for 1.4 million km^2 in Central Africa, 35.1 million population for 1.2 million km^2 in the Western Pacific, and 70.1 million population for 0.7 million km^2 in Southeast Asia [30, 31]. The fight against malaria in these forested areas of the world, and particularly in Africa, is a major challenge due to their uneven land forms, presence of streams, and dense vegetation and requires new approaches [32].

4 Correlates of Interventions

4.1 Vector Elimination Program

The last decade is characterized by the significant progress made in malaria control in view of its elimination, defined as the reduction to the level of zero of the incidence of infection caused by a specific malaria parasite in a defined geographical area as a result of deliberate efforts. Increased financial support for malaria programmes has enabled impressive reductions in transmission in many endemic regions. The most commonly used methods to prevent mosquito bites are sleeping under an insecticide-treated net (ITN) and spraying the inside walls of houses with insecticide, an intervention known as indoor residual spraying (IRS). Use of ITNs has been shown to reduce malaria case incidence rates by 50% in a range of settings and to reduce malaria mortality rates by 55% in children under 5 years of age in sub-Saharan Africa [2, 33]. These two-core vector-control interventions, that is, the use of ITNs and IRS, are considered to have made a major contribution to the reduction in malaria burden since 2000 [34].

In sub-Saharan African countries, the long-lasting insecticidal nets (LLINs) are the predominant type of ITNs used (with an estimated effective life span of 3 years) as a method of malaria vector control [35]. Recently, the data provided by World Malaria reports 2017 and 2018 shows that in this part of the African continent, there is a real and ever increasing percentage of the population at risk that sleeps under an ITN, from 30% (95% CI: 28–32) in 2010 to 54.10% (95% CI: 50–58) in 2016 with a slight decrease in 2017 (50%); the percentage of households with at least one ITN, from 50% (95% CI: 48–52) in 2010 to 79.70% (95% CI: 76–84) in 2016; and at the individual level, access to the ITN also increased from 34% (95% CI: 32–35) in 2010 to 61.20% (95% CI: 58–65) in 2016, compared to at least one ITN for every two people in 2017 [15], demonstrating that the policies and strategies developed by the national malaria control programs (NMCP) to distribute ITNs in most households can indeed reach most households and need to be strengthened.

4.2 Bed Nets and Drug Coverage

According to the data provided by the World malaria reports 2017 and 2018, the proportions of population at risk with access to an ITN in sub-Saharan Africa in 2016 were: less than 50% for

Mauritania, Gabon, Equatorial Guinea, Republic of the Congo, Angola, North Sudan, South Sudan Eritrea, Somalia, Tanzania, Zimbabwe, and Djibouti; between 50% and 80% access to ITNs for Gambia, Guinea-Bissau, Guinea, Sierra Leone, Cote d'Ivoire, Burkina Faso, Togo, Benin, Nigeria, Cameroon, Chad, Niger, Central African Republic, Democratic Republic of the Congo, Malawi, Uganda, Kenya, Ethiopia, Zambia, Mozambican, Comoros, and Madagascar; and more than 80% access to ITNs for Rwanda, Liberia, Ghana, Senegal, and Mali. The proportion of households with sufficient nets also rose from just 19% (95% CI: 18–20) in 2010 to 43.40% (95% CI: 40–47) in 2016. In the period 2015–2017, 459 million (83%) were distributed in sub-Saharan Africa with very few countries (Ethiopia, Niger, Nigeria, and Sudan) below the operational universal coverage target of one ITN per two persons at risk by 2017 [15]; a good increase but still substantially lower than the universal coverage targets. This relatively low level of net adequacy is partly responsible for relatively low utilization rates.

4.3 Combination of IRS and ITNs

In sub-Saharan Africa, between 2010 and 2016, the use of IRS and ITNs for malaria prevention, when considered separately, showed a significant increase in the proportion of the population using only ITNs, from 20% in 2010 to 45% in 2016; by combining all these data obtained from ITNs coverage model from Malaria Atlas Project, after multiple analyses by the WHO, an increase was found in the proportion of the population benefiting from protection against the malaria vector from 27% in 2010 58% in 2016 in this WHO region [36].

4.4 Universal Health Coverage

Universal health coverage will be effective if all people have access to the health services they need, when and where they need them, regardless of where they live or their financial condition. In 2016, just 54% of people at risk of malaria in sub-Saharan Africa were sleeping under an ITN, which is the primary prevention method. This level of coverage represents a considerable increase since 2010, but is far from the goal of universal access. At the same time of period, the number of people using IRS declined in this region since 2010.

In the WHO African region, most people who seek treatment for malaria in the public health system receive an accurate diagnosis and effective medicines. However, access to the public health system remains far too low. National-level surveys in the WHO African region show that only about one-third (34%) of children with fever are taken to a medical provider in this sector.

5 The Economics of Malaria

5.1 Social and Economic Toll

In Africa today, malaria is a disease of poverty and a cause of poverty, with significant measurable direct and indirect costs, which has been shown to be a major constraint to economic development. On the economic front, malaria is now responsible for a growth penalty, which can be estimated in terms of loss of GDP to more than 1.3% in African countries. Accumulated over the years, this loss results in a substantial difference in GDP between countries with and without malaria and severely restrains the economic growth of the entire region. There are two categories of malaria costs, direct costs and indirect costs. The direct costs are those related to individual and public expenditures for disease prevention and treatment, the indirect costs are those related to lost productivity or income associated with illness or death. In the event of death, these costs include the discounted future income of the deceased. All this has a very pronounced negative effect on the human resources of the African continent.

Another indirect cost of malaria is the human pain and suffering caused by the disease. Malaria also hampers children's schooling and social development through both absenteeism and permanent neurological and other damages associated with severe episodes of the disease. The simple presence of malaria in a community or country also hampers individual and national prosperity due to its influence on social and economic decisions. The risk of contracting malaria in endemic areas can deter investment, both internal and external, and affect individual and household decision-making in many ways, which have a negative impact on economic productivity and growth.

5.2 Malaria Burden

In 2015 and 2016, 91 countries reported an increase in the number of malaria cases, from 211 to 216 million, respectively, with a constant number of 445,000 deaths. Mortality rates have followed a similar pattern. The major proportion (90%) of these malaria cases and deaths worldwide are still from the WHO African Region, with 15 countries—all in sub-Saharan Africa except India—carrying 80% of the global malaria burden.

In order to meet the 2030 objectives of the WHO global malaria strategy, a minimum investment of 6.5 billion US dollars are required annually by 2020. However, in 2016 an inadequate amount of 2.7 billion US dollars, representing less than half of the required amount, was invested to this end. This observation started in 2014, where this amount allocated for malaria control on average declined in the majority of the high-burden countries.

5.3 Vulnerable Populations and Poverty

Complex situations, resulting of natural factors such as excessive rains, flooding or earthquakes, or of human-made ones such as conflict and political crises, often disrupt service delivery and the implementation of interventions. Where the ecological conditions are suitable for malaria, such situations often result in increased malaria transmission, disease and deaths. The burden of disease can be exceptionally high among the most vulnerable, such as children and pregnant women, especially when worsening nutritional conditions impair their capacity to fight the disease.

6 Malaria Advisory

Recently, in 2017, the WHO Malaria Policy Advisory Committee created the Malaria Elimination Oversight Committee (MEOC) and the Malaria Elimination Certification Panel (MECP) to further assist countries to achieve malaria elimination goals. The first provides independent operational and programmatic advice as well as oversight monitoring of malaria elimination globally and the second reviews country applications for elimination certification, and recommends whether countries should receive WHO certification [37]. Based on these, recommendations were made: (a) To protect all nonimmune travelers and migrants, as indicated in the global technical strategy for malaria 2016–2030 delivered in 2018, chemoprophylaxis should be given to individuals exposed to a high risk of contracting malaria in combination with advice about measures (ITN, IRS) to reduce vector bites—particularly in nonimmune travelers (who are more susceptible to malaria illness and death) [37]; (b) to prevent the reestablishment of local malaria transmission, easy access to diagnostic facilities and free treatment of malaria must be given to travelers from endemic areas. Vector control must continue to be used to contain local outbreaks and protect areas that are known to be receptive to the resumption of transmission as well as exposed to frequent importation of malaria parasites The patterns of vigilance that need to be applied in order to ensure the successful maintenance of the malaria-free status depend on the vulnerability and receptivity of an area. The program for preventing the reestablishment of transmission has an unlimited duration; thus, surveillance should be maintained in countries that no longer have transmission. For the children under the age of 5, the Malaria Policy Advisory Committee suggested an additional analysis of changing endemicity and all-cause under-5 mortality. Malaria Policy Advisory Committee recommended the inclusion of the burden of malaria in pregnancy and its indirect effect on neonatal mortality, in addition to the consequences of malaria-related anemia [37].

7 Certification of Malaria Elimination, Current Situation

Globally, the number of countries that were malaria endemic in 2000 and reported fewer than 10,000 malaria cases, and are therefore nearing elimination, increased from 37 in 2010 to 44 in 2016. These countries are distributed across the WHO regions as follows: the Americas (14), European (8), African (7), Southeast Asia (6), Western Pacific (5), and Eastern Mediterranean (4).

The WHO certification of malaria elimination is acquired by a country if it has reported no indigenous case of malaria for at least the last three consecutive years. Between 2000 and 2016, only 18 countries worldwide (Egypt, United Arab Emirates, Oman, Kazakhstan, Morocco, Syrian Arab Republic, Armenia, Turkmenistan, Iraq, Georgia, Argentina, Paraguay, Azerbaijan, Algeria, Turkey, Kyrgyzstan, Sri Lanka, and Uzbekistan) reached zero indigenous cases for 3 years or more. The majority (10 of these 18 countries) achieved this target between 2011 and 2016. This WHO certification of the elimination of malaria during this period from 2000 to 2016 has been validated only for 6 countries, United Arab Emirates (2007), Morocco (2010), Armenia (2011), Kyrgyzstan (2016), Sri Lanka (2016), and Turkmenistan (2010). This certification process is initiated for two other countries, Argentina and Paraguay, with Uzbekistan having formally given it to the WHO in 2017. In Africa, Morocco alone has achieved this feat and so far none in sub-Saharan Africa.

8 Risk Assessment

8.1 Antimalarial Drug Resistance

Antimalarial drug resistance is a threat to malaria control and has important implications for global public health. In particular, when chloroquine resistance emerged in Africa in the 1980s, there were documented increases in hospital admissions and mortality, mainly due to severe malaria and increased transmission. Resistance to antimalarial drugs has had a significant impact on the cost of global malaria control (due to the need for new drugs, and the social and health costs of treatment failure). Artemether-lumefantrine (AL) and artesunate-amodiaquine (ASAQ) are the first-line treatment policies used in most African countries, with some countries adding dihydroartemisinin-piperaquine (DP). Between 2010 and 2016, the overall average efficacy of DP, ASAQ, and AL were 98.7%, 98.3%, and 97.9%, respectively. When the failure rates of all three treatments were analyzed separately by year, it was found that their high efficacy remained constant over time. In studies of AL, treatment failure rates above 10% occurred in three countries (Angola, Gambia, and Malawi), although lumefantrine resistance could not be confirmed by molecular marker, in vitro test or blood dosage levels. In Africa, artemisinin resistance was not confirmed. Studies of *P. vivax* were conducted in Ethiopia, Madagascar (both of which had previously reported CQ resistance) and Mauritania. In Ethiopia, treatment failure rates ranged from 3% to 22% (median: 5.1%). Treatment failure rates of 0% for ASAQ were reported in Madagascar and for Chloroquine in Mauritania.

8.2 Vector Resistance

Malaria prevention and control strategies are increasingly threatened by resistance of malaria vectors to the four insecticide classes (pyrethroids, organochlorines, carbamates and organophosphorus) commonly used in household ITNs or in IRS. Resistance to at least one of these insecticides from a collection site was detected in 61 of the 76 malaria-endemic countries that reported standard monitoring data for 2010–2016. Although the duration of this monitoring varied between regions, the WHO Europe region did not detect any resistance; however, it was detected for at least two or more insecticide classes in 50 of the 61 countries. As described by the WHO or Centers for Disease Control and Prevention, for the 6-year period (from 2010 to 2016), more than 70% of the data were reported by the African countries where there is a known recent resistance status of multiple insecticide classes or types, mosquito species or time points were tested. The proportion of malaria endemic countries that reported pyrethroid resistance increased from 71% to 81% in this period; added to this, from the 72 countries monitored, only 16 did not detect any pyrethroid resistance. In more than two-thirds of the monitored sites in Africa and the WHO Eastern Mediterranean Region, resistance to pyrethroids acquired by malaria vectors was higher than in other regions.

Concerning organochlorines (mainly DDT), carbamates and organophosphates (three other insecticide classes), which are used in adult malaria vector control, resistance is also detected in all WHO regions except Europe. Between 2010 and 2016, resistance to at least one of these three insecticides was confirmed in 80% of the monitored countries for organochlorines, 65% for carbamates and 51% for organophosphorus. This last insecticide group (organophosphorus) presenting a resistance by at least one malaria vector species at almost two-thirds of the sites tested in the four WHO regions, with a low prevalence in the WHO Region of the Americas. Compared to carbamate, this resistance was detected in one-third of the monitored sites worldwide. While in the WHO regions of the Eastern Mediterranean, Southeast Asia, and the Western Pacific, organophosphate resistance has been detected in more than half of the monitored sites, it was less prevalent in malaria vectors in the Americas and Africa.

8.3 Therapy-Seeking Behavior

In 2016, 37 out of 46 countries in the WHO African region indicated that at least 80% of public health facilities had reported data on malaria through their national health information system.

Effective surveillance of malaria cases and deaths is essential for identifying the areas or population groups that are most affected by malaria, and for targeting resources for maximum impact. A strong surveillance system requires high levels of access to care and case detection, and complete reporting by all health sectors, whether public or private. However, prompt and accurate diagnosis of malaria (by microscopy or malaria rapid diagnostic test in all patients) followed by treatment is the most effective means of preventing a mild case of malaria from developing into a severe disease and thus leading to death. More febrile children sought care in the public sector (34%, IQR: 28–44) than in the private sector (22%, IQR: 14–34). However, data provided by the World Malaria Report (2018) shows that African surveys also indicate that a high proportion (36%, IQR: 30–46) of febrile children in sub-Saharan Africa attended public health facilities but, a considerable proportion of these children were not brought for care (40%, IQR: 28–45). Possible reasons included poor access to healthcare providers or lack of awareness among caregivers. In 2017, among national-level surveys completed in 19 countries in sub-Saharan Africa between 2015 and 2017 (representing more than 65% of the population at risk), a median of 52% (IQR: 38–56) of febrile children was taken to a trained medical provider for care. This includes public sector hospitals and clinics, formal private sector facilities and community health workers.

9 Salutogenesis and Malaria: Looking Towards Malaria Control and Elimination Through Different Lenses in Africa

The heavy burden posed on the world by poverty related diseases (PRDs) like malaria has made it an international fight and has kept it on the global political agenda of international bodies such as the United Nations (UN). In the year 2000 for example, the world united to set a number of goals called the millennium development goals (MDG) to be achieved by 2015, among which was the goal to eradicate the infamous trio of poverty-related diseases (PRDs), namely malaria, HIV and TB. Even though this effort registered some success, the goal was not fully achieved and the fight against PRDs continues in a new set of sustainable development goals (SDG) slated for 2030 [38]. Seemingly, malaria and other PRDs have remained as fixed points on the global agenda and the focus of many global initiatives because the goals to eliminate it have so far been hard to achieve.

9.1 Malaria Coherence

So far, the attention, understanding, and the funding in the fight against malaria has been disease-focused. This means that emphasis was placed mainly on prevalence studies, identification of risk factors, the development of new drugs, of insecticides (including how to overcome resistance), and of more effective diagnostic techniques, as well as discovery of novel vaccine candidates [39]. This posture is also taken by many governments in Africa. Health initiatives and ministries of public health and scientific research and innovation respond to malaria with a focus on infection. This disease-focused approach is important and has helped to reduce the malaria burden. However, malaria is still a public health problem.

9.2 Coping with Malaria: The Salutogenic Model of Health

From the abovementioned scenario, complementary approaches to tackle the malaria problem are therefore necessary. There is need for an integrated approach on critical health issues such as malaria in developing countries [40]. Approaches that investigate what factors help people to cope well with malaria are complementary and necessary [41]. Antonovsky's salutogenic model of health (SMH) [42] comes in as a theoretical vision of health development and it focuses of investigating ways to create, enhance and improve physical, mental and social health. Salutogenesis asks "what creates health" instead of "what creates disease" (the pathogenic model of health). The salutogenic model of health situates health as a result of a multifactorial and context-dependent process [43]. Focusing on people's perceptions of malaria and how they cope with it, would reveal new insights and challenges about understanding malaria in health and development.

In malaria salutogenesis, malaria is not a state but a movement along a continuum. This continuum also referred to as the ease-dis (ease) continuum has at one end "total absence of health" and at the other end "total health" [43]. According to Antonovsky, people, because of the stressors in their lives, are always moving on this continuum. A stressor is defined as a demand made upon a person by his internal or external environment for which he lacks an immediate response [39]. Coping successfully with stressors will enable a person to maintain his/her health or move towards the ease end of the continuum. On the other hand, failure to successfully handle stressors may lead to breakdown or a movement towards the *dis*ease end of the continuum [44, 45]. The SMH in malaria therefore highlights processes through which people move toward the ease end of the continuum in the context of their daily lives and experiences with malaria. Malaria as a stressor requires that people move to the ease end of the continuum to overcome it. In order to do this, people need to employ resources.

The SMH has two pivotal concepts, which are the Generalized Resistance Resources (GRRs) and Sense of Coherence (SOC) [46]. These two elements are essential for coping with malaria and creating health. Antonovsky defined GRRs as "physical, biochemical, artefactual-material, cognitive, emotional, valuative attitudinal, interpersonal, relational, macro-sociocultural characteristics of an individual, primary group, subculture, society, which are effective in avoiding or combatting a wide variety of stressors" [42]. GRRs can be material or immaterial attributes found within people or their immediate or remote environments (e.g., knowledge, genetic qualities, intelligence, or control) [44]. In the fight against malaria, it is important that people not only have GRRs but also their ability to recognize and reuse resources in a way that promotes health. A study carried out on camp-dwellers in Cameroon identified knowledge about malaria and free healthcare services as potential GRRs employed to combat malaria [47]. The important aspect was for the camp-dwellers to be able to identify these as resources before they can be available for use. Being able to identify potential resources is based on the second element of salutogenesis, which is SOC. SOC is defined as "a global orientation that expresses the extent to which one has a pervasive, enduring though dynamic feeling of confidence that: (a) the stimuli from one's internal and external environments in the course of living are structured, predictable and explicable (comprehensibility); (b) the resources are available to meet the demands posed by these stimuli (meaningfulness); and (c) these demands are challenges worthy of investment and engagement (manageability)" [43]. SOC accurately reflects a person's capacity to respond to stressful situations. In the case of malaria, therefore, a person with a strong SOC will be better able to identify resources and apply them to combat malaria. In the aforementioned camp-dweller study, SOC was a predictor for coping. Camp-dwellers with stronger SOC were most likely to use the free healthcare services offered by CDC or their knowledge about malaria to stay healthy in situations of malaria [48].

9.3 Health Despite Malaria

The salutogenic model of health explores malaria at a hitherto unexplored angle and should enable a holistic and more integrated approach to malaria control and elimination [49, 50]. The fight against malaria explored this way will bring out individual, social and environmental aspects related to coping with malaria. Such findings are important for successful and sustainable health promotion interventions that aim to eradicate or reduce the devastating effects of malaria. Salutogenesis highlights people as vital instruments to be included in matters that concern them because they are responsible for decisions about their health and welfare. Instead of focusing therefore on only the causes of disease, the SMH will shift the focus towards people's agency and capabilities in dealing with malaria. This approach will highlight the different resistance resources that people identify and use to deal with malaria and therefore contribute to people maintaining their health despite malaria.

References

1. World Health Organization (2016) World malaria report. World Health Organization, Geneva
2. Lengeler C (2004) Insecticide-treated bed nets and curtains for preventing malaria. Cochrane Database Syst Rev (2):CD000363
3. Hawley WA, Phillips-Howard PA, ter Kuile FO et al (2003) Community-wide effects of permethrin-treated bed nets on child mortality and malaria morbidity in western Kenya. Am J Trop Med Hyg 68:121–127
4. Howard SC, Omumbo J, Nevill C et al (2009) Evidence for a mass community effect of insecticide-treated bed nets on the incidence of malaria on the Kenyan coast. Trans R Soc Trop Med Hyg 94:357–360
5. Midzi N, Mtapuri-Zinyowera S, Mapingure MP et al (2011) Knowledge attitudes and practices of grade three primary schoolchildren in relation to schistosomiasis, soil transmitted helminthiasis and malaria in Zimbabwe. BMC Infect Dis 11:169
6. Abate A, Degarege A, Erko B (2013) Community knowledge, attitude and practice about malaria in a low endemic setting of Shewa Robit Town, northeastern Ethiopia. BMC Public Health 13:312
7. Mutua EN, Bukachi SA, Bett BK et al (2016) Lay knowledge and management of malaria in Baringo county, Kenya. Malar J 15:486
8. Adongo PB, Kirkwood B, Kendall C (2005) How local community knowledge about malaria affects insecticide-treated net use in northern Ghana. Trop Med Int Health 10:366–378
9. O'Neill S, Gryseels C, Dierickx S et al (2015) Foul wind, spirits and witchcraft: illness conceptions and healthseeking behaviour for malaria in the Gambia. Malar J 14:167
10. Njama D, Dorsey G, Guwatudde D et al (2003) Urban malaria: primary caregivers' knowledge, attitudes, practices and predictors of malaria incidence in a cohort of Ugandan children. Trop Med Int Health 8:685–692
11. Krezanoski PJ, Tsai AC, Hamer DH et al (2014) Household malaria knowledge and its association with bed net ownership in settings without large-scale distribution programs: evidence from rural Madagascar. J Glob Health 4:10401
12. Shimaponda-Mataa NM, Tembo-Mwase E, Gebreslasie M et al (2017) Knowledge, attitudes and practices in the control and prevention of malaria in four endemic provinces of Zambia. S Afr J Infect Dis 32:29–39
13. Kanyangarara M, Hamapumbu H, Mamini E et al (2018) Malaria knowkedge and bed net use in three transmission settings in Southern Africa. Malar J 17:41
14. World malaria report (2017) Geneva: World Health Organization. Licence: CC BY-NC-SA 3.0 IGO
15. World malaria report (2018) Geneva: World Health Organization. Licence: CC BY-NC-SA 3.0 IGO
16. Panter-Brick C, Clarke SE, Lomas H et al (2006) Culturally compelling strategies for behaviour change: a social ecology model and case study in malaria prevention. Soc Sci Med 62:2810–2825
17. Shililu J, Ghebremeskel T, Mengistu S et al (2003) High seasonal variation in entomologic inoculation rates in Eritrea, a semi-arid region of unstable malaria in Africa. Am J Trop Med Hyg 69:607–613
18. Okello PE, Van Bortel W, Byaruhanga AM et al (2006) Variation in malaria transmission intensity in seven sites throughout Uganda. Am J Trop Med Hyg 75:219–225
19. Carter R, Mendis KN, Roberts D (2000) Spatial targeting of interventions against malaria. Bull World Health Organ 78:1401–1411
20. Mabaso ML, Craig M, Ross A et al (2007) Environmental predictors of the seasonality of malaria transmission in Africa: the challenge. Am J Trop Med Hyg 76:33–38
21. Kelly-Hope LA, McKenzie FE (2009) The multiplicity of malaria transmission: a review of entomological inoculation rate measurements and methods across sub-Saharan Africa. Malar J 8:19
22. de Souza D, Kelly-Hope L, Lawson B et al (2012) Environmental factors associated with the distribution of *Anopheles gambiae* s.s in Ghana; an important vector of lymphatic filariasis and malaria. PLoS One 5:e9927
23. Charlwood JD, Kihonda J, Sama S et al (1995) The rise and fall of *Anopheles arabiensis* (Diptera: Culicidae) in a Tanzanian village. Bull Entomol Res 85:37–44
24. Drakeley C, Schellenberg D, Kihonda J et al (2003) An estimation of the entomological inoculation rate for Ifakara: a semi-urban area in a region of intense malaria transmission in Tanzania. Trop Med Int Health 8:767–774
25. Cairns M, Roca-Feltrer A, Garske T et al (2012) Estimating the potential public health impact of seasonal malaria chemo-prevention in African children. Nat Commun 3:881

26. Zhou G, Munga S, Minakawa N et al (2007) Spatial relationship between adult malaria vector abundance and environmental factors in western Kenya highlands. Am J Trop Med Hyg 77:29–35
27. Manda H, Gouagna LC, Foster WA et al (2007) Effect of discriminative plant-sugar feeding on the survival and fecundity of *Anopheles gambiae*. Malar J 6:113
28. Okech BA, Gouagna LC, Yan G et al (2007) Larval habitats of *Anopheles gambiae* s.s. (Diptera: Culicidae) influences vector competence to *Plasmodium falciparum* parasites. Malar J 6:50
29. Guerra CA, Snow RW, Hay SI (2006) A global assessment of closed forests, deforestation and malaria risk. Ann Trop Med Parasitol 100:189–204
30. Achard F, Eva HD, Stibig HJ et al (2002) Determination of deforestation rates of the world's humid tropical forests. Science 297:999–1002
31. Mayaux P, Holmgren P, Achard F et al (2005) Tropical forest cover change in the 1990s and options for future monitoring. Philos Trans R Soc Lond Ser B Biol Sci 360:373–384
32. Erhart A, Ngo DT, Phan VK et al (2005) Epidemiology of forest malaria in central Vietnam: a large scale cross-sectional survey. Malar J 4:58
33. Eisele TP, Larsen D, Steketee RW (2010) Protective efficacy of interventions for preventing malaria mortality in children in *Plasmodium falciparum* endemic areas. Int J Epidemiol 39: i88–i101
34. Bhatt S, Weiss DJ, Cameron E et al (2015) The effect of malaria control on *Plasmodium falciparum* in Africa between 2000 and 2015. Nature 526:207–211
35. World Health Organization (2013) WHO recommendations for achieving universal coverage with long-lasting insecticidal nets in malaria control (revised March 2014). WHO, Geneva. (http://www.who.int/malaria/publications/atoz/who)
36. Bhatt S, Gething P (2014) Insecticide-treated nets (ITNs) in Africa 2000–2016: coverage, system efficiency and future needs for achieving international targets. Malar J 13(Suppl 1):029
37. World Health Organization (2018) Global Malaria Programme, Malaria Policy Advisory Committee (MPAC) meeting report, April 2018. http://www.who.int/malaria/mpac/meeting_reports/en/
38. Alnazly E (2016) Coping strategies and socio-demographic characteristics among Jordanian caregivers of patients receiving hemodialysis. Saudi J Kidney Dis Transpl 27:101
39. Antonovsky A (1979) Health, stress, and coping, 1st edn. Jossey-Bass, San Francisco
40. Antonovsky A (1987) The Jossey-Bass social and behavioral science series and the Jossey-Bass health series. In: Unraveling the mystery of health: how people manage stress and stay well. Jossey-Bass, San Francisco, CA
41. Dardet CA, Tomas AB, Boonekamp G, Breton E, Contu P, Fosse E, Hofmeister A, Juvinya D, Kennedy L, Koelen M, Lindström B, Masanot G, Pavlekoviç G, Pocetta G, Vaandrager L, Wagemakers A (2016). Twenty-five years of capacity building. ETC-PHHP Team 2016
42. Eriksson M, Lindström B, Lilja J (2007) A sense of coherence and health. Salutogenesis in a societal context: Aland, a special case? J Epidemiol Community Health 61:684–688
43. Lindstrom B, Eriksson J (2010) The hitchhiker's guide to salutogenesis: salutogenic pathways to health promotion. Helsinki, Folkhalsan Research Centre
44. Makoge V, Hogeling L, Maat H et al (2017) Poverty-related diseases: factors that predict coping in two Cameroonian settings. Health Promot Int. https://doi.org/10.1093/heapro/dax088
45. Makoge V, Maat H, Vaandrager L et al (2017) Health-seeking behaviour towards poverty-related disease (PRDs): a qualitative study of people living in camps and on campuses in Cameroon. PLoS Negl Trop Dis 11:e0005218
46. Makoge V, Maat H, Vaandrager L et al (2017) Poverty-related diseases (PRDs): unravelling complexities in disease responses in Cameroon. Trop Med Health 45:2
47. Marmot M (2005) Social determinants of health inequalities. Lancet 365:1099–1104
48. Mittelmark MB et al (2017) The handbook of salutogenesis. Springer Open, Heidelberg. https://doi.org/10.1007/978-3-319-04600-6
49. Ntonifor NH, Veyufambom S (2016) Assessing the effective use of mosquito nets in the prevention of malaria in some parts of Mezam division, Northwest Region Cameroon. Malar J 15:390
50. Sachs JD (2012) From millennium development goals to sustainable development goals. Lancet 379:2206–2211

Chapter 3

Current Malaria Situation in Asia-Oceania

Chansuda Wongsrichanalai, Rossitza Kurdova-Mintcheva, and Kevin Palmer

Abstract

Asia-Oceania is a diverse region that comprises roughly 65% of the global population at risk for malaria. In 2016 WHO estimated the number of malaria cases across the Asia-Oceania to be 17 million, which is only a small part (8%) of the total global malaria burden, and the number of cases is shrinking rapidly. Most countries have brought their cases down to the point where elimination is in sight. *Plasmodium vivax* (*P. vivax*) is becoming the dominant malaria species in many of those countries, where malaria occurs in hot spots of transmission frequently along international borders. The challenge is now to concentrate on those areas. This chapter reviews the situation in various areas of the Region and focuses on a number of important issues, including the prevalence of *P. vivax* and drug-resistant malaria.

Key words Malaria, South West Asia, South East Asian Region, Western Pacific Region, Elimination, *Plasmodium vivax*, Resistance

1 Introduction

Geographically, Asia-Oceania includes a total of 24 malaria-endemic countries in three WHO regions: five countries in the southwest Asia (SWA) part of the Eastern Mediterranean Region (EMR), nine countries in the Southeast Asia Region (SEAR), and ten in the Western Pacific Region (WPR). It is a diverse Region that stretches from Vanuatu in the southeast to Afghanistan in the west with a total population of 4 billion, which represents 72% of the global population. It comprises roughly 65% of the population at risk for malaria in the world. The WHO estimate of the total malaria cases in this region in 2016 is 17 million (Table 1).

Overall there has been a significant decline in malaria incidence combined with a sharp drop in malaria mortality to the point where, by 2015, 21 countries had adopted the goal of malaria

Electronic supplementary material: The online version of this chapter (https://doi.org/10.1007/978-1-4939-9550-9_3) contains supplementary material, which is available to authorized users.

Frédéric Ariey et al. (eds.), *Malaria Control and Elimination*, Methods in Molecular Biology, vol. 2013, https://doi.org/10.1007/978-1-4939-9550-9_3, © Springer Science+Business Media, LLC, part of Springer Nature 2019

Table 1
The countries grouped by WHO Regions showing total population, population-at-risk of malaria, the number of confirmed malaria cases, and WHO point estimate of malaria cases in 2016 (World Health Organization, 2017)

Region/country	Total population (UN) (in million)	Population-at-risk (low + high) (in million)	Population-at-risk (high) (in million)	Confirmed malaria cases[a] (reported)	WHO point estimate of malaria cases
Southwest Asia (SWA)					
Afghanistan	34.7	26.7	9.4	392,551	556,000
Iran	80.3	<0.5	–	705 Mostly imported	≤100
Pakistan	193.2	189.9	55.9	2,115,941	1,307,000
Saudi Arabia	32.3	<0.1	–	5382 Mostly imported	270
Yemen	27.6	21.5	6.9	144,628 37% imported	433,000
SWA Total	368.1	238.6		**2,659,207**	**989,370**
WHO Southeast Asia (SEAR)					
Bangladesh	163.0	17.5	2.1	4787	6000
Bhutan	0.8	<0.1	–	74 Mostly imported	≤100
Democratic Republic of Korea (DPRK)	25.4	9.5	–	5113	2700
India	1324.2	1237.3	160.6	1,090,724	13,170,000
Indonesia	261.1	261.1	16.7	218,450	1,281,000
Myanmar	52.9	31.5	8.4	110,146	142,600
Nepal	29.0	8.4	1.5	10,687	4000
Thailand	69.0	13.1	1.5	11,522	11,520
Timor-Leste	1.3	0.2	<0.1	95	140
SEAR Total	1926.7	1578.6		**1,451,598**	**14,618,060**
WHO Western Pacific (WPR)					
Cambodia	15.8	11.1	7.6	23,492	83,300
China	1411.4	<0.01	–	3143 Almost all imported	≤10

(continued)

Table 1 (continued)

Region/country	Total population (UN) (in million)	Population-at-risk (low + high) (in million)	Population-at-risk (high) (in million)	Confirmed malaria cases[a] (reported)	WHO point estimate of malaria cases
Lao PDR	6.8	3.5	3.5	11,223	27,390
Malaysia	31.2	<0.1	–	2302 (mostly *P. knowlesi*)	270[b]
Papua New Guinea	8.1	8.1	7.6	728,798	1,407,000
The Philippines	103.3	60.0	7.0	6690	16,630
Republic of Korea (RoK)	50.8	–	–	673	600
Solomon Islands	0.6	0.6	0.6	84,513	86,000
Vanuatu	0.3	0.3	0.2	2147	4000
Viet Nam	94.6	69.7	6.4	10,446	6000
WPR Total	**1722.9**	153.3		**867,267**	**1,631,200**
Asia-Oceania Regional total	4017.7 (71.8% of global total	1970.5 (65.1% of global total)		**4,978,072**	**17,220,630** 8.0% of global total
Global total	5592.6	3025.8			**215,900,000**

[a]Reported cases (different from WHO estimate, which is 17 million for regional total)
[b]*P. knowlesi* not included

elimination in line with the global goal of eliminating malaria in 35 countries by 2030 [1]. In the recent past, two countries were WHO-certified malaria-free: Maldives in 2015, and Sri Lanka in 2016. Other countries are at various stages along the path to elimination as defined by WHO [2].

Malaria incidence in the Asia-Oceania Region is highlighted by its diversity. A few countries still have high levels of transmission, including Afghanistan, Pakistan, India, Indonesia, and Papua New Guinea, but the majority has an annual parasite incidence (API) of less than five cases per thousand. In those countries, remaining cases are localized in hot spots, and the challenge is how to reach those areas. Below, we consider the importance of malaria depending on areas in the Region and specific issues including population movements and ongoing conflict situations. The epidemiology of malaria at the country level is available in Supplementary Files 1–3. We also consider the problem of resistance to antimalarials.

2 A Glance at the Region

2.1 Southwest Asia (SWA)

Countries of SWA with malaria transmission are Afghanistan, Islamic Republic of Iran, Pakistan, Saudi Arabia, and Yemen. Of these, Iran and Saudi Arabia are in the elimination phase. Incidence rates decreased by >75% from 2000 to 2015 in Afghanistan, Iran, and Saudi Arabia. Most areas of Iran (except the border with Pakistan) and of Saudi Arabia (except the border with Yemen) are free of malaria [3]. Access to diagnosis and treatment is very good in Iran and Saudi Arabia, at the level of universal coverage. In other countries, access has improved but remains a problem in peripheral areas, where access to malaria prevention and case management is still poor. Figure 1 shows the overall trend of confirmed cases and deaths for the region (presumed cases and imported cases excluded). Country-specific trends vary. In some countries especially Pakistan and Yemen, there are fluctuations in confirmed cases, and therefore it is not possible to conclude whether malaria incidence is actually increasing, decreasing, or constant [3].

Among the SWA countries, key obstacles to malaria control and elimination are population movements, political instability, and civil conflicts leading to security concerns and humanitarian emergency conditions. Limited capability of surveillance, insufficiency of trained healthcare staff, reliance on external resources, and, in some endemic areas, the rising insecticide resistance further limit the ability to sustain the gains achieved to date. The Region experienced the reemergence of malaria following the conflicts in Afghanistan and Yemen.

2.2 Southeast Asia Region (SEAR)

SEAR accounts for 70% of the global malaria burden outside of Africa (14.6 million out of 21 million). Among the nine endemic countries, India, Indonesia, and Myanmar together contribute

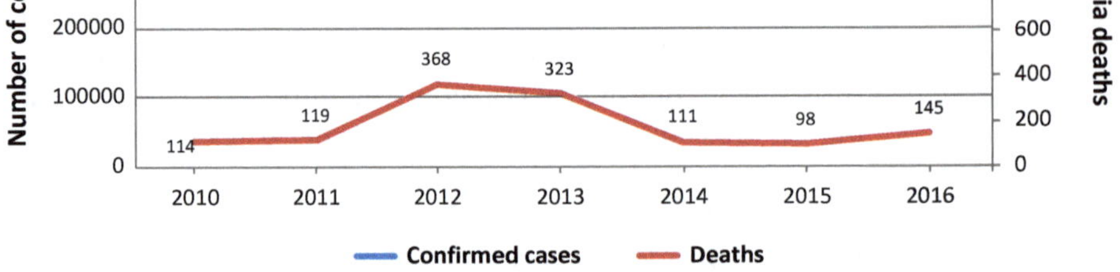

Fig. 1 Southwest Asia—malaria cases and deaths, 2010–2016 (Presumed cases and imported cases excluded)

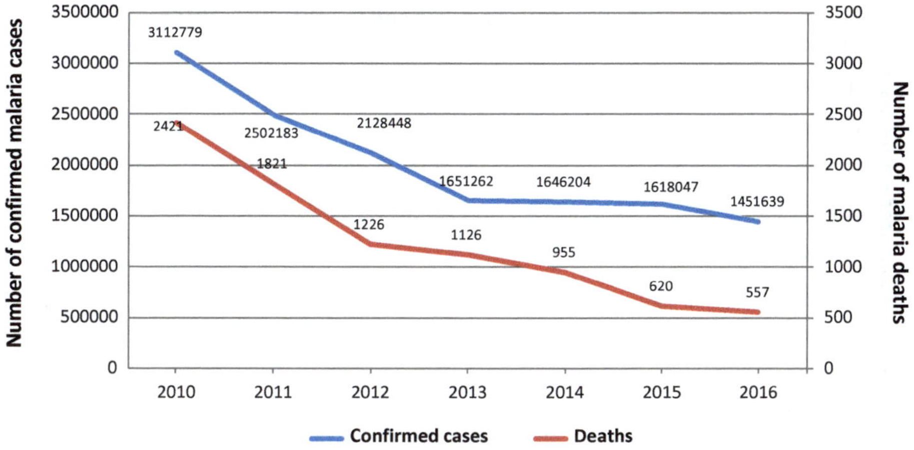

Fig. 2 Southeast Asia—malaria cases and deaths, 2010–2016

almost all the cases. Importantly, there has been a steady decline in the annual malaria incidence and deaths since 2000 in the Region, with a 48% reduction in cases and a 77% reduction in malaria deaths between 2010 and 2016 (Fig. 2). The Region has set an elimination target of 2030, and already two countries have been certified malaria-free: Maldives in 2015 (malaria-free since 1984) and Sri Lanka in 2016 [4].

Plasmodium vivax (*P. vivax*) has increasingly become dominant in the Region and is accounting for >70% of *P. vivax* cases globally [5]. The proportion of cases due to *P. falciparum* varies greatly, ranging from 91% in Bangladesh to 0 in the Democratic People's Republic of Korea (DPRK). The major challenges that stand in the way of malaria elimination in the Region include *P. falciparum* parasites resistant to artemisinin combinations and vector mosquitoes resistant to pyrethroids. Migration both internally and across international borders results in constant re-introduction of parasites from high-transmission to highly receptive, malaria-free areas. Reducing the high disease burdens in India, Indonesia, and Myanmar is now the major challenge, as the other countries are moving toward malaria-free status. Weak reporting systems, limited capacity of case-based surveillance in some countries, and the sustainability of funding all complicate efforts to eliminate the disease.

2.3 Western Pacific Region (WPR)

The total population of WPR is approximately 1.7 billion, of which 153 million (9%) live in areas with some risks (Table 1). Excluding Papua New Guinea, malaria cases in the Region decreased by 37% and malaria death by 88% between 2010 and 2016 (Fig. 3). In 2016, 92% of all cases in the Region were attributed to two countries: 85% to Papua New Guinea (PNG) and 10% to Solomon Islands. Since 2014 both countries as well as nearby Vanuatu have

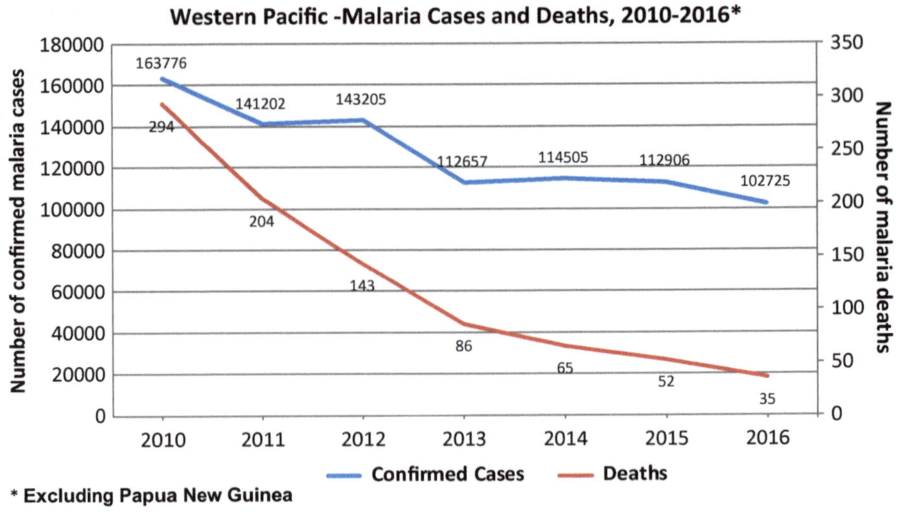

Fig. 3 Western Pacific—malaria cases and deaths, 2010–2016

reported a steady increase in cases, whereas in all other countries, malaria cases and deaths have continued to decline [6].

Malaria epidemiology exhibits enormous geographical and group-related heterogeneity throughout the Region and even within countries. Countries generally conform to one of the three epidemiological subgroups, based on their malaria transmission risk and underlying social and demographic factors [7]: (1) the three Melanesian countries where transmission is generally most intense, i.e., PNG, the Solomon Islands, and, to a lesser extent, Vanuatu; (2) Cambodia, Lao PDR, the Philippines, and Viet Nam, where transmission is often more focal and the disease affects ethnic minorities, migrant workers, and other mobile populations disproportionately; and (3) three countries where malaria elimination is within reach [China, Republic of Korea (ROK) and Malaysia]. China reported zero indigenous case in 2017 and Malaysia in 2018.

3 Malaria Parasites and Human Hosts

3.1 Parasite Species

Although globally only 7% of malaria cases are due to *P. vivax*, this species is increasingly important in Oceania and Asia. According to WHO, *P. vivax* accounts for 35% and 26% of all cases in SEAR and WPR, respectively (WHO 2017). The percentage of malaria deaths due to *P. vivax* were estimated at 7% in SEAR and 17% in WPR, while *P. vivax* is responsible for less than 1% of malaria deaths globally [8].

In southwest Asia, *P. falciparum* is still the dominant species among locally transmitted malaria cases in the Arabian Peninsula (Saudi Arabia and Yemen), while in Afghanistan, Iran, and Pakistan,

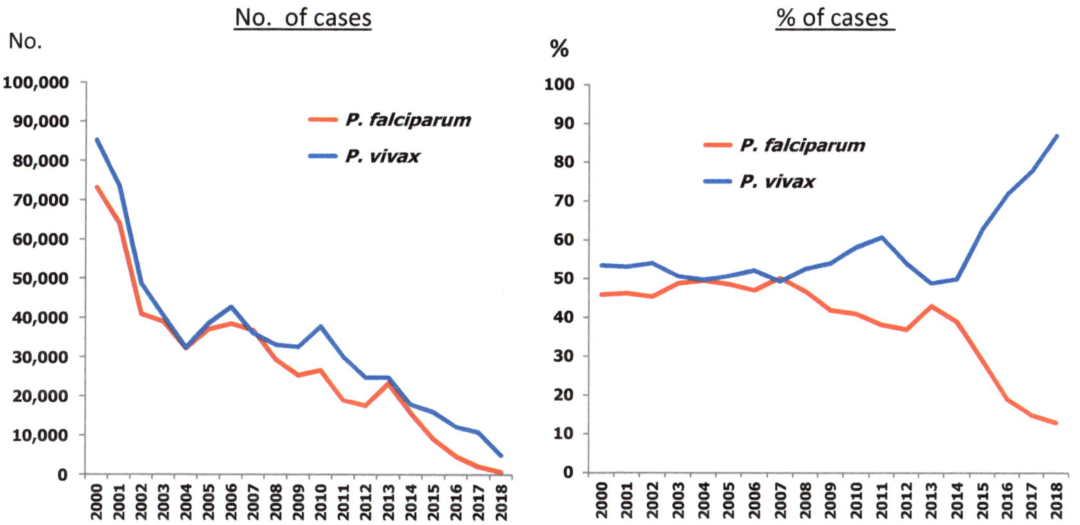

Fig. 4 Trend of malaria prevalence in Thailand by species, 2000–2018. Source: Bureau of Vector Borne Disease Control, Department of Disease Control, Thai Ministry of Public Health

over 80% of reported cases are caused by *P. vivax*. Both *P. falciparum* and *P. vivax* are common in SEAR, but there has been an increase in the proportion of *P. vivax* in recent years as malaria incidence declines. A good example is Thailand (Fig. 4), where *P. vivax* is now responsible for >80% of cases [9]. *P. falciparum* remains the dominant species in Bangladesh, India, Myanmar, and Timor-Leste. *P. vivax* is predominant among locally transmitted infections in Vanuatu and Viet Nam and accounts for all cases on the Korean Peninsula, i.e., ROK and the Democratic Republic of Korea (DPRK).

P. knowlesi, a parasite "of macaques", accounts for 88% of human cases in Malaysia. A large focus of human infections was identified over a decade ago in Sarawak State (northwestern part of Borneo Island) [10]. Since then, small pockets have been found elsewhere in the Region [11]. The pathogenesis of this species in humans, its epidemiology, the true disease burden, and transmission patterns are still not well understood [12].

3.2 Treatment of *P. vivax* and G6PD Deficiency in Populations in Endemic Areas

In SWA, chloroquine with primaquine (14 daily doses or 8 weekly doses) is the regimen of choice for *P. vivax* infection in all five countries. Chloroquine remains the first-line schizonticide drug for *P. vivax* malaria in several other Asian countries, but there are reports of chloroquine-resistance *P. vivax* from wide geographic areas [13]. High-grade resistance in Indonesia and Papua New Guinea led to the use of ACT as *P. vivax* schizonticide in those countries, as well as in other Oceania countries (Solomon Islands and Vanuatu). Based on evidence of reduced chloroquine efficacy in therapeutic efficacy surveillance, Cambodia also adopted ACT to replace chloroquine for treating *P. vivax* [14, 15]. In Lao PDR, the ACT first-line therapy (artemether-lumefantrine) is used against both *P. falciparum* and *P. vivax* to simplify the treatment practice.

Despite the increasing proportion of *P. vivax*, radical therapy with primaquine is not implemented in most countries even though it is part of most national treatment guidelines. Fear of hemolysis in G6PD-deficient patients and the lack of access to point-of-care G6PD testing have made many healthcare personnel reluctant to administer primaquine. Exceptions are the ROK and Malaysia, where most *P. vivax* patients can be hospitalized or well monitored to ensure compliance of the extended (14-day) primaquine radical therapy and to allow observation/notification of any adverse events.

There are a number of variants of G6PD deficiency, some of which have a deadly reaction to primaquine, while others produce no or minor hemolysis. The frequency of G6PD deficiency varies among ethnic groups. For example, in Afghanistan, 9% of the population of the Pashtun/Pashai ethnic group is deficient, which is much higher than the rest of the country, where roughly 2.0% of the population is deficient. In Pakistan, the prevalence was found to be 8% in Peshawar, but among the Pathan ethnic group, the prevalence varied from 7% to 16% [16]. In Indonesia, the Mediterranean, Vanua Lava, and Viangchan variants that can be highly reactive to primaquine are common in the East, suggesting that caution must be taken when considering giving primaquine without a G6PD test [17]. In Cambodia, the common G6PD Viangchan, known for its association with severe hemolysis, has led to removal of primaquine from the country for decades.

4 Malaria Treatment and Drug Resistance

4.1 SWA

In southwest Asia, Iran and Saudi Arabia use artesunate + sulfadoxine + pyrimethamine (AS-SP). Afghanistan and Pakistan have just switched to artemether-lumefantrine. Yemen is using artemether-lumefantrine as an interim therapy (2018) while anticipating a formal policy adoption that will include a single-dose primaquine. Adeel and collaborators studied AS-SP and artemether-lumefantrine efficacy in Yemen during 2009–2013. Both were highly efficacious, but as expected, artemether-lumefantrine had better efficacy in clearing gametocytemia [18].

4.2 SEAR

All countries have used ACT for uncomplicated *P. falciparum* infection, with artemether-lumefantrine being the drug of choice for Bangladesh, Bhutan, Nepal, and Timor-Leste. Myanmar mainly uses artemether-lumefantrine (Government health facilities) but also includes in the National Treatment Guidelines (NTG) dihydroartemisinin-piperaquine and artesunate-mefloquine as options in some settings. Thailand switched from artesunate-mefloquine to dihydroartemisinin-piperaquine during 2016/2017. India has primarily used AS-SP, but according to the latest NTG, India has switched to artemether-lumefantrine in the north-eastern states [19], where the efficacy of AS-SP had been shown to be poor [20]. Indonesia uses dihydroartemisinin-piperaquine for both *P. falciparum* and *P. vivax* infections.

4.3 WPR

All countries have adopted ACT as the first-line regimen for uncomplicated *P. falciparum* malaria. Artemether-lumefantrine is used in Lao PDR, PNG, Solomon Islands, Vanuatu, and the Philippines, while dihydroartemisinin-piperaquine is used in Viet Nam. Malaysia uses artesunate-mefloquine. China's NTG include four choices of first-line ACTs for *P. falciparum* malaria: dihydroartemisinin-piperaquine, artemisinin-naphthoquine, artemisinin-piperaquine, and artesunate-amodiaquine.

4.4 Greater Mekong Subregion (GMS) Is a Hot Spot of Antimalarial Drug Resistance

The GMS is the core area of multidrug-resistant malaria. Cambodia and Thailand, in particular, have adopted more antimalarial regimens in their treatment policies than any of the other countries. Chloroquine, sulfadoxine-pyrimethamine (SP), quinine, artesunate-mefloquine, atovaquone-proguanil (Malarone), and dihydroartemisinin-piperaquine have all been used. After the emergence of artemisinin resistance in the early 2000s, Cambodia has experienced a series of multidrug resistance issues necessitating repetitive changes in their first-line therapy for *P. falciparum* [21–24]. The characteristics of drug resistance in Mekong are independent emergence of artemisinin partial resistance in multiple locations and the emergence of multidrug resistance, including partial artemisinin resistance and partner drug resistance causing ACT failure [24].

In 2016, Cambodia had to switch back to artesunate-mefloquine due to high treatment failures of dihydroartemisinin and piperaquine combination [25, 26]. Most recently, piperaquine resistance was also documented in Viet Nam along with a decline in the susceptibility of *P. falciparum* to dihydroartemisinin-piperaquine [27]. After almost two decades of using artesunate-mefloquine as the first-line therapy, Thailand had to replace it with dihydroartemisinin-piperaquine recently due to high treatment failure rates in some parts of the countries. Thailand is also in the process of introducing pyronaridine-artesunate in selected endemic areas. The trend of declining artemether-lumefantrine efficacy has also been documented in Lao PDR [24].

Multidrug-resistant malaria, especially resistance to artemisinin compounds, continues to be a key obstacle to malaria control and a threat to the progress in malaria elimination in Asia. Resistance to one or more ACTs has been documented in the Mekong countries with therapeutic efficacy surveillance data suggesting resistance to multiple WHO-recommended ACTs in Cambodia, Thailand, Lao PDR, and Viet Nam [24].

Recent identification of the PfKelch13 (K13) mutations enables a more refined definition of artemisinin resistance [23]. A large number of K13 mutants have been reported in Asia and elsewhere. Distinct alleles with K13 mutations are common and widely distributed in Southeast Asia especially in the GMS, where artemisinin resistance first emerged [24, 28]. Several of them are candidate resistance markers (correlate with delayed parasite clearance in clinical trials), but to date less than a dozen have been "validated" as markers of resistance (correlated with slow parasite clearance and also with reduced in vitro drug sensitivity) [24]. It should be noted that the prevalence of the K13 mutation cannot be used as an indicator of ACT treatment outcomes. In Cambodia, where 95% of *P. falciparum* parasites carry the K13 C580Y mutation (a validated marker) and previous ACT failures were known, a certain ACT may still be highly efficacious. Despite the presence of delayed parasite clearance (partial artemisinin resistance), patients are still cured if the partner drug of that ACT remains efficacious. In Lao PDR, artemisinin resistance was confirmed in 2013 with the detection of K13 C580Y mutants in southern Laos. In Myanmar, the predominant K13 mutant does not appear to have spread from Cambodia but is more likely to be of independent origin [29]. Because of the need to eliminate artemisinin-resistant parasites as soon as possible, a separate, species-specific, earlier target for the elimination of *P. falciparum* has been set by some countries, e.g., Cambodia by 2020.

5 Conclusion: The Path to Regional Elimination

The malaria burden across the Asia-Oceania Region is only 8% of the total global malaria burden, and it is shrinking rapidly. At one end of the spectrum are Afghanistan, Pakistan, Yemen, India, Papua New Guinea, and the Solomon Islands, where the disease burden is still high and elimination is still far in the future. At the other end are Sri Lanka and the Maldives that are already certified malaria-free. For the rest, the so-called eliminating countries can be put into two groups: those that have set targets of 2021 or before and those that are targeted for between 2022 and 2029. In the first group are Bhutan, Timor-Leste, China, Malaysia, and the ROK. China recorded no locally acquired cases in 2017 and 2018, and Malysia in 2018 All other countries are well on track to meet their targets. In the second group are DPRK, Nepal, Thailand, Cambodia, Lao PDR, the Philippines, Vanuatu, and Viet Nam. In addition, interim targets for eliminating *P. falciparum* by 2020 have been set by Cambodia, Iran, and Saudi Arabia and by 2025 for Myanmar. Also by 2025, APIs are expected to be reduced to <1/1,000 population in all subnational-level administrative units in Bangladesh and Indonesia.

The goals are ambitious and will require long-term political commitment on the part of the countries and continuing commitment on the part of key partners to provide the necessary financial and technical support to finish the job. This is going to be especially important for those countries that currently have high malaria burdens, civil and political unrest, weak health systems, and lack of political commitment that prevent the effective implementation of the control strategies that we now have. The path to elimination of malaria is not easy, but the goal is for the first time in sight in Asia-Oceania.

Acknowledgments

The following individuals have contributed to this manuscript: Ghasem Zamani, Mohammad Sami Nahzat, Mya S. Ngon, Preecha Prempree, Dysoley Lek, and Akira Kaneko. We are also grateful to the Bureau of Vector Borne Disease Control, Department of Disease Control, Thai Ministry of Public Health, for their support.

References

1. Newby G, Bennett A, Larson E et al (2016) The path to eradication: a progress report on the malaria-eliminating countries. Lancet 387:1775–1784
2. World Health Organization (2015) Global Technical Strategy for Malaria 2016–2030. World Health Organization, Geneva
3. World Health Organization Regional Office for the Eastern Mediterranean (2017) Regional Malaria Action Plan 2016–2020—Towards a Malaria-Free Region. WHO Regional Office for the Eastern Mediterranean, Cairo
4. World Health Organization South-East Asia Regional Office (2017) Regional Action Plan 2017-2013. World Health Organization, New Delhi
5. World Health Organization (2015) World Malaria Report 2015. World Health Organization, Geneva
6. World Health Organization (2017) World Malaria Report 2017. World Health Organization, Geneva
7. World Health Organization Regional Office for the Western Pacific (2017) Regional Framework for Malaria Control and Elimination in the Western Pacific (2016-2020). World Health Organization, Manila, Philippines
8. World Health Organization (2016) World Malaria Report 2016. World Health Organization, Geneva
9. Department of Disease Control Ministry of Public Health Thailand. Thailand Malaria Elimination Program; online statistics. http://203.157.41.215/malariaR10/index_newversion.php
10. Singh B, Kim Sung L, Matusop A et al (2004) A large focus of naturally acquired *Plasmodium knowlesi* infections in human beings. Lancet 363:1017–1024
11. Singh B, Daneshvar C (2013) Human infections and detection of *Plasmodium knowlesi*. Clin Microbiol Rev 26:165–184
12. Barber BE, Grigg MJ, William T et al (2017) The treatment of *Plasmodium knowlesi* malaria. Trends Parasitol 33:242–253
13. Price RN, von Seidlein L, Valecha N et al (2014) Global extent of chloroquine-resistant *Plasmodium vivax*: a systematic review and meta-analysis. Lancet Infect Dis 14:982–991

14. Leang R, Barrette A, Bouth DM et al (2013) Efficacy of dihydroartemisinin-piperaquine for treatment of uncomplicated *Plasmodium falciparum* and *Plasmodium vivax* in Cambodia, 2008 to 2010. Antimicrob Agents Chemother 57:818–826
15. Leang R, Ros S, Duong S et al (2013) Therapeutic efficacy of fixed dose artesunate-mefloquine for the treatment of acute, uncomplicated *Plasmodium falciparum* malaria in Kampong Speu, Cambodia. Malar J 12:343
16. Moiz B (2013) A review of G6PD deficiency in Pakistani perspective. J Pak Med Assoc 63 (4):501–503
17. Surjadjaja C, Surya A, Baird JK (2016) Epidemiology of *Plasmodium vivax* in Indonesia. Am J Trop Med Hyg 95:121–132
18. Adeel AA, Saeed NA, Aljasari A et al (2015) High efficacy of two artemisinin-based combinations: artesunate + sulfadoxine-pyrimethamine and artemether-lumefantrine for falciparum malaria in Yemen. Malar J 14:449
19. Ministry of Health and Welfare India (2013) Diagnosis and treatment of malaria Directorate of National Vector Borne Disease Control Programme (NVBDCP). Directorate General Health Services
20. Mishra N, Kaitholia K, Srivastava B et al (2014) Declining efficacy of artesunate plus sulphadoxine-pyrimethamine in northeastern India. Malar J 13:284
21. Wongsrichanalai C, Pickard AL, Wernsdorfer WH et al (2002) Epidemiology of drug-resistant malaria. Lancet Infect Dis 2:209–218
22. Vijaykadga S, Rojanawatsirivej C, Cholpol S et al (2006) *In vivo* sensitivity monitoring of mefloquine monotherapy and artesunate-mefloquine combinations for the treatment of uncomplicated falciparum malaria in Thailand in 2003. Tropical Med Int Health 11:211–219
23. Ariey F, Witkowski B, Amaratunga C et al (2014) A molecular marker of artemisinin-resistant *Plasmodium falciparum* malaria. Nature 505:50–55
24. World Health Organization Global Malaria Programme (2018) Artemisinin resistance and artemisinin-based combination therapy efficacy. Status report. Geneva. https://apps.who.int/iris/bitstream/handle/10665/274362/WHO-CDS-GMP-2018.18-eng.pdf?ua=1
25. Amaratunga C, Lim P, Suon S et al (2016) Dihydroartemisinin-piperaquine resistance in *Plasmodium falciparum* malaria in Cambodia: a multisite prospective cohort study. Lancet Infect Dis 16:357–365
26. Duru V, Witkowski B, Menard D (2016) *Plasmodium falciparum* resistance to artemisinin derivatives and piperaquine: A major challenge for malaria elimination in Cambodia. Am J Trop Med Hyg 95:1228–1238
27. Thanh NV, Thuy-Nhien N, Tuyen NT et al (2017) Rapid decline in the susceptibility of *Plasmodium falciparum* to dihydroartemisinin-piperaquine in the south of Vietnam. Malar J 16:27
28. Menard D, Khim N, Beghain J et al (2016) A worldwide map of *Plasmodium falciparum* K13-Propeller polymorphisms. N Engl J Med 374:2453–2464
29. Takala-Harrison S, Jacob CG, Arze C, Cummings MP, Silva JC, Dondorp AM et al (2015) Independent emergence of artemisinin resistance mutations among Plasmodium falciparum in Southeast Asia. J Infect Dis 211 (5):670–679. https://doi.org/10.1093/infdis/jiu491

Chapter 4

Malaria Situation in Latin America and the Caribbean: Residual and Resurgent Transmission and Challenges for Control and Elimination

Marcelo U. Ferreira and Marcia C. Castro

Abstract

Despite recent progress toward malaria elimination in Latin America and the Caribbean, with an overall 62% decrease in incidence between 2000 and 2015, malaria remains endemic to 21 countries and territories in the region, where 120 million people are exposed to some risk of infection. Here we review recent epidemiologic trends, highlight current challenges, and briefly discuss the relative role of traditional and novel strategies for better malaria control and elimination across the continent.

Key words Malaria, Latin America, Epidemiology, Control, Elimination

1 Introduction

Although sub-Saharan Africa and South and Southeast Asia account for a disproportionately larger fraction of the global burden of malaria, this disease remains endemic to 21 countries in Latin America and the Caribbean, where 120 million people are exposed to some risk of infection. Malaria is responsible for limited mortality, but causes considerable morbidity in rural populations of the continent. Transmission is heterogeneously distributed in Latin America and nine countries, and territories in northern South America, namely, Bolivia, Brazil, Colombia, Ecuador, Guyana, French Guyana, Peru, Suriname, and Venezuela, currently account for 93.2% of the region's malaria burden [1].

As a former field officer of the Institute of Inter-American Affairs observed in 1947, "in a considerable number of countries of Latin America, real progress has been made in the control of malaria about the important cities and larger towns. (...) Less attention has been given to the smaller towns and rural areas" [2]. Since then, the 1955 Global Malaria Eradication Campaign brought transmission in Latin America to very low levels between

Frédéric Ariey et al. (eds.), *Malaria Control and Elimination*, Methods in Molecular Biology, vol. 2013,
https://doi.org/10.1007/978-1-4939-9550-9_4, © Springer Science+Business Media, LLC, part of Springer Nature 2019

the late 1950s and the early 1970s, especially in the major cities and most developed areas [3]. Six decades later, the main malaria hotspots map to relatively remote rural sites across the Amazon, which contributes approximately 90% of the malaria burden in South America, on the Pacific Coast of Peru, Ecuador, and Colombia, on the Atlantic Coast of Central America, as well as in Haiti. These hotspots are intermingled with areas of low or moderate risk (Fig. 1).

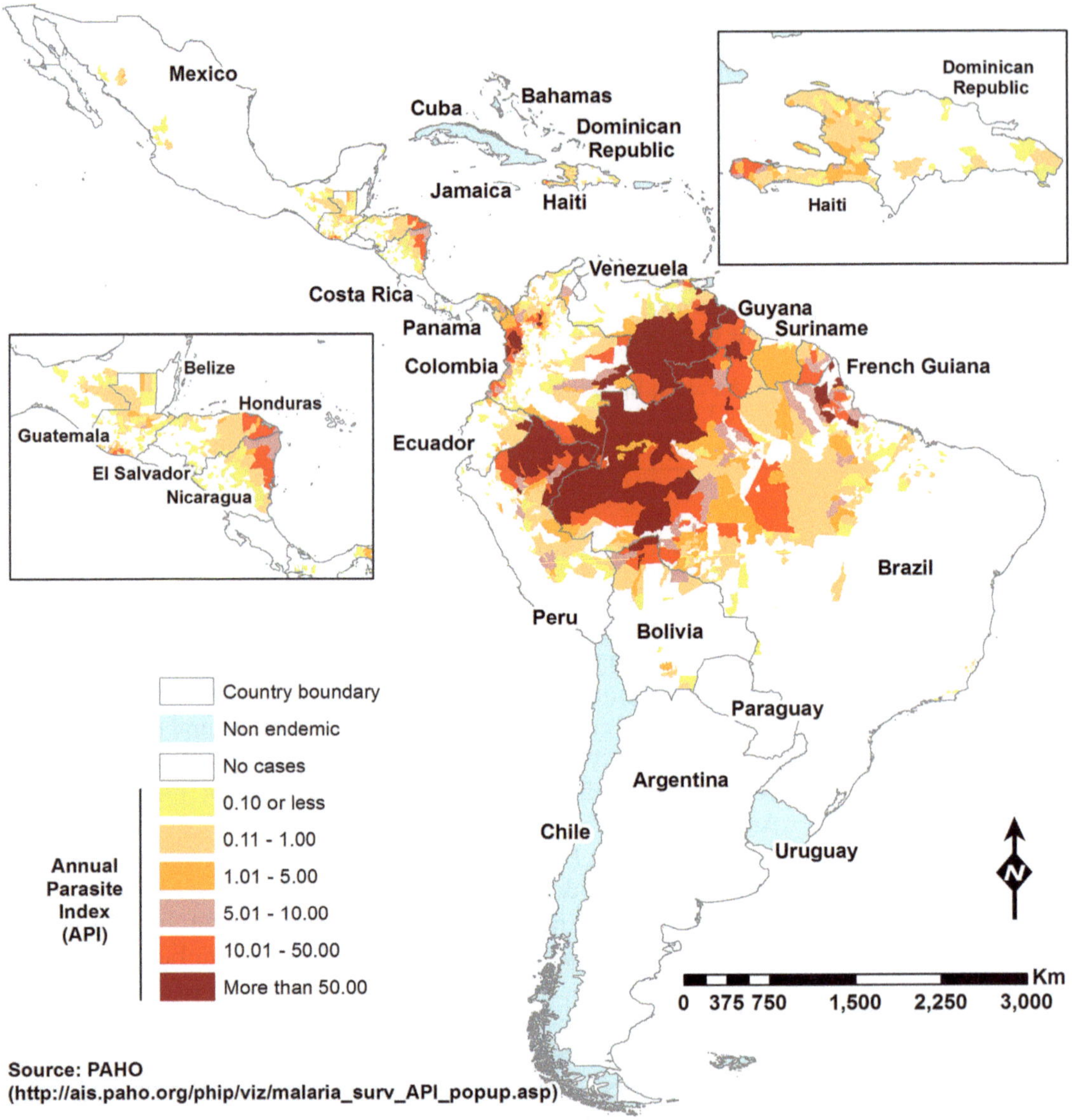

Fig. 1 Malaria Annual Parasite Index in Latin America and the Caribbean, 2015. Data extracted from the Pan American Health Organization (PAHO) Interactive Malaria Statistics [4]

2 Recent Epidemiologic Trends

Malaria incidence in the Americas has decreased by 62% between 2000 and 2015, when 451,242 laboratory-confirmed cases and 159 malaria-related deaths were officially reported to the Pan American Health Organization (PAHO). There was, however, a 16% increase in cases in 2015 compared to 2014, the year with the lowest malaria burden in the region over the past four decades [1]. Fourteen endemic countries achieved a ≥75% reduction in their case incidence rates between 2000 and 2015, as called for by the United Nations' Millennium Development Goals (MDGs) target 6.C [1]. Brazil alone contributed over half of the regional malaria burden in the early 2000s, but now reports only 31.7% of the microscopically confirmed cases and 22.0% of malaria-related deaths in the Americas [1, 5, 6]. The 143,162 cases recorded in Brazil in 2015 represent the lowest malaria incidence in this country in 36 years. Yet, foci of residual malaria remain entrenched across the Amazon Basin, which accounts for >99% of the country's malaria cases, and represent a major challenge for the Plan for Malaria Elimination launched by the Brazilian Ministry of Health in November 2015 [5].

A decrease in transmission in Haiti and major increases in Peru and Venezuela were the main changes in malaria epidemiology observed in the region over the past few years. Malaria was eliminated in most of the Caribbean islands nearly five decades ago, except for the Hispaniola, an island shared between Haiti and the Dominican Republic. The number of locally acquired malaria cases reported yearly in the Dominican Republic remained consistently below 1000 since 2012, while that in Haiti increased from 10,871 in 2001 to 86,635 after the devastating 2010 earthquake [7]. Most transmission in Haiti occurs in the Grand'Anse and Ouest departments, which together report approximately 72% of all cases in this country [1]. Rapid diagnostic tests (RDTs) for malaria were adopted countrywide following the 2010 earthquake [8], and the number of cases reported by the Ministry of Public Health and Population of Haiti, virtually all of them due to *Plasmodium falciparum* [9], decreased from 32,969 in 2011 [10] to 21,430 cases in 2016 [8]. These figures, however, underestimate total infections, since asymptomatic and subpatent infections appear to be very common in the main endemic sites [11]. Improved access to laboratory diagnosis and treatment, as well as enhanced surveillance and ability to respond to outbreaks, were the main factors explaining the downward trend of malaria in Haiti [8].

Currently, resurgent malaria is a major public health concern in Peru and Venezuela, where incidence has doubled and tripled, respectively, between 2010 and 2015 [1]. Most infections are acquired in small villages, rural settlements, and gold mining camps within the Amazon rainforest [12]. The department of Loreto, in the northern Peruvian Amazon region, has only 4% of total country's population but has consistently concentrated most of the malaria burden in Peru [13]; it currently accounts for 96% of the malaria cases diagnosed countrywide [1]. Malaria incidence in Peru had decreased to 10–20 cases per 100,000 inhabitants in the mid-1960s, as a result of intensive indoor residual (IRS) spraying campaigns with dichlorodiphenyltrichloroethane (DDT) and improved case management during the 1955 eradication campaign. However, after DDT use was discontinued in 1988, incidence in Loreto increased 50-fold over the next decade [14]. The country failed to achieve the $\geq$75% reduction in malaria morbidity between 2000 and 2015 set by the MDGs target 6.C [1]; indeed, malaria incidence decreased by only 12% over this time frame, from 249.57 cases per 100,000 inhabitants in 2000 to 220.58 cases per 100,000 inhabitants in 2015 [15]. Moreover, incidence in Loreto rose from 9306 *P. vivax* and 2473 *P. falciparum* cases reported in 2011 to 46,924 and 12,425 cases, respectively, registered in 2015, with a constant vivax/falciparum ratio of approximately 3.8:1 [16]. A large proportion of parasite carriers is asymptomatic, with submicroscopic parasite densities that remain undiagnosed and untreated and are likely to represent important reservoirs for maintaining local malaria transmission [17]. There is a wide variation of entomological inoculation rates for the main vector, *Anopheles darlingi*, across Loreto region [18].

With regard to Venezuela, over two-thirds of its territory was declared malaria-free by the World Health Organization (WHO) in 1961, following a massive DDT spraying campaign that started one decade earlier [19]. However, malaria transmission now occurs in 16 of the 24 country states [20], and incidence has increased steadily since 2008 [12]. The heaviest burden of disease associated with malaria infection is shared between the states of Bolivar and Amazonas, which border with northernmost Brazil. A total of 136,402 laboratory-confirmed cases were reported in 2015 – the largest malaria burden in this country since 1937 [19], corresponding to 30.2% of all cases in the Americas [1]. The number of reported cases further increased to 240,613 in 2016 [20], when Venezuela surpassed Brazil as the country reporting the most malaria cases in the Americas. Most (75%) infections are due to *P. vivax*, with 19% of *P. falciparum* infections and 6% of mixed-species infections [20]. The explosion of gold mining activities, mostly illegal, across the Amazon Basin is the major driver of malaria transmission, especially in Sifontes municipality in Bolivar state, which alone contributed 52.7% of the country's malaria cases in 2015 [1]. Gold miners, who account for an estimated 80% of malaria cases in Venezuela, typically live in temporary huts with incomplete walls and have limited access to antimalarial drugs.

Local microscopists are often overburdened, and RDTs are not available in mining camps [20].

Malaria associated with gold mining is not limited to Venezuela. In fact, Brazil, Colombia, Suriname, French Guiana, and Peru all have significant gold extraction activities leading to increased malaria transmission [12, 17]. The situation is particularly dramatic in the Guiana Shield, which comprises Suriname, Guyana, and French Guiana and parts of Brazil, Colombia, and Venezuela [21]. Suriname, a country reaching the malaria pre-elimination phase and where <100 locally acquired cases were officially reported in 2015 [1], has an estimated 15,000 illegal immigrants, mainly from Brazil, working in gold mines in the eastern and central parts of the country [22]. They live in temporary and remote settlements where health infrastructure and compliance with national malaria treatment policies are typically very poor [23]. In Guyana, where malaria transmission remains intense, with 9984 cases registered in 2015 [1], there is molecular evidence that artemisinin-resistant parasites currently comprise 5% of the local *P. falciparum* population [24]. In French Guyana, between 5000 and 20,000 undocumented gold prospectors, the vast majority of them from Brazil [25], work in outbreak-prone remote areas in the Amazon rainforest [26]. Symptomless carriage of subpatent parasitemias, which are missed by conventional microscopy, is common among miners [25, 27], who typically use erratic and substandard artemisinin-based drug regimens to treat malaria episodes, facilitating the long-term persistence of low-level parasitemias and favoring the selection of drug-resistant strains [28]. Not surprisingly, miners from French Guiana represent a significant source of imported malaria into Brazil and Suriname [1]. Therefore, malaria in mining camps across the Guiana Shield poses a major threat to elimination efforts in French Guiana, Suriname, Guyana, and the northernmost areas in Brazil [29].

Lastly, major progress toward elimination has recently been made by selected countries in Latin America. Indeed, no locally acquired malaria cases were reported in Argentina, Paraguay, and Costa Rica in 2015 [1]. In the Southern Cone of South America, malaria has been a public health concern in parts of Paraguay and Argentina bordering Bolivia and Brazil, where population movements are intense and where dams and reservoirs for agricultural developments have created suitable breeding sites for mosquitoes [3]. Argentina has already requested WHO to initiate the process of certification of elimination, while three countries in Central America (Belize, Costa Rica, and El Salvador), Mexico, and three in South America (Ecuador, Paraguay, and Suriname) are on track to eliminate malaria by 2020 [1, 7].

3 Malaria Parasite Species

Plasmodium vivax caused 72% of malaria cases in the Americas in 2015. In Belize, El Salvador, Mexico, and Panama, local malaria is virtually restricted to *P. vivax*, while in Haiti and the Dominican Republic, it is almost exclusively caused by *P. falciparum*, which also predominates in Guyana. *Plasmodium malariae* is also transmitted in the Americas, but accounts for less than 0.1% of laboratory-confirmed infections [1].

The overall contribution of *P. falciparum* to the malaria burden in the continent changed significantly over time. In Brazil, for example, *P. falciparum* accounted for nearly half of the infections diagnosed countrywide in the 1980s. However, *P. falciparum* incidence declined steadily since the 1990s, and the proportion of falciparum malaria reached only 11.7% in 2015 [1, 5]. Malaria-related deaths, mostly caused by *P. falciparum*, followed a similar downward trend countrywide [5]. There is little documented transmission (<0.1% of all cases) of *P. malariae* in Brazil, although molecular techniques have revealed the presence of this species in 9–12% of malaria patients in selected settings [5].

However, the opposite trend has been observed in some countries in the region. Colombia, Ecuador, and Venezuela, for example, reported an increase in the proportion of *P. falciparum* cases between 2015 and 2016 [20]. In Colombia, two-thirds of the cases diagnosed in 2013 were due to *P. vivax*, while 57% of those in 2016 were due to *P. falciparum*, with 40% due to *P. vivax*, and 3% were mixed-species infections [12, 20]. The vast majority (84%) of these *P. falciparum* infections reported in 2016 came from the states of Choco, Nariño, Antioquia, Buenaventura, and Cauca [20].

The predominance of *P. vivax* in most of the Americas has several implications for malaria control and elimination. First, low-density *P. vivax* infections are common, especially in areas approaching elimination, rendering laboratory diagnosis more difficult [30]. Second, *P. vivax* persists in human hosts for several months as hypnozoites, the dormant liver stages that may eventually cause relapses [31]. Primaquine (PQ), the only licensed antimalarial with hypnozoitocidal activity, requires a relatively long treatment course and can cause severe hemolysis in patients with glucose-6-phosphate dehydrogenase (G6PD) deficiency [32]. Third, although severe and sometimes fatal *P. vivax* infections have been documented in the region [33–35], the overall lethality of vivax malaria remains low. Fourth, *P. vivax* transmission is favored by the early production of infective stages, by mature gametocytes, and by the shorter duration of sporogony in mosquito vectors, further complicating control efforts. Finally, large-scale interventions, such as mass drug administration and immunization, are more likely to select for escape variants in a highly diverse parasite population [36]. Somewhat surprisingly, genome-wide analyses have revealed an extensive genetic diversity in *P. vivax* circulating in the Americas [37, 38], much higher than that of *P. falciparum* from the same region [39–41], and comparable with *P. vivax* from South and Southeast Asia, where transmission is typically more intense [42, 43]. These findings are consistent with separate introductions of geographically and genetically diverse *P. vivax* lineages into the Americas, followed by extensive admixture among parasites from different source populations. Yet, this demographic scenario remains to be formally tested [37].

4 Case-Finding Strategies

Routine case-finding strategies in most endemic settings in Latin America target only patients who present with fever or with a history of recent fever, who are screened for malaria parasites by conventional microscopy or RDTs, and who receive prompt antimalarial treatment if found to be infected. These strategies have several limitations. First, conventional microscopy often overlooks very low parasite loads, which are revealed by polymerase chain reaction (PCR) or other nucleic acid-based diagnostic methods. A series of PCR-based studies across the Amazon challenge the persisting view that subjects exposed to relatively low malaria transmission are unlikely to harbor low parasitemias, due to the lack of acquired immunity [44–48]. To the contrary, the proportion of subpatent infections tends to increase as malaria transmission declines in the Amazon [45], as previously shown in Africa [49], further complicating case finding in the context of malaria elimination.

Malaria RDTs, which detect soluble parasite antigens using specific monoclonal antibodies, do not appear to be a feasible alternative for population-based screening of low-level parasitemias in some areas with substantial *P. falciparum* transmission in the region. The most commonly used RDTs target the *P. falciparum* histidine-rich protein 2 (PfHRP2), for species-specific diagnosis, and conserved epitopes in parasite lactate dehydrogenase (pLDH), for detection of all human malaria parasite species [50]. However, a substantial proportion of *P. falciparum* isolates from Peru, Colombia, and northwestern Brazil, but less commonly in Bolivia, fail to express HRP2, remaining potentially undetected by most RDTs [51, 52].

Second, asymptomatic parasite carriage is quite common across the continent [12, 17, 27, 44, 45, 53] and creates a clinically silent reservoir, overlooked by routine surveillance, that maintains ongoing malaria transmission. For example, 56.6% of all *P. vivax* infections diagnosed over 3 years in farming settlements in the rural

Amazon were found to be asymptomatic; one-third of them were both subpatent and asymptomatic [45]. Apparently healthy subjects accounted for half of the total *P. vivax* biomass circulating in the local population, and nearly all asymptomatic *P. vivax* carriers had mature gametocytes detected with molecular techniques. Only 17.0% of the asymptomatic *P. vivax* carriers developed clinical symptoms over 6 weeks of follow-up, becoming detectable by routine surveillance of febrile illnesses [45]. The infectiousness of asymptomatic carriers of low-grade parasitemias to Amazonian malaria vectors remains understudied, but one study described an infection rate of 1.2% after feeding *An. darlingi* with blood from asymptomatic *P. vivax* carriers and of 22% for the mosquitoes fed with blood from symptomatic carriers [54].

Third, malaria diagnosis and treatment routinely offered by the National Malaria Control Programs is often unavailable to hard-to-reach populations, including illegal miners scattered in the interior of the Guiana Shield. Not only is access to health services severely limited in remote mining camps, but also undocumented migrants are very unlikely to actively seek for health care in government-run facilities in larger towns and cities, where they face the risk of deportation [25].

Eliminating residual foci of transmission in countries reaching pre-elimination is the next major challenge in Latin America. As malaria transmission declines, populations must be routinely screened to diagnose the relatively few remaining infections, most of them subpatent and asymptomatic. Mass blood screening is unlikely to be cost-effective as a case-finding strategy in pre-elimination settings in Latin America, but reactive case detection strategies may play a role in areas with substantial spatial clustering of malaria episodes [55]. For example, subjects living in close proximity to malaria cases detected by routine passive surveillance (termed "index cases") were found to carry symptomatic and asymptomatic infections much more frequently than randomly selected inhabitants in the same farming settlements in the rural Amazon of Brazil, where only *P. vivax* is currently transmitted [56]. The increased risk of infection in the proximity of index cases extended over the next few months, due to the relapsing nature of *P. vivax*. Four rounds of microscopy-based screening for malaria parasites targeted at these high-risk subjects, carried out between 0 and 180 days after index case enrollment, identified 76.8% of the total *P. vivax* biomass circulating in the proximity of index cases [56]. These findings suggest that reactive case detection, even with imperfect diagnostics such as conventional microscopy, may be a component of elimination strategies in selected low-endemicity settings in the region.

5 Treatment Regimens

Chloroquine (CQ) resistance in *P. falciparum* emerged in the Americas in the early 1960s, independently in Brazil and Colombia [57], and became widespread across the Amazon Basin by the mid-1980s [58]. Currently, artemisinin-based combination therapies (ACTs) – either artesunate-mefloquine or artemether-lumefantrine – are the first-line treatment for uncomplicated falciparum malaria in all countries in South America [1]. Resistance to ACTs has not been unequivocally documented in this region [59, 60], but there is some concern that artemisinin-resistant parasites may emerge as a result of the widespread use of substandard drug regimens in mining camps across the Guiana Shield [21, 23, 24, 29].

Surprisingly, CQ remains highly efficacious for *P. falciparum* infections acquired in Mexico and Central America, including the Hispaniola. Nevertheless, a small clinical study has recently documented late parasitological failures following CQ treatment in Haiti [61]. Therefore, CQ remains as the current first-line treatment for falciparum malaria in Mexico and most of Central America, except for Panama [1], but continued in vitro and in vivo monitoring of *P. falciparum* responses to CQ is crucial in this part of the continent.

CQ and PQ are co-administered for vivax malaria treatment in all countries in Latin America [1]. Although CQ-resistant vivax malaria remains relatively infrequent in South America [62], convincing reports of treatment failure following CQ alone or CQ-PQ combination are available from Guyana [63], Peru [64], Brazil [65, 66], and Bolivia [67]. No evidence is currently available for *P. vivax* resistance to CQ in Mexico and Central America.

The current anti-relapse efficacy of PQ and the extent to which PQ metabolism is affected by cytochrome P450 (CYP) 2D6 polymorphisms in the Americas remain largely undetermined. PQ is essentially an inactive prodrug that depends on the CYP 2D6 enzyme to generate hydroxylated metabolites that are toxic to hypnozoites. Therefore, PQ failure may be caused by poor PQ metabolism in patients, rather than drug resistance. Recent evidence also indicates that blood schizonticidal antimalarials that are routinely co-administered with PQ to clear asexual blood stage parasites, including CQ, can inhibit CYP2D6 activity [68]. However, true PQ resistance has been conclusively demonstrated in a *P. vivax* strain from Brazil used to experimentally infect owl and squirrel monkeys [69]. If PQ is indeed failing, a substantial proportion of *P. vivax* infections in the region may actually be relapses, placing improved anti-relapse treatment as a top research priority for ongoing malaria elimination efforts.

6 Vector Control

Vector control efforts in Latin America and the Caribbean reflect the feeding, biting, resting, and breeding behavior of *Anopheles* in the region. Six dominant vector species, with varied behavior and distinct geographical coverage, have been identified: *Anopheles albimanus*, the *Albitarsis* complex, *An. aquasalis*, *An. darlingi*, *An. nuneztovari*, and *An. pseudopunctipennis* [70–73].

Anopheles albimanus is found mainly along the Atlantic and Pacific coast of Central America, in the Caribbean, and in Venezuela, Colombia, Ecuador, and Peru [73]. The *Albitarsis* complex comprises eight recognized species (*An. albitarsis* s.s., *An. albitarsis* F, *An. albitarsis* G, *An. albitarsis* I, *An. deaneorum*, *An. janconnae*, *An. marajoara*, *An. oryzalimnetes*) and one lineage (*An. albitarsis* H). Its geographical distribution is quite widespread in Central America, in the Caribbean, and in South America, except for the Southern Cone [73]. *Anopheles aquasalis* is mainly found in salty water along the Pacific coast, up to Ecuador, and the Atlantic coast up to southern Brazil [70, 73]. *Anopheles darlingi* is one of the most efficient vectors in the Neotropical region and the most important vector in the Amazon basin [70, 73]. *Anopheles nuneztovari* is present in the northern part of South America, including the Amazon basin [70]. Lastly, *An. pseudopunctipennis* is found in Central America and along the Andes, up to Bolivia, surviving in higher altitudes than the other vectors [71, 72].

All those species were found to be both anthropophilic and zoophilic, with the exception of *An. darlingi*, which is mainly anthropophilic. The biting behavior is mainly exophagic, with endophagic biting observed with less frequency. In addition, the resting behavior is predominantly exophilic, although geographic variation is observed, both before and after feeding, with the exception of *An. pseudopunctipennis*, which can have an endophilic post-feeding resting behavior. Most species bite at dusk and at night, and *An. darlingi* also bites at dawn [70, 72, 73].

IRS and the use of long-lasting insecticide-treated nets (LLINs) played an important role in the recent decline of malaria in Africa [74]. In Latin America and the Caribbean, the use of IRS was widespread during the 1955 Global Malaria Eradication Campaign and contributed to important declines in transmission [5, 19, 75]. However, the use of IRS and of ITNs may lead to vector behavior shifts, as it has been largely documented worldwide [76]. Regardless of the reasons for the predominantly exophagic and exophilic behavior of the dominant vector species in Latin America and the Caribbean, three issues are critical in regard to vector control. First, the effect of ITNs and IRS in reducing malaria transmission in the region is limited by vector behavior; depending on the vector species composition and on the prevalence of indoor biting/resting, these interventions may render infeasible. Second, other control strategies that target outdoor biting and resting behavior are needed in order to reduce the human-vector contact. Third, environmental management and larval control, although largely neglected by national malaria control programs, could potentially be adopted in specific settings.

Therefore, characterizing the local species composition and behavior to inform the most appropriate and effective use of all vector control strategies currently available and pursuing novel strategies that target outdoor behavior are critical steps to facilitate the path to malaria elimination in the region.

7 Prospects

Malaria incidence in Latin America and the Caribbean has shown a declining trend in the past two decades, and many countries are aiming at eliminating the disease. Yet, history has shown that the path to elimination can suffer setbacks for varied reasons [77, 78]. Recently, an economic crisis resulted in dramatic increases of malaria in Venezuela [20], a country certified by the WHO for eradicating malaria in its most populated areas in 1961 [19]. Austerity measures have been progressively implemented in Brazil since 2016, and, after a steady decline since 2010, the number of cases reported in 2017 (up to September) is already larger than that reported in 2014. Besides political and economic instability, climatic conditions may also affect transmission [79]. Future trends will depend on a variety of biological, social, and environmental factors but will also reflect countries' commitment to the goal of eliminating malaria and ability to manage crisis.

Acknowledgments

The authors' malaria-related studies have been funded by the National Institute of Allergy and Infectious Diseases, the National Institutes of Health (U19 AI089681 to Joseph M. Vinetz), and the Fundação de Amparo à Pesquisa do Estado de São Paulo (FAPESP, 2016/18740-9 to MUF), Brazil. MUF receives a senior researcher scholarship from the Conselho Nacional de Desenvolvimento Científico e Tecnológico of Brazil; MCC received a visitor researcher scholarship from FAPESP (2013/17259-7).

References

1. Pan American Health Organization (2016) Report on the Situation of Malaria in the Americas, 2000–2015. Regional Malaria Program, Pan American Health Organization, Washington, D.C.
2. Hinman EH (1947) Recent trends in malaria control in Latin America. Mosq News 7:144–151
3. Prothero RM (1995) Malaria in Latin America: Environmental and human factors. Bull Latin Am Res 14:357–365
4. Pan American Health Organization (2017) Interactive Malaria Statistics. Pan American Health Organization, Washington. http://ais.paho.org/phip/viz/malaria_surv_API_popup.asp
5. Ferreira MU, Castro MC (2016) Challenges for malaria elimination in Brazil. Malar J 15:284
6. Oliveira-Ferreira J, Lacerda MV, Brasil P et al (2010) Malaria in Brazil: an overview. Malar J 9:115
7. Herrera S, Ochoa-Orozco SA, González IJ et al (2015) Prospects for malaria elimination in Mesoamerica and Hispaniola. PLoS Negl Trop Dis 9:e0003700
8. Lemoine JF, Boncy J, Filler S et al (2017) Haiti's commitment to malaria elimination: progress in the face of challenges, 2010-2016. Am J Trop Med Hyg 97(4 Suppl):43–48
9. Weppelmann TA, Carter TE, Chen Z et al (2013) High frequency of the erythroid silent Duffy antigen genotype and lack of *Plasmodium vivax* infections in Haiti. Malar J 12:30
10. Carter KH, Singh P, Mujica OJ et al (2015) Malaria in the Americas: trends from 1959 to 2011. Am J Trop Med Hyg 92:302–316
11. Elbadry MA, Al-Khedery B, Tagliamonte MS et al (2015) High prevalence of asymptomatic malaria infections: a cross-sectional study in rural areas in six departments in Haiti. Malar J 14:510
12. Recht J, Siqueira AM, Monteiro WM et al (2017) Malaria in Brazil, Colombia, Peru and Venezuela: current challenges in malaria control and elimination. Malar J 16:273
13. Griffing SM, Gamboa D, Udhayakumar V (2013) The history of 20th century malaria control in Peru. Malar J 12:303
14. Quispe AM, Llanos-Cuentas A, Rodriguez H et al (2016) Accelerating to Zero: Strategies to eliminate malaria in the Peruvian Amazon. Am J Trop Med Hyg 94:1200–1207
15. Failoc-Rojas VE, Molina-Ayasta C (2016) Malaria in South America: the target is close. Am J Trop Med Hyg 95:735–735
16. Ministerio de Salud del Perú (2015) Boletín Epidemiológico (Lima): Ministerio de Salud del Perú. http://www.dge.gob.pe/boletin.php
17. da Silva-Nunes M, Moreno M, Conn JE et al (2012) Amazonian malaria: asymptomatic human reservoirs, diagnostic challenges, environmentally driven changes in mosquito vector populations, and the mandate for sustainable control strategies. Acta Trop 121:281–291
18. Reinbold-Wasson DD, Sardelis MR, Jones JW et al (2012) Determinants of *Anopheles* seasonal distribution patterns across a forest to periurban gradient near Iquitos, Peru. Am J Trop Med Hyg 86:459–463
19. Griffing SM, Villegas L, Udhayakumar V (2014) Malaria control and elimination, Venezuela, 1800s–1970s. Emerg Infect Dis 20:1691
20. Pan American Health Organization (2017) Epidemiological Alert: Increase in cases of malaria. Pan American Health Organization, Washington, D.C.. http://www.paho.org/hq/index.php?option=com_docman&task=doc_download&Itemid=&gid=38146&lang=pt
21. Musset L, Pelleau S, Girod R et al (2014) Malaria on the Guiana Shield: a review of the situation in French Guiana. Mem Inst Oswaldo Cruz 109:525–533
22. Hiwat H, Hardjopawiro LS, Takken W et al (2012) Novel strategies lead to pre-elimination of malaria in previously high-risk areas in Suriname, South America. Malar J 11:10
23. Adhin MR, Labadie-Bracho M, Vreden S (2014) Gold mining areas in Suriname: reservoirs of malaria resistance? Infect Drug Resist 7:111–116
24. Chenet SM, Akinyi Okoth S, Huber CS et al (2016) Independent emergence of the *Plasmodium falciparum* kelch propeller domain mutant allele C580Y in Guyana. J Infect Dis 213:1472–1475
25. Douine M, Mosnier E, Le Hingrat Q et al (2017) Illegal gold miners in French Guiana: a neglected population with poor health. BMC Public Health 18:23
26. Pommier de Santi V, Dia A, Adde A et al (2016) Malaria in French Guiana linked to illegal gold mining. Emerg Infect Dis 22:344–346
27. Pommier de Santi V, Djossou F, Barthes N et al (2016) Malaria hyperendemicity and risk for artemisinin resistance among illegal gold miners, French Guiana. Emerg Infect Dis 22:903–906

28. Douine M, Lazrek Y, Blanchet D et al (2017) Predictors of antimalarial self-medication in illegal gold miners in French Guiana: a pathway towards artemisinin resistance. J Antimicrob Chemother 73:231–239
29. Nacher M, Guerin PJ, Demar-Pierre M et al (2013) Made in Europe: will artemisinin resistance emerge in French Guiana? Malar J 12:152
30. Cheng Q, Cunningham J, Gatton ML (2015) Systematic review of sub-microscopic *P. vivax* infections: prevalence and determining factors. PLoS Negl Trop Dis 9:e3413
31. White NJ, Imwong M (2012) Relapse. Adv Parasitol 80:113–150
32. Luzzatto L, Seneca E (2014) G6PD deficiency: a classic example of pharmacogenetics with ongoing clinical implications. Br J Haematol 164:469–480
33. Alexandre MA, Ferreira CO, Siqueira AM et al (2010) Severe *Plasmodium vivax* malaria, Brazilian Amazon. Emerg Infect Dis 16:1611–1614
34. Lacerda MV, Fragoso SC, Alecrim MG et al (2012) Postmortem characterization of patients with clinical diagnosis of *Plasmodium vivax* malaria: to what extent does this parasite kill? Clin Infect Dis 55:e67–e74
35. Quispe AM, Pozo E, Guerrero E et al (2014) *Plasmodium vivax* hospitalizations in a monoendemic malaria region: severe vivax malaria? Am J Trop Med Hyg 91:11–17
36. Arnott A, Barry AE, Reeder JC (2012) Understanding the population genetics of *Plasmodium vivax* is essential for malaria control and elimination. Malar J 11:14
37. de Oliveira TC, Rodrigues PT, Menezes MJ et al (2017) Genome-wide diversity and differentiation in New World populations of the human malaria parasite *Plasmodium vivax*. PLoS Negl Trop Dis 11:e0005824
38. Winter DJ, Pacheco MA, Vallejo AF et al (2015) Whole genome sequencing of field isolates reveals extensive genetic diversity in *Plasmodium vivax* from Colombia. PLoS Negl Trop Dis 9:e0004252
39. Anderson TJ, Haubold B, Williams JT et al (2000) Microsatellite markers reveal a spectrum of population structures in the malaria parasite *Plasmodium falciparum*. Mol Biol Evol 17:1467–1482
40. Griffing SM, Mixson-Hayden T, Sridaran S et al (2011) South American *Plasmodium falciparum* after the malaria eradication era: clonal population expansion and survival of the fittest hybrids. PLoS One 6:e23486
41. Machado RL, Povoa MM, Calvosa VS et al (2004) Genetic structure of *Plasmodium falciparum* populations in the Brazilian Amazon region. J Infect Dis 190:1547–1555
42. Hupalo DN, Luo Z, Melnikov A et al (2016) Population genomics studies identify signatures of global dispersal and drug resistance in *Plasmodium vivax*. Nat Genet 48:953–958
43. Pearson RD, Amato R, Auburn S et al (2016) Genomic analysis of local variation and recent evolution in *Plasmodium vivax*. Nat Genet 48:959–964
44. Alves FP, Durlacher RR, Menezes MJ et al (2002) High prevalence of asymptomatic *Plasmodium vivax* and *Plasmodium falciparum* infections in native Amazonian populations. Am J Trop Med Hyg 66:641–648
45. Barbosa S, Gozze AB, Lima NF et al (2014) Epidemiology of disappearing *Plasmodium vivax* malaria: a case study in rural Amazonia. PLoS Negl Trop Dis 8:e3109
46. da Silva-Nunes M, Codeco CT, Malafronte RS et al (2008) Malaria on the Amazonian frontier: transmission dynamics, risk factors, spatial distribution, and prospects for control. Am J Trop Med Hyg 79:624–635
47. Ladeia-Andrade S, Ferreira MU, Carvalho ME (2009) Age-dependent acquisition of protective immunity to malaria in riverine populations of the Amazon Basin of Brazil. Am J Trop Med Hyg 80:452–459
48. Roshanravan B, Kari E, Gilman RH et al (2003) Endemic malaria in the Peruvian Amazon region of Iquitos. Am J Trop Med Hyg 69:45–52
49. Okell LC, Bousema T, Griffin JT et al (2012) Factors determining the occurrence of submicroscopic malaria infections and their relevance for control. Nat Commun 3:1237
50. Maltha J, Gillet P, Jacobs J (2013) Malaria rapid diagnostic tests in travel medicine. Clin Microbiol Infect 19:408–415
51. Gamboa D, Ho MF, Bendezu J et al (2010) A large proportion of *P. falciparum* isolates in the Amazon region of Peru lack *pfhrp2* and *pfhrp3*: implications for malaria rapid diagnostic tests. PLoS One 5:e8091
52. Rachid Viana GM, Akinyi Okoth S, Silva-Flannery L et al (2017) *Histidine-rich protein 2* (*pfhrp2*) and *pfhrp3* gene deletions in *Plasmodium falciparum* isolates from select sites in Brazil and Bolivia. PLoS One 12:e0171150
53. Douine M, Musset L, Corlin F et al (2016) Prevalence of *Plasmodium spp.* in illegal gold miners in French Guiana in 2015: a hidden but critical malaria reservoir. Malar J 15:315

54. Alves FP, Gil LH, Marrelli MT et al (2005) Asymptomatic carriers of *Plasmodium spp.* as infection source for malaria vector mosquitoes in the Brazilian Amazon. J Med Entomol 42:777–779
55. Moonen B, Cohen JM, Snow RW et al (2010) Operational strategies to achieve and maintain malaria elimination. Lancet 376:1592–1603
56. Fontoura PS, Finco BF, Lima NF et al (2016) Reactive case detection for *Plasmodium vivax* malaria elimination in rural Amazonia. PLoS Negl Trop Dis 10:e0005221
57. Wootton JC, Feng X, Ferdig MT et al (2002) Genetic diversity and chloroquine selective sweeps in *Plasmodium falciparum*. Nature 418:320–323
58. Cortese JF, Caraballo A, Contreras CE (2002) Origin and dissemination of *Plasmodium falciparum* drug-resistance mutations in South America. J Infect Dis 186:999–1006
59. Ladeia-Andrade S, de Melo GN, de Souza-Lima Rde C et al (2016) No clinical or molecular evidence of *Plasmodium falciparum* resistance to artesunate-mefloquine in northwestern Brazil. Am J Trop Med Hyg 95:148–154
60. Montenegro M, Neal AT, Posada M et al (2017) K13-propeller alleles, mdr1 polymorphism, and drug effectiveness at day 3 after artemether-lumefantrine treatment for *Plasmodium falciparum* malaria in Colombia, 2014-2015. Antimicrob Agents Chemother 61: e01036–e01017
61. Raccurt CP, Brasseur P, Ciceron M et al (2017) *In vivo* study of *Plasmodium falciparum* chloroquine susceptibility in three departments of Haiti. Malar J 16:313
62. Goncalves LA, Cravo P, Ferreira MU (2014) Emerging *Plasmodium vivax* resistance to chloroquine in South America: an overview. Mem Inst Oswaldo Cruz 109:534–539
63. Phillips EJ, Keystone JS, Kain KC (1996) Failure of combined chloroquine and high-dose primaquine therapy for *Plasmodium vivax* malaria acquired in Guyana, South America. Clin Infect Dis 23:1171–1173
64. Ruebush TK, Zegarra J, Cairo J et al (2003) Chloroquine-resistant *Plasmodium vivax* malaria in Peru. Am J Trop Med Hyg 69:548–552
65. de Santana Filho FS, Arcanjo AR, Chehuan YM et al (2007) Chloroquine-resistant *Plasmodium vivax*, Brazilian Amazon. Emerg Infect Dis 13:1125–1126
66. Marques MM, Costa MR, Santana Filho FS et al (2014) *Plasmodium vivax* chloroquine resistance and anemia in the western Brazilian Amazon. Antimicrob Agents Chemother 58:342–347
67. Anez A, Moscoso M, Laguna A et al (2015) Resistance of infection by *Plasmodium vivax* to chloroquine in Bolivia. Malar J 14:261
68. Marcsisin SR, Reichard G, Pybus BS (2016) Primaquine pharmacology in the context of CYP 2D6 pharmacogenomics: current state of the art. Pharmacol Ther 161:1–10
69. Nayar JK, Baker RH, Knight JW et al (1997) Studies on a primaquine-tolerant strain of *Plasmodium vivax* from Brazil in *Aotus* and *Saimiri* monkeys. J Parasitol 83:739–745
70. Conn JE, Quiñones ML, Póvoa MM (2013) Phylogeography, vectors and transmission in Latin America. In: Manguin S (ed) *Anopheles* mosquitoes—new insights into malaria vectors. InTech, London, pp 145–172
71. Pimenta PF, Orfano AS, Bahia AC et al (2015) An overview of malaria transmission from the perspective of Amazon *Anopheles* vectors. Mem Inst Oswaldo Cruz 110:23–47
72. Sinka ME, Rubio-Palis Y, Manguin S et al (2010) The dominant *Anopheles* vectors of human malaria in the Americas: occurrence data, distribution maps and bionomic précis. Parasit Vectors 3:72
73. Sinka ME (2013) Global distribution of the dominant vector species of malaria. In: Manguin S (ed) *Anopheles* mosquitoes - new insights into malaria vectors. InTech, London, pp 109–143
74. Bhatt S, Weiss DJ, Cameron E et al (2015) The effect of malaria control on *Plasmodium falciparum* in Africa between 2000 and 2015. Nature 526:207–211
75. PAHO, WHO (1966) Report on the Status of Malaria Eradication in the Americas. XIV Report. Pan American Health Organization, World Health Organization, Washington, D.C.
76. Durnez L, Coosemans M (2013) Residual transmission of malaria: an old issue for new approaches. In: Manguin S (ed) *Anopheles* mosquitoes—new insights into malaria vectors. InTech, London, pp 671–704
77. Cohen JM, Smith DL, Cotter C et al (2012) Malaria resurgence: a systematic review and assessment of its causes. Malar J 11:122
78. Smith DL, Cohen JM, Chiyaka C et al (2013) A sticky situation: the unexpected stability of malaria elimination. Philos Trans R Soc Lond B Biol Sci 368:20120145
79. Castro MC (2017) Malaria transmission and prospects for malaria eradication: the role of the environment. Cold Spring Harb Perspect Med 7:a025601

Part II

Methods

Chapter 5

Diagnosing Malaria: Methods, Tools, and Field Applicability

Lawrence Ayong, Carole Else Eboumbou Moukoko, and Wilfred Fon Mbacham

Abstract

Diagnosing malaria is a key component of effective case management and monitoring of antimalarial programs worldwide. This chapter features the different diagnostic approaches currently in use or under testing for use in case management and/or epidemiological studies of malaria. Emphasis is laid on the basic principles of each diagnostic approach as well as their operational limits under different malaria endemicity settings. The discussed methods are defined as "conventional" or "unconventional" depending on their widespread use in malaria case management. The chapter therefore provides a practical guide to students, health practitioners, and field researchers involved in the fight against malaria through community-based interventions.

Key words Malaria diagnosis, Conventional tools, Unconventional approaches, Drawbacks

1 Introduction

Diagnosing malaria involves the use of one or several clinical, parasitological, or immunological methods to identify individuals with active infection by malaria parasites or those whose medical condition results from recent exposure to malaria parasites. Malaria is a mosquito-borne disease caused by parasitic protozoans of the genus *Plasmodium*. At least five *Plasmodium* species are reported to cause malaria in humans, the most virulent being *Plasmodium falciparum*. The other four species include *Plasmodium vivax*, *Plasmodium ovale*, *Plasmodium malariae*, and *Plasmodium knowlesi* that sometimes cause severe malaria although at low mortality rates. An estimated 3.3 billion people are at risk of malaria infection globally, with over 200 million reported cases and 400,000 deaths each year. Reported annual malaria cases, however, are often considered a gross underestimation of actual numbers of annual cases, as more than triple the number of cases may remain unreported or exist as asymptomatic infections [1]. In the absence of any approved antimalarial mass treatment or vaccination program in the majority

Frédéric Ariey et al. (eds.), *Malaria Control and Elimination*, Methods in Molecular Biology, vol. 2013, https://doi.org/10.1007/978-1-4939-9550-9_5, © Springer Science+Business Media, LLC, part of Springer Nature 2019

of endemic countries, early diagnosis remains key to effective management of new cases. Indeed, prompt and accurate diagnosis is critical to prevent significant morbidity and mortality due to malaria parasites, curb misuse of antimalarial drugs, promote appropriate management of non-malarial fevers, and monitor the impact of implemented antimalarial interventions. Spurred by the global impact of malaria in recent years, significant effort has been made to develop better tools for malaria diagnosis, some of which are deemed suitable in malaria control settings, whereas others are most appropriate in areas undergoing malaria elimination. In this chapter, we review the different methods in current use for malaria diagnosis, while outlining the merits and limitations of each approach in the context of malaria control or elimination.

2 Conventional Methods for Malaria Diagnosis

The conventional methods for malaria diagnosis include both clinical- and microscopy-based approaches as well as various strip-based immunochromatographic techniques (ICTs) [2].

2.1 Clinical Diagnosis

Clinical diagnosis is based on patients' signs and symptoms and routinely practiced by highly trained healthcare personnel. The clinical presentation of malaria is highly variable and includes fever, headache, chills, anorexia, body itches, abdominal pain, diarrhea, nausea, vomiting, anemia, arrhythmia, general weakness, convulsion, and coma. These signs and symptoms overlap considerably with other common and potentially life-threatening diseases, including various viral and bacterial infections. Thus, clinical diagnosis alone is only recommended in high transmission zones in resource-limited countries, where laboratory diagnosis may be nonexistent. To improve management, especially of severe malaria by minimally trained healthcare personnel, clinical diagnostic algorithms have been established with aims to increase diagnostic sensitivity of clinical methods [3]. However, such highly sensitive but often weakly specific algorithms may lead to overdiagnosis, resulting in excessive use of antimalarial drugs that may favor the emergence of drug resistance while compromising the quality of care for patients with non-malarial fevers. Another limitation of clinical diagnosis is the inability to detect asymptomatic malaria cases that often adopt a non-healthcare-seeking attitude, thereby serving as important human reservoirs of malaria, necessitating the use of specialized diagnostic tools to ensure their elimination.

2.2 Microscopy-Based Diagnosis

Traditionally, malaria is diagnosed by microscopic examination of stained blood smears that have been prepared on glass slides. Two types of blood smears are available for use in malaria diagnosis: (1) thick blood smear, which is a parasite concentration method commonly used for estimating infection loads, particularly in patients with low parasite densities ($\leq$16,000 parasites/µl), and (2) thin blood smears that are routinely used for identifying parasite species and for more accurate determination of infection loads in heavily infected persons (>16,000 parasites/µl). Generally in most endemic areas, both thick and thin smears are prepared on routine basis, with thick smears used to screen for parasite presence, whereas thin smears are used to identify parasite species. The difference between thick and thin blood smears lies in the volume of blood spotted on each glass slide as well as the smear preparation process. In thin blood smear microscopy, the red blood cells are fixed to preserve cell morphology. This allows species identification on the basis of parasite sizes and shapes.

To prepare a thin smear, approximately 2 microliters of blood is spotted on a central position of a glass slide and spread using the ground edge of the spreader slide. For thick smears, approximately 6 microliters of peripheral blood is deposited on a glass slide and spread in a circular pattern using the beveled corner of a spreader slide until a diameter of about 12 mm is evenly covered. Lower or higher blood volumes may be used to prepare thick smears, but it is necessary to adjust the diameter of the smear to maintain staining consistency. Upon drying the smears for about 1 h at 37–40 °C or overnight at room temperature in a dehumidified chamber, the thin smear is fixed by dipping in absolute methanol for a few seconds and air-dried to eliminate water artifacts. Both the fixed thin smear and unfixed thick smears are then stained using one of Giemsa, Wright's, or Field's stains, which are variations of a mixture of different basic and acidic dyes. The commonly used basic dyes are methylene blue (azure) and its oxidative products (azure A, azure B, azure C, and thionin), whereas the most widely used acidic dye is eosin. Under appropriate pH conditions, the basic dye reacts with acidic cellular elements such as nucleic acids and nucleoproteins, conferring a characteristic basic dye color that is distinguishable from the acidic dye that preferentially binds acidophilic cellular components such as hemoglobin and various cytoplasmic constituents. The recommended and most widely used stain for both thick and thin blood smear microscopy in malaria endemic areas is Giemsa, which is composed of methylene blue and eosin. At pH 7.2, the methylene blue component stains the parasite cytoplasm blue, while the eosin component stains the nucleus red. The wide acceptance of the Giemsa technique for malaria diagnosis can be attributed to its simplicity, low cost, and dye stability under variable temperature conditions.

Following dye staining, the slides are washed by brief dipping in and out of buffered water and air-dried for at least 30 min at room temperature prior to microscopic examination using an immersion oil 100× objective. As the thick smear is unfixed, the smeared red cells would lyse upon staining with any water-based dye leaving mostly the naked parasites and white cells on the slide.

Quantification of parasites (asexual or sexual forms) in the thick smear is made by counting the number of identifiable parasites against a recommended number of white blood cell count (WBC) or high-power microscopic fields (HPFs), whereas parasite quantification on the thin smear is by determining the proportion of infected red blood cells (blood parasitemia) after examining over 100 microscopic fields. The number of parasites per μl of whole blood (parasite density) is then calculated on the basis of the patient's own white cell count or using an estimated average white blood cell count of 8000/μl. Because the presence of malaria parasites in peripheral blood proves ongoing infection, microscopic diagnosis has long been considered the "gold standard" method for malaria diagnosis. As such, it is widely used in the evaluation and validation of new malaria diagnostic methods. However, microscopic diagnosis is laden with several shortcomings, including the fact that detection of parasites in peripheral blood films may not be conclusive evidence for cause of disease. Furthermore, the staining and slide reading processes are labor-intensive, are time-consuming, and require considerable expertise. The method is prone to significant observer-related variations and lacks sensitivity when performed by non-expert microscopists. Its estimated sensitivity limit is 5–10 parasites/μl for expert microscopists, 50–100 parasites/μl for average microscopists, and lower for the majority of microscopists in malaria endemic areas. Microscopy diagnostic errors are most frequent for patients with low parasitemias (<200 parasites/μl of whole blood), although parasite quantification errors are also common for parasite densities >20,000 parasites/μ l. In general, microscopic diagnosis of malaria necessitates continuous training of medical laboratory technicians to minimize misdiagnosis and improve case management, especially of non-malarial fevers. With the advent of several automated computer-based technologies, it is expected that some of the above shortcomings will be addressed to improve malaria diagnostic quality, particularly in resource-limited environments.

2.3 Immunochromatographic Methods

The existing ICT-based methods for malaria diagnosis are based on the detection of parasite-specific proteins in infected whole blood using both soluble and immobilized antibody species on a chromatographic test strip. Various dipstick formats of ICTs, also known as rapid diagnostic tests (RDTs), are commercially available and exhibit variable degrees of sensitivity and specificity potentials depending on the analyte antigen. Malaria antigens that are currently targeted by RDTs include histidine-rich protein 2 (HRP-2), lactate dehydrogenase (LDH), and aldolase. HRP-2 proves to be a highly sensitive and specific marker for detecting *P. falciparum* infections and as such represents the most targeted *P. falciparum* antigen in the current RDTs [4]. However, HRP-2 antigens exhibit long half-lives and persist in the peripheral blood during several weeks after successful clearance of blood parasite antimalarial drugs. This is of particular concern in moderate to high transmission areas where false-positive tests may frequently result in provision of antimalarial treatment to healthy individuals [5, 6]. LDH, on the other hand, is short-lived, and it is often tested in parallel with HRP-2 to confirm an active infection. The existing LDH-based RDTs have been designed to detect all five human malaria species (pan-*Plasmodium*) or are species-specific (PfLDH or PvLDH). Due to the rapidity of RDTs (<10 min operation time) and instant availability of results at point of care, RDTs have been positively recommended by the World Health Organization (WHO) for use in clinical care of malaria when reliable microscopy is not available. A major limitation of the current RDTs is the lack of sensitivity (detection limits >100 parasites/μl whole blood) especially in low-density parasitemic patients, necessitating the use of more sensitive parasitological or molecular approaches. Test false negatives may also occur due to deletion of targeted protein sequences in circulating parasite strains or as a result of the so-called "hook" or "prozone" effect in high-antigenemic patients that arise from saturation of immobilized antibody sites by free antigens, preventing the binding and concentration of required antigen-gold-labeled antibody complexes on the test bands. On the other hand, a false-positive RDT result could arise from antibody cross-reactivity with non-malarial antigens including reactions with host rheumatoid factors.

3 Unconventional Methods for Malaria Diagnosis

The alternative methods for malaria diagnosis include those that are based on fluorescence microscopy and antigen or antibody detection methods (ELISA, IFA, flow cytometry) and those that are based on amplification of parasite-specific nucleic acids (PCR, LAMP) or detection of certain metabolites.

3.1 Fluorescence Microscopy

As a way of overcoming some of the limitations of light microscopy, methods based on parasite staining with fluorescence dyes and signal visualization using a fluorescence microscopy have been developed. These include the quantitative buffy coat (QBC) technique that is based on capillary tube technology and various slide-based Cyscope® microscopy techniques. The QBC method involves staining parasites in micro-hematocrit tubes by using fluorescent DNA dyes, notably acridine orange, and detection by epi-fluorescence microscopy. Briefly, test blood is taken up by capillarity in a hematocrit tube containing an anticoagulant and acridine orange as fluorochrome. The tube is centrifuged at 12,000 × g for 5 min to separate different cell layers on the basis of their buoyant densities and immediately examined under a fluorescent microscope. Parasite and leucocyte nuclei fluoresce yellowish green, whereas cytoplasm appears yellow-orange. The parasitized red blood cells separate alongside the buffy coat but at different levels depending on their life cycle stages and the parasite density. In fact, at low parasite densities, the parasitized red blood cells form the upper brown layer of RBCs, whereas in heavily infected blood, the parasites may be found anywhere in the tube. The QBC technique is easy to use, rapid, sensitive, and specific, particularly for *P. falciparum* diagnosis. However, both its sensitivity and specificity are reduced in the case of non-falciparum malaria due to the predominance of mature forms of such parasites in the peripheral blood that co-separate with host leucocytes in the buffy coat. Cyscope® microscope is a mobile, battery-operated system with readily prepared and ready-to-use slides that have been labeled with unspecific nucleic acid-binding dyes such as DAPI (4′-6-diamidino-2-phenylindole). Malaria diagnosis using the Cyscope® microscope involves placing a drop of blood on the labeled area of the slide followed by a coverslip and visualization under ultraviolet light (365 nm) using a 40× objective. The presence of bright tiny dots indicates presence of malaria parasites. Cyscope® fluorescence microscopy is easy to use, relatively cheap, and highly sensitive for malaria diagnosis. However, it is prone to DAPI artifacts that might lead to misdiagnosis of some individuals. The method is also incapable of distinguishing between the infecting species, thereby requiring the use of other species detection techniques.

3.2 Antigen- and Antibody-Based Assays

Immunological methods that are based on the detection of malaria parasite-specific antigens or antibodies in body fluids play a key role in malaria diagnosis. Depending on test formats, immunological diagnostic assays can provide information on past exposure to malaria parasites (antibody tests) or reveal ongoing infections (antibody and antigen detection assays). Among the conventional immunological methods that have been tested for malaria diagnosis, those based on indirect immunofluorescence assay (IFA) and enzyme-linked immunosorbent assay (ELISA) have received the greatest attention.

For IFA-based methods, parasitized erythrocytes are used as capture antigen, permitting the detection of specific antibody-antigen reactions by flow cytometry or fluorescence microscopy techniques. The use of such techniques is limited to reference laboratory settings, given the need for high technical expertise, their labor-intensiveness, and operational costs. ELISA-based methods rely on the use of crude parasite extracts, heterologously expressed single antigens or peptide antigens for antibody detection, or the use of target-specific antibodies (monoclonal or polyclonal antibodies) to detect circulating parasite antigens in the patient's blood. The main limitations of ELISA-based methods have been labor-intensiveness, long turnaround times, and the lack of standardized reagents. These limit the use of ELISA-based methods mostly to specialized diagnostic laboratories or for research purposes. However, ELISA methods are very useful as primary screening assays in population-based studies, given their medium-throughput potentials, and often exhibit high sensitivities detecting as little as 1–10 parasites per 1000,000 red blood cells.

3.3 Molecular Diagnosis

Nucleic acid amplification techniques represent the most accurate and sensitive method for detecting malaria parasites. These molecular techniques include PCR-based methods such as nested, real-time, multiplex, and reverse transcription-based PCRs and isothermal approaches such as nucleic acid sequence-based amplification (NASBA) and loop-mediated nucleic acid amplification (LAMP)-based methods [7]. PCR is based on the use of a DNA polymerase such as *Taq* polymerase, as well as a pair of sequence-specific primers to amplify target DNA sequence from extracted parasite DNA. This approach involves temperature cycling between template denaturation, primer annealing, and strand synthesis steps. Detection of the resulting amplicon is achieved either by agarose gel electrophoresis or by using a real-time format in which a DNA-binding fluorescent dye or target-specific probe is added to the reaction mix and its fluorescence emission monitored over time. PCR methods may be used simply as an infection detection test (traditional PCR), for quantifying the infection density (quantitative real-time PCR), or for parasite speciation (multiplex PCR).

For RNA templates, one of several known reverse transcriptase enzymes is used to generate the corresponding cDNA strands prior to conventional PCR. The advantage of using RNA is that it is much more abundant in cells than DNA, with up to 1000-fold RNA copies as some DNA sequences per parasite. As such, RT-PCR-based methods exhibit higher sensitivities (detection limits of 0.002–5 parasites/μl) when compared to their corresponding PCR techniques (detection limits of 0.7–10 parasites/μl) and thus are more suitable for use in settings with extremely low peripheral blood parasite densities. RNA targets, because of their instability and short half-lives, are also more suitable for distinguishing between a recent and ongoing infection. Although PCR-based techniques are extremely sensitive and specific when compared with gold standard microscopy, they are limited by their high costs, absolute need for electricity and expensive equipment, labor-intensiveness, long turnaround times (2–4 h), as well as susceptibility to common laboratory contamination [8]. As such, the use of PCR-based techniques is limited to reference laboratory settings and for research purposes.

Isothermal nucleic acid amplification techniques such as NASBA and LAMP are quite promising as point-of-care malaria diagnostic approaches, as they eliminate the need for costly and power-intensive thermocyclers, are rapid (~1 h for NASBA and

<30 min for LAMP), and are capable of detecting infections of <1 parasites/μl of whole blood. NASBA is a nucleic acid amplification method that amplifies RNA in a manner similar to the replication of retroviruses. It involves the use of oligonucleotide primers and the three enzymes avian myeloblastosis virus reverse transcriptase (AMV-RT), RNase H, and T7 RNA polymerase for target-specific amplification, usually at 41 °C constant temperature. This approach generates high numbers of RNA copies per cycle, enabling it to generate detectible amounts of RNA products in a shorter time frame than PCR-based methods. Detection of NASBA products can be by probe-capture hybridization, by electro-chemiluminescence, or, more recently, by real-time analysis using molecular beacons that fluoresce when bound to a target sequence. The commonly used diagnostic target for malaria NASBA techniques is the 18S rRNA, with a detection limit of 0.1–0.01 parasites/μl of whole blood. In general, NASBA is a quantitative technique that can produce results in just 1 h, and it is highly sensitive and specific. However, it is expensive, labor-intensive, and prone to frequent laboratory contamination and false-positive amplifications. Of the existing molecular tests for malaria diagnosis, LAMP appears to be the most attractive in terms of its field applicability, cost-effectiveness, diagnostic performances, and rapidity. LAMP is a one-step amplification technique that is based on the use of strand displacement polymerases, notably *Bst* DNA polymerase to amplify target DNA with high sensitivity and specificity under isothermal conditions (65 °C) [9]. The method necessitates four specially designed oligonucleotide primers that recognize six distinct regions within the target DNA sequence. The high specificity of LAMP reactions is attributable to the requirement for all six regions to be recognized for amplification to occur. The addition of two other primers, known as loop forward and loop backward primers, enables sequence amplification at multiple loop sites, resulting in the accumulation of up to 10^9 copies of target sequence in just under 1 h. The addition of a reverse transcriptase makes it possible to amplify DNA from RNA targets (RT-LAMP) [10].

4 Conclusion

Diagnosing malaria has proven extremely valuable for preventing widespread fatalities due to malaria parasites and for monitoring approved intervention programs. However, several operational challenges exist with the current tools warranting a careful selection of methods based on the type of intervention and guided by the working principle of each diagnostic method [11]. Table 1 summarizes the attributes of each malaria diagnostic method and the recommended use in areas with high- or low-level transmission of malaria parasites.

Table 1
Diagnostic attributes of commonly used malaria diagnostic approaches

Attribute	Clinical	Microscopy	RDT	PCR	RT-PCR	LAMP	RT-LAMP	NASBA
Field use	Yes	Possible	Yes	No		Possible		No
Parasite detection limit	Undetermined	5–200/μl, depending on skill level	>100/μl	1–5/μl	0.1–5/μl	0.2–5/μl	<0.2	0.01–0.1/μl
Species identification	No	Yes, if expert microscopist	Yes, species-specific and pan-species RDTs	Multiplex PCRs	Possible	Possible	Possible	Yes
Skill requirement	High	High	Minimal	High	High	Minimal	Minimal	High
Turnaround time	Depends on physician's skill	>60 min per slide	15–20 min per sample	>5 h per 96-well plate	>5 h per 96-well plate	0.5–2 h, depending on sample processing needs	0.5–2 h, depending on sample processing needs	>5 h per 96-well plate
Throughput (samples per assay)	Low	Low (<25 slides per day)	Low (<10 tests per run)	Medium	Medium	Medium	Medium	Medium
Instrument cost	None	Low-moderate	Low	Expensive	Expensive	Low-moderate	Low-moderate	Expensive
Cost per test	–	$0.12–0.40 for a test	$0.55–3.22	$1.5–4.0 (reagents only)	~$5.0 (reagents only)	<$3.0	<$3.0	Unknown

(Ayong et al., Chapter. 5)

References

1. Koram KA, Molyneux ME (2007) When is "malaria" malaria? The different burdens of malaria infection, malaria disease, and malaria-like illnesses. Am J Trop Med Hyg 77 (6 Suppl):1–5
2. Wilson ML (2013) Laboratory diagnosis of malaria conventional and rapid diagnostic methods. Arch Pathol Lab Med 137:805–811
3. Chandramohan D, Jaffar S, Greenwood B (2002) Use of clinical algorithms for diagnosing malaria. Tropical Med Int Health 7:45–52
4. Ahmed MU, Hossain MA, Khan AH et al (2013) Efficacy of immunodiagnosis of falciparum malaria at different levels of parasitemia. J Enam Med Col 3:88–90
5. Ali IM, Bigoga JD, Forsah DA et al (2016) Field evaluation of the 22 rapid diagnostic tests for community management of malaria with artemisinin combination therapy in Cameroon. Malar J 15:31
6. Hendriksen IC, Mtove G, Pedro AJ et al (2011) Evaluation of a PfHRP2 and a pLDH-based rapid diagnostic test for the diagnosis of severe malaria in 2 populations of African children. Clin Infect Dis 52:1100–1107
7. Britton S, Cheng Q, McCarthy JS (2016) Novel molecular diagnostic tools for malaria elimination: a review of options from the point of view of high-throughput and applicability in resource limited settings. Malar J 15:88
8. Khan SA, Ahmed S, Mushahid N et al (2013) Comparison of real time polymerase chain reaction with microscopy and antigen detection assay for the diagnosis of malaria. J Coll Physicians Surg Pak 23:787–792
9. Chander Y, Koelbl J, Puckett J et al (2014) A novel thermostable polymerase for RNA and DNA loop-mediated isothermal amplification (LAMP). Front Microbiol 5:395
10. Kemleu S, Guelig D, Eboumbou MC et al (2016) A field-tailored reverse transcription loop-mediated isothermal assay for high sensitivity detection of *plasmodium falciparum* infections. PLoS One 11:e0165506
11. Kasetsirikul S, Buranapong J, Srituravanich W et al (2016) The development of malaria diagnostic techniques: a review of the approaches with focus on dielectrophoretic and magnetophoretic methods. Malar J 15:358

Chapter 6

Serological Profiling for Malaria Surveillance Using a Standard ELISA Protocol

Linda M. Murungi, Rinter K. Kimathi, James Tuju, Gathoni Kamuyu, and Faith H. A. Osier

Abstract

The enzyme-linked immunosorbent assay (ELISA) is a reliable and relatively low-cost method for measuring soluble ligands such as antibodies and proteins in biological samples. For analysis of specific antibodies in serum, a capture antigen is immobilized onto a solid polystyrene surface from which it can capture the antibodies. The captured antibodies are subsequently detected using a secondary antibody conjugated to an enzyme. Detection is accomplished by addition of a colorimetric substrate, and the readout is absorbance (optical density). Here, we provide a detailed standardized ELISA protocol for the quantification of antibodies against malaria antigens.

Key words ELISA, Antibodies, Optical density, Serum, Antigens

1 Introduction

Quantification of malaria-specific antibodies is important for the identification of correlates of protection or potential vaccine candidates, for surveillance of malaria transmission, and for evaluating the immunogenicity of malaria vaccines. The enzyme-linked immunosorbent assay (ELISA)-based approach has been used widely to quantify antibodies, replacing traditional methods such as the radioimmunoassay. The method is reliable, sensitive, reproducible, and relatively low-cost but is limited to measurement of one analyte at a time. Moreover, the volume of serum required increases in proportion with the number of antigens measured: a concern for field studies and clinical trials where serum volume may be limited.

Multiplexed assays are alternatives to the ELISA that can be used to simultaneously measure antibody responses to several antigens. Multiple antigens can be immobilized onto microspheres, beads (multiplexed bead array assay) or immobilized onto a solid matrix such as microarray slides or nitrocellulose membranes. In

Frédéric Ariey et al. (eds.), *Malaria Control and Elimination*, Methods in Molecular Biology, vol. 2013, https://doi.org/10.1007/978-1-4939-9550-9_6,

malaria, the multiplex bead and protein microarrays have been utilized for serological testing of up to 46 synthetic peptides [1] and over 1000 unique *P. falciparum* antigens [2, 3], respectively. A major advantage of the multiplex platform is that much more data can be obtained from a comparable volume of sample. The quantity of antigen utilized per assay is also considerably less than that in the ELISA. In addition, some studies have shown that these assays exhibit a wider dynamic range compared to the conventional ELISA [4, 5]. This linearity range is several orders of magnitude higher because of the wide dynamic range of fluorescence intensity compared with absorbance. As antibodies to different antigens occur at varying concentrations, a wide linear range is ideal for optimal quantification of concentrations. However, a major limitation of the multiplex bead-based assay is the need to have specialized technology to measure fluorescence of the beads such as flow cytometry or the Luminex system. Coupled to this is the expense: separate bead sets have to be purchased for each protein that is tested in a multiplex format. These costs can become prohibitive when both the number of samples and proteins to be tested is large. Protein microarrays are attractive with regard to high-throughput, minimal sample and antigen requirements [6]. However, as with the multiplexed assays, specialized equipment is required for slide printing and processing, as well as for data acquisition. The assay readout is based on advanced scanning technology, and the data have to undergo rigorous normalization processes before analysis.

With regard to ease of use and feasibility in resource-limited settings, ELISAs are widely accepted as the "gold standard." The ELISA method was developed simultaneously and independently in 1971 by Engvall and Perlmann [7] and by van Weemen and Schuurs [8]. In its basic format, an antigen is immobilized onto a solid polystyrene surface from which it can capture soluble ligands such as antibodies. The captured ligand is subsequently detected using a secondary antibody conjugated to an enzyme. Detection is accomplished by addition of a colorimetric substrate, and the readout is absorbance (optical density) on a plate spectrophotometer. Here, we describe a standardized ELISA method for quantification of antibodies against malaria antigens.

2 Materials

1. Coating buffer: 15 mM Na_2CO_3, 35 mM $NaHCO_3$, pH 9.6. Weigh 1.59 g of Na_2CO_3 and 2.93 g $NaHCO_3$ in 1 L of distilled water. Mix and adjust pH to 9.6. Store at room temperature.

2. Wash buffer: 0.05% Tween 20 in 1× PBS. Dissolve ten tablets of PBS in 1 L of distilled water, and add 500 μL of Tween 20.
3. Blocking buffer: 1% skimmed milk in wash buffer. Dissolve 1 g skimmed milk in 100 mL of wash buffer.
4. Secondary antibody: HRP-conjugated rabbit antihuman IgG.
5. Substrate solution: 0.1 M citric acid, 0.2 M Na_2HPO_4, *o*-phenylenediamine dihydrochloride tablets, hydrogen peroxide, and distilled water. To make up sufficient volume for one plate, dissolve 4 mg *o*-phenylenediamine dihydrochloride tablets in 5 mL distilled water. Add 2.4 mL of 0.1 M citric acid, 2.56 mL of 0.2 M Na_2HPO_4, and 8 μL of hydrogen peroxide.
6. Stop solution: 2 M H_2SO_4,
7. ELISA plates.
8. Microdilution tubes.
9. ELISA plate washer.
10. ELISA plate reader.

3 Methods

3.1 ELISA

1. Coat ELISA plates with 100 μL of the antigen. The appropriate coating concentration of the antigen is determined by titrating out the antigen (Fig. 1) (*see* **Notes 1a, 2,** and **3**).
2. Incubate plates overnight at 4 ° C.

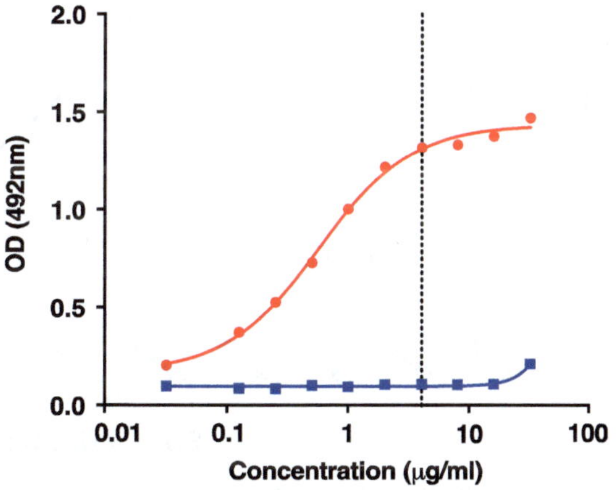

Fig. 1 The graph shows the optical density readings of pools of sera from malaria-exposed (red) and nonexposed donors (blue) at different concentrations of the coating antigen. The optimal coating concentration is shown by the black dotted line and corresponds to the maximum OD reading with low background and least antigen concentration

3. Wash the plates four times using an ELISA plate washer (*see* **Notes 4** and **5**).
4. Block the plates for 5 h with 200 μL of blocking buffer. Incubate the plates at room temperature (*see* **Note 6**).
5. Wash plates four times as above.
6. Incubate test samples; 100 μL/well at 1/1000 dilution in blocking buffer and leave overnight at 4 ° C. The appropriate serum dilution is determined by titration (Fig. 2) (*see* **Note 1b**).
7. Wash plates four times as above.
8. Incubate with 100 μL secondary antibody (1/5000, dilution in blocking buffer) for 3 h at room temperature. Determination of the optimal secondary antibody and serum dilutions can be performed simultaneously as shown in Fig. 2 (*see* **Note 1c**).
9. Wash plates four times as above.
10. Add 100 μL/well of substrate solution, and incubate for 15 min in the dark at room temperature.

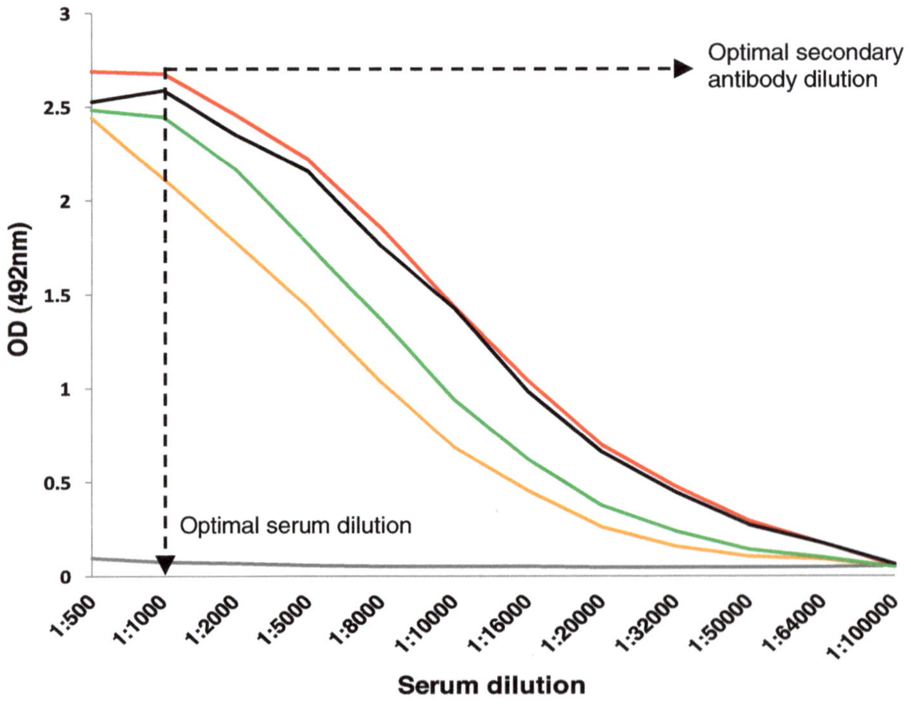

Fig. 2 A checkerboard titration of a pool of malaria-exposed sera (1:500–1:100,000) and four secondary antibody dilutions: 1:5000 (red), 1:4000 (black), 1:2500 (green), and 1:1000 (orange). Serial dilutions of a pool of malaria nonexposed sera were also tested at 1:5000 secondary antibody dilution (gray). The appropriate serum dilution is shown by the vertical dotted line and clearly differentiates between the positive and the negative sera. The optimal secondary antibody dilution (horizontal dotted line) corresponds to the OD reading where the signal is strongest and the background is low

11. Stop the reaction using 25 μL/well of 2 M H_2SO_4.
12. Promptly read the optical density (OD) at 492 nm.

3.2 Data Quality and Analysis

1. Each plate includes blank wells, negative and positive controls (at least two blanks; two wells for positive controls; and a variable number on negative controls (2–20) depending on the total number of samples being tested and the purpose of the assay). Blank wells are used to establish the background or non-specific reactivity; ideally the reading of the blank well should be below 0.05 ELISA OD. If this is high, consider further optimization or subsequent subtraction of this reading from all wells. Negative controls are samples taken from malaria-nonexposed individuals. These samples are used to set threshold for seropositivity (usually mean plus three standard deviations of non-malaria-exposed sera). Positive controls include a pool of sera from long-term residents of a malaria endemic area. This pool allows for standardization of data across plates (plate to plate variation) and across days (day to day variation).
2. Serial dilutions of a pool of sera from malaria-exposed adults are included on every plate to generate a standard curve that allows for conversion of ELISA OD values to relative antibody units. Arbitrary units are assigned to this pool of serum.
3. Generate the standard curve using a five- or four-parameter logistic regression equation, and interpolate the concentration of the samples from this curve. Samples that fall outside the linear range of the standard curve (those with ODs above and below this range) are repeated at higher and lower dilutions, respectively.
4. All assays are conducted in duplicate. Once plate data are acceptable based on blank, negative, and positive controls, the coefficient of variation (CV) between duplicate test samples is calculated using the formula:

$$CV = (\text{standard deviation}/\text{mean}) \times 100\%.$$

   Samples with a CV of less than 20% are accepted, while those with a higher CV are retested.
5. For antigens that have a purification tag, e.g., maltose-binding protein (MBP) and glutathione *S*-transferase (GST), the final OD result is obtained by subtracting the OD result of the purification tag from that of the fusion protein.

3.3 Interpretation of Results

1. Samples are deemed seropositive if the ELISA OD value exceeds the cutoff, usually defined as the mean plus three standard deviations of non-malaria exposed sera.

2. Analysis and interpretation are dependent on the expected application of the results; the above represents the "standard" routinely used in studies of malaria immuno-epidemiology.

3.4 Data Reporting/ Presentation

The magnitude of responses can be presented as raw ELISA optical density (OD) values [9, 10], end point titers [11, 12], or relative antibody units with reference to the units assigned to a pool of sera from malaria-exposed individuals [13] or a standard commercial reagent [14, 15]. Others have reported absolute antibody concentrations with reference to an antigen-specific standard [16] or using a mathematical conversion factor that converts arbitrary units to actual protein concentrations (in μg/mL) [17]. Calibration-free concentration analysis (CFCA) which measures the rate of binding of specific antibodies to their target antigens by surface plasmon resonance (SPR) also provides an absolute measure of antibody titers without using a standard [18, 19]. A standardized method of measurement and reporting of antibody responses would allow better comparison of data from different studies.

4 Notes

1. Titrations should be performed to determine the optimal antigen-coating concentration, serum dilution, and secondary antibody concentration to use in the assay:
   (a) The optimal antigen-coating concentration should be at a point where there's maximum OD reading with low background but with the least antigen concentration (Fig. 1).
   (b) For serum, the optimal dilution factor should clearly differentiate between the positive and the negative controls (Fig. 2).
   (c) The secondary antibody should be used at a dilution factor where the signal is strong and the background is low (Fig. 2).
2. The ELISA plate used to coat the antigen may need to be adapted for specific antigens; for example, if the antigen is biotinylated, one would need to use pre-coated streptavidin plates.
3. The coating buffer PH is crucial for effective immobilization on the plate; thus, for new assays it is important to test a number of coating buffers side by side for optimal antigen immobilization.
4. Do not allow the plate to dry completely at any step.
5. The plates can be washed manually.
6. Dilution of samples can be performed during this incubation period.

Acknowledgments

This paper is published with the permission of the director of KEMRI. F.H.A.O. is supported by an MRC/DFID African Research Leader Award jointly funded by the UK Medical Research Council (MRC) and the UK Department for International Development (DFID) under the MRC/DFID Concordat agreement (MR/L00450X/1); an EDCTP Senior Fellowship (TMA 2015 SF—1001); and a Sofja Kovalevskaja Award from the Alexander von Humboldt Foundation (3·2—1184811—KEN—SKP). L.M.M. is supported by the DELTAS Africa Initiative [DEL-15-003]. The DELTAS Africa Initiative is an independent funding scheme of the African Academy of Sciences (AAS)'s Alliance for Accelerating Excellence in Science in Africa (AESA) and supported by the New Partnership for Africa's Development Planning and Coordinating Agency (NEPAD Agency) with funding from the Wellcome Trust [107769/Z/10/Z] and the UK government. The views expressed in this publication are those of the author (s) and not necessarily those of AAS, NEPAD Agency, Wellcome Trust, or the UK government. RKK and JT are supported by a Wellcome Trust Strategic Award (107499/Z/15/Z). GK was jointly supported by the MRC/DFID African Research Leader Award (MR/L00450X/1) and the DELTAS Africa Initiative [DEL-15-003].

References

1. Fonseca AM, Quinto L, Jimenez A et al (2017) Multiplexing detection of IgG against *Plasmodium falciparum* pregnancy-specific antigens. PLoS One 12:e0181150
2. Finney OC, Danziger SA, Molina DM et al (2014) Predicting antidisease immunity using proteome arrays and sera from children naturally exposed to malaria. Mol Cell Proteomics 13:2646–2660
3. Crompton PD, Kayala MA, Traore B et al (2010) A prospective analysis of the Ab response to *Plasmodium falciparum* before and after a malaria season by protein microarray. Proc Natl Acad Sci U S A 107:6958–6963
4. Tighe PJ, Ryder RR, Todd I et al (2015) ELISA in the multiplex era: potentials and pitfalls. Proteomics Clin Appl 9:406–422
5. Vignali DA (2000) Multiplexed particle-based flow cytometric assays. J Immunol Methods 243:243–255
6. Kingsmore SF (2006) Multiplexed protein measurement: technologies and applications of protein and antibody arrays. Nat Rev Drug Discov 5:310–320
7. Engvall E, Perlmann P (1971) Enzyme-linked immunosorbent assay (ELISA). Quantitative assay of immunoglobulin G. Immunochemistry 8:871–874
8. Van Weemen BK, Schuurs AH (1971) Immunoassay using antigen-enzyme conjugates. FEBS Lett 15:232–236
9. Osier FH, Fegan G, Polley SD et al (2008) Breadth and magnitude of antibody responses to multiple *Plasmodium falciparum* merozoite antigens are associated with protection from clinical malaria. Infect Immun 76:2240–2248
10. Polley SD, Conway DJ, Cavanagh DR et al (2006) High levels of serum antibodies to merozoite surface protein 2 of *Plasmodium falciparum* are associated with reduced risk of clinical malaria in coastal Kenya. Vaccine 24:4233–4246
11. Dodoo D, Hollingdale MR, Anum D et al (2011) Measuring naturally acquired immune responses to candidate malaria vaccine antigens in Ghanaian adults. Malar J 10:168
12. Dutta S, Sullivan JS, Grady KK et al (2009) High antibody titer against apical membrane

antigen-1 is required to protect against malaria in the Aotus model. PLoS One 4:e8138

13. Corran PH, Cook J, Lynch C et al (2008) Dried blood spots as a source of anti-malarial antibodies for epidemiological studies. Malar J 7:195
14. Nebie I, Diarra A, Ouedraogo A et al (2008) Humoral responses to *Plasmodium falciparum* blood-stage antigens and association with incidence of clinical malaria in children living in an area of seasonal malaria transmission in Burkina Faso, West Africa. Infect Immun 76:759–766
15. Sirima SB, Tiono AB, Ouedraogo A et al (2009) Safety and immunogenicity of the malaria vaccine candidate MSP3 long synthetic peptide in 12-24 months-old Burkinabe children. PLoS One 4:e7549
16. Yoon IK, Angov E, Larson D et al (2005) Characterization of a human reference standard for antibody to *Plasmodium falciparum* merozoite surface protein 1(42). Am J Trop Med Hyg 72:714–718
17. Miura K, Zhou H, Diouf A et al (2009) Anti-apical-membrane-antigen-1 antibody is more effective than anti-42-kilodalton-merozoite-surface-protein-1 antibody in inhibiting *Plasmodium falciparum* growth, as determined by the *in vitro* growth inhibition assay. Clin Vaccine Immunol 16:963–968
18. Pol E, Karlsson R, Roos H et al (2007) Biosensor-based characterization of serum antibodies during development of an anti-IgE immunotherapeutic against allergy and asthma. J Mol Recognit 20:22–31
19. Williams AR, Douglas AD, Miura K et al (2012) Enhancing blockade of *Plasmodium falciparum* erythrocyte invasion: assessing combinations of antibodies against PfRH5 and other merozoite antigens. PLoS Pathog 8:e1002991

Chapter 7

Controlled Human Malaria Infection (CHMI) Studies: Over 100 Years of Experience with Parasite Injections

Kai Matuschewski and Steffen Borrmann

Abstract

Human experimentation by deliberate infection with malarial parasites seems unethical yet has a long history in infectious disease research. After rigorous screening, volunteers are inoculated with *Plasmodium* sporozoites or blood stages and monitored under strict clinical supervision until they are treated with a licensed malaria drug and the infection is completely resolved. Historically, experimental *Plasmodium* challenge infections were applied to confirm that *Anopheles* mosquitoes were the malaria vector and to treat neurosyphilis in *Treponema pallidum*-infected patients. The lifesaving treatment with reliable parasite inoculation, monitoring, and drug cure was awarded with a Nobel Prize in 1927 and paved the way for human trials for clinical tests of candidate drugs and vaccines. Importantly, controlled human malaria infection (CHMI) studies are indispensable to bridge the major gap between phase I safety and phase II field trials. Here, we describe the biological basis, historical experiences, applications, and ethical considerations for CHMI studies. Acceleration of antimalarial drug and vaccine development remains a priority in medical research and critically depends on capacity building for CHMI studies.

Key words Malaria, *Plasmodium*, Human trials, Clinical monitoring, Adverse effects, Sporozoite, Asexual blood stage, Vaccines, Drugs

1 Introduction

Controlled human malaria infections (CHMI) are a unique and powerful research tool for accelerating the development of antimalarial interventions, be it vaccines or novel drugs. CHMI is an intentional infection with *Plasmodium* parasites and, hence, a research procedure that has to be carefully designed and to undergo stringent review by ethics committees and regulatory authorities. CHMI starts with the inoculation of defined numbers of drug-sensitive parasites either by exposure to *Plasmodium*-infected female *Anopheles* mosquitoes or by syringe injection of defined numbers of parasites. The former route of parasite challenge closely mimics the natural course of infection, where sporozoites inside the mosquito salivary glands are injected intradermally during the

Frédéric Ariey et al. (eds.), *Malaria Control and Elimination*, Methods in Molecular Biology, vol. 2013,
https://doi.org/10.1007/978-1-4939-9550-9_7,

probing phase, followed by subsequent intradermal migration and transmigration of a capillary to enter the bloodstream. This important skin phase of infection contributes to modulation of antimalarial immunity and is bypassed by syringe injection of purified, aseptic sporozoites. Direct sporozoite inoculation has, however, multiple advantages, including large-scale production and characterization of defined parasite challenge lots. Moreover, injection of defined parasite numbers tends to improve reproducibility and to reduce variations in clinical trial outcomes. Similarly, transfusion of *Plasmodium*-infected red blood cells is an effective inoculation scheme and bypasses the otherwise obligatory first parasite expansion phase in the liver.

Decades of experience at dedicated research centers have proved that the success of CHMI rests on the rigorous standardization of procedures and a cooperative spirit between all participants, i.e., clinicians, parasitologists, entomologists, ethics review boards, and volunteers. For the safety of volunteers, it is mandatory to carry out daily monitoring to detect: (a) typical malaria symptoms, mostly fever, chills, fatigue, nausea or headache, and (b) exponentially proliferating asexual blood stages as the earliest possible time point. Fast-acting, curative treatment can thus be immediately initiated, in most cases prior to the first disease symptoms. Most importantly, curative treatment must occur before pathogenic blood-stage infections could trigger life-threatening complications, such as deep coma, metabolic acidosis, multi-organ failure, or severe anemia. Accordingly, every volunteer has to understand and approve that the experimental infection can potentially lead to a lethal outcome and that full cooperation with the clinical research team is essential to minimize morbidity. It follows that of utmost concern is whether patients are exposed to disproportionate risks or even exploited and whether adequate consent can be obtained. Luckily, the breadth of clinical experience that accumulated over 100 years of experimental *Plasmodium* infections and the successful record of multiple malaria clinical trials centers makes CHMI a standard procedure that can be readily adapted, provided that the necessary clinical infrastructure, including access to emergency care, is in place.

Because CHMI with sporozoites mimics natural transmission yet allows detailed and full control over exposure and course of infection, this highly controlled setup allows unbiased assessment of central clinical development objectives: (a) level of protection after immunization with vaccine candidates and (b) chemoprophylactic efficacy of drug candidates. Moreover, CHMI may be critical for the discovery of immunological correlates of protection and advancement of our understanding of antimalarial immunology in general. In a special use case, CHMI is at the core of some of the most promising whole-parasite vaccine approaches. In this chapter, we describe the unique parasite biology and research opportunities that together make CHMI one of the most encouraging tools in clinical malaria research. The interested reader is also encouraged to consult recent excellent reviews on this topic [1–3].

2 A Brief History of over 100 Years of CHMI

The history of CHMI starts with a groundbreaking experiment in malaria research, "the experimental proof of the mosquito-malaria theory" by Giovanni Battista Grassi and Amico Bignami, who exposed *Anopheles* mosquitoes to hospitalized malaria patients and then infected naive individuals by mosquito bite [4]. Manson subsequently confirmed these findings by performing an experiment in which his son, a medical student in London at that time, exposed himself to *Anopheles* mosquitoes that had been fed on *Plasmodium vivax* patients in Rome [5]. Shortly thereafter in the 1910s, CHMI was pioneered by Julius Wagner-Jauregg, who worked in Vienna and employed iatrogenic *Plasmodium* inoculations as pyrogenic treatment of paralysis in late-stage syphilis. In the absence of curative drugs against *Treponema pallidum* at that time, the characteristic, regular, and painful high fever bouts of *Plasmodium* infections led to the heat-induced killing of the spirochete pathogen and ultimately resolution of neurosyphilis, hence the term pyrotherapy. This highly unusual cure of a pathogen by infection with another pathogen became common practice in the 1920s and was swiftly recognized with a Nobel Prize in 1927. Tens of thousands of patients received CHMI with *P. vivax*. This *Plasmodium* species typically elicits the highest fever of all malarial parasites and is self-limiting when administered by blood transfusion. Occasional infections with the lethal *P. falciparum* parasite and even less frequently and mostly depending on availability of parasite sources, *P. malariae* or *P. ovale*, have been documented. For pyrotherapy parasites were inoculated via infected mosquito bites or injection of infected blood. The advent and commercialization of penicillin in the 1940s immediately replaced CHMI for treating syphilis.

Thirty years later, in the 1970s, CHMI made a comeback, this time as a research tool following the successful demonstration of sterilizing protection induced by attenuated sporozoites transmitted by bites from hundreds of irradiated mosquitoes [6]. Since then, thousands of volunteers across different continents have been safely challenged by CHMI. Most importantly, over the course of 45 years, not a single case of severe malaria or death, related to CHMI, has been reported. Standardized CHMI protocols with only slight modifications are now in use in several clinical trial centers in the United States, Europe, and Africa.

3 *Plasmodium* Biology: Gradual Population Expansion and Parasite Stage Conversion as the Basis for CHMI

Parasites of the genus *Plasmodium* are vector-borne obligate intracellular pathogens that display remarkable host specificity. As single-cell eukaryotes, they have the exceptional capacity to invade, remodel, and replicate within erythrocytes, the only nonnucleated, terminally differentiated cell population in mammals. Intracellular replication and formation of a dozen new merozoites are synchronized within a population and last between 24 h (*P. knowlesi*) and 72 h (*P. malariae*). All malaria-related symptoms, ultimately leading to morbidity and mortality, are strictly linked to the asexual replication phase in the blood. Although asexual blood-stage propagation is exponential and results in an approximately tenfold increase in population size at every replication round, this pathogen proliferation is confined to blood, relatively modest in semi-immune individuals, and can be readily monitored by classical microscopy of Giemsa-stained blood films. In naive volunteers additional precautions are essential, and quantitative PCR is now the benchmark for sensitive detection of emerging *Plasmodium* blood stages. Progression of a *Plasmodium* infection to mild malaria and further to severe malaria is only partly understood and the result of a complex interplay of multiple factors, including size of initial parasite inoculum, parasite virulence factors, gene expression dynamics, host factors, coinfections, innate immunity, and adaptive immune responses. Nevertheless, malarial parasite density is a useful and acceptable proxy for risk of morbidity in nonimmune volunteers. Since the course of infection follows standard patterns, monitoring the initial onset of a malarial infection after CHMI generates robust data of high predictive value, including for vaccine and drug efficacy.

A distinct hallmark of parasitic infections is stage conversion, whereby the pathogen adopts purpose-built cell shapes and expresses characteristic molecular repertoires during progression through its life cycle. *Plasmodium* is no exception, and sporozoites and merozoites are profoundly different cells that are tailored for their respective tasks: mosquito salivary gland colonization, intradermal and intrahepatic migration, and successful invasion of a suitable hepatocyte *versus* erythrocyte invasion. The preerythrocytic phase encompasses the entire period from sporozoite inoculation during the bite of an infected female *Anopheles* mosquito to emergence of first-generation merozoites. Merozoites are eventually formed after transformation of intrahepatic sporozoites to liver trophozoites followed by the subsequent obligate first population expansion phase. This period is inaccessible to diagnostic detection of the parasite. Blood stage infections, however, can be readily detected, and the time to demonstration of an infection in blood samples is termed prepatent period. The rule of parasite stage conversion has important implications for CHMI with sporozoites. The massive expansion of the *Plasmodium* population size in the liver is considered benign to volunteers and allows for up to 6–7 days of interventions against *P. falciparum*, e.g., chemoprophylaxis, to inhibit or, ideally, completely eliminate preerythrocytic parasites.

A specific and robust anti-sporozoite or anti-liver-stage activity can be readily established from an absence of blood infection in comparison to the control group. A delay of parasite detection in the blood signifies considerably reduced anti-preerythrocytic efficacy, typically excluding further consideration of the intervention strategy. This is because the exponential expansion of blood-stage parasites, even if delayed, will generally result in morbidity, including lifethreatening manifestations in non-immune individuals. In other words, preerythrocytic interventions need to be repeatedly 100% effective in CHMI studies, unless an inhibitory effect is also unequivocally demonstrated against blood-stage propagation. In contrast, the information gained from monitoring of CHMI of *Plasmodium*-infected erythrocytes is limited to anti-blood stage activities. Finally, in CHMI trials with *P. vivax* sporozoites, but not blood stages, curative treatment with primaquine, a demanding once-daily 14-day regimen, is essential to firmly eliminate dormant forms, termed hypnozoites, which can cause frequent tertian malaria relapses well beyond the clinical trials. Accordingly, all trial participants of *P. vivax* sporozoite CHMI studies need to have a particularly clear understanding of the trial design and implications. In conclusion, the first silent *Plasmodium* expansion phase in the liver offers ample opportunities for efficacy testing of drug and vaccine candidates, but strict parasite monitoring and careful interpretation of the course of infection are prerequisites for successful translation and product development.

4 Methods and Technology of CHMI Studies

The conduct of CHMI is guided by two major criteria: predictability of infection and safety of the volunteers. Several milestone improvements in these two areas have contributed to the general acceptance of CHMI as a safe and valuable malaria research tool. An early breakthrough was the adoption of continuous blood-stage culture protocols in the 1970s [7], followed by the identification of gametocyte-producing *P. falciparum* strains, namely, NF54, its clone 3D7, and 7G8, which can be cultured and used for reliably infecting female *Anopheles* mosquitoes to be used for transmitting *Plasmodium falciparum* infections to volunteers. These advances have freed CHMI from the vagaries of finding suitable *Plasmodium*-infected human donors.

Only a small proportion of salivary gland sporozoites are being transmitted during a single mosquito bite, and estimates vary between a dozen and a few hundreds. Therefore, at least five infected mosquitoes are allowed to feed on a volunteer to produce an infection in close to 100% of cases. Infected mosquito batches are verified before inoculation of volunteers by scoring midgut oocysts (around 7 days after the blood meal) and/or salivary gland sporozoites (around 14 days post feeding). The latter procedure is also carried out on all mosquitoes after they have fed on a volunteer. Any mosquito found to be either not blood-engorged or with a salivary gland infection score of less than 2 (corresponding to less than ten residual sporozoites) is replaced until a volunteer has received bites from a minimum of five mosquitoes with confirmed infection status. Replacing mosquitoes that are not blood engorged is a conservative approach since sporozoites are being injected during probing. The size of the sporozoite inoculum correlates with the probability of detectable blood-stage infections but the biological basis of the apparent stochastic nature of the infectivity of low-inoculum infections, e.g., CHMI with less than five mosquito bites, even in completely nonimmune individuals, is poorly understood. It is possible that these barely infective inocula reflect an evolutionary hardwired immune evasion strategy of the parasite. Whatever the biological or immunological basis of the five-mosquito requirement, by-bite CHMI necessitates a well-functioning, safety three-level insectary for maintaining *Plasmodium falciparum*-infected *Anopheles* mosquitoes colonies.

Since the early 1980s, *An. stephensi* has proven to be a reliable and comparatively robust vector. Nonetheless, the conduct of by-bite CHMI has been largely confined to small cohorts of volunteers and to a slowly growing but still exclusive club of dedicated research institutions—mainly due to the complexity of protocols and dedicated infrastructures necessary for generating "flying syringes," i.e., infected *Anopheles* mosquitoes. Thus, the availability of aseptic, cryopreserved sporozoites that can be inoculated with simple medical syringes and needles even in large phase IIb-type clinical trial cohorts has led to another major expansion of CHMI trial activities—this time including clinical trials in malaria-endemic countries. Over the last 7 years, more than 2,000 individuals have received injections with cryopreserved sporozoites. These efforts were spearheaded at a commercial company (Sanaria) that uses proprietary protocols for isolating and cryopreserving *P. falciparum* sporozoites from aseptically raised mosquitoes under stringent GMP regulations. Initially, cryopreserved *P. falciparum* sporozoites were inoculated intradermally in an attempt to mimic the natural route of transmission. However, not all volunteers developed subsequent blood-stage infections, plateauing at around 80% of challenged volunteers even with high sporozoite doses of 25,000 per intradermal injection [8]. The predictability of by-needle CHMI improved dramatically when sporozoites were injected intravenously. As pointed out above, this rather unusual route of administration of a live pathogen enabled successful CHMI challenge in 100% of volunteers with defined doses of around 3,000 sporozoites. Currently, only two strains, NF54 of West African origin and 7G8 of South American origin, are available for CHMI in the form of cryopreserved, vialed sporozoites. Two more strains, NF135.C10 of Southeast Asian origin and NF166.C8 of West African origin, are available for conventional by-bite CHMI [9, 10]. This limited diversity of strains can be attributed to the long-standing challenge of identifying culture-adapted strains that support robust production of mosquito-infective gametocytes. In addition, for GMP-grade production of vialed sporozoites, each new strain requires new approval. Conventional by-bite CHMI does not require regulatory approval for a biological product and, thus, offers far more experimental flexibility.

Besides the different approaches for inoculating live sporozoites, the CHMI protocols currently in use are fairly, if not entirely, standardized. Because infections cannot be detected during the liver-stage phase, the follow-up of volunteers focuses on the accurate and timely detection of blood-stage infections. The primary parasitological endpoint of CHMI protocols in nonimmune volunteers, especially when used as challenge for assessing vaccine efficacy, is asexual parasite patency. As pointed out above, the predictable nature of the cyclical proliferation of blood stages in nonimmune volunteers also allows for more nuanced secondary parasitological endpoints such as the replication rate for assessing potential vaccine-induced, anti-blood-stage immunity. Asexual parasites in the peripheral blood can be detected either by using conventional light microscopy or by significantly more sensitive molecular techniques. The microscopic examination of Giemsa-stained thick blood smears has been the gold standard due to a general confidence in directly observed data ("seeing is believing"). However, its elevated detection threshold heralds two major drawbacks: (a) volunteers often develop symptoms before smear positivity; and by extension, (b) curative therapy has to be initiated immediately, preventing detailed assessments of parasite replication kinetics. Both points are addressed by much more sensitive quantitative real-time PCR reactions (qPCR), for instance, targeting the multi-copy 18S small subunit ribosomal RNA gene [11] that increases the detection threshold from 10^4 parasites/mL by microscopy to 1–10 parasites/mL by qPCR. On average, detection by qPCR precedes thick blood smear patency by 2–4 days, corresponding to one or two additional rounds of replication. In fact, qPCR protocols can reliably detect even "first-wave" asexual parasites after hepatocyte egress on days 6–8 in nonimmune volunteers [12]. The dramatically improved sensitivity of qPCR thus also

(a) permits the specific assessment of potential preerythrocytic immunity, whether vaccine-induced or naturally acquired, and (b) can reveal strain-specific differences in preerythrocytic development.

Parasite kinetics upon CHMI demonstrates a fairly predictable pattern in nonimmune or unvaccinated individuals, especially when using the highly standardized doses for intravenous injections [13, 14]. In partially immune individuals or in vaccinees, the pattern depends on the degree and stage specificity of anti-parasitic immunity [15].

In conclusion, CHMI by needle injection, in particular when using the intravenous route, offers superior options for the standardization of trials. Indeed, GMP production of aseptic, cryopreserved infectious sporozoites has been a prerequisite for the active clinical development of whole-parasite vaccine protocols using CHMI as vehicle for antigen delivery. CHMI by infective mosquito bites, precisely because it does not fall under GMP regulation, remains an attractive alternative that offers more experimental flexibility. This could be an advantage for rapidly testing different *P. falciparum* or even, non-*P. falciparum* strains for CHMI, including regional parasite isolates.

Finally, CHMI with parasite-infected red blood cells provides an alternative route for inducing *Plasmodium* infections [16]. Experiences with blood-stage inoculations also go back to its use as "malaria therapy" for late-stage syphilis. No inoculation-related serious adverse events have been reported, but the risk of inadvertent inoculation of blood-borne pathogens requires particular attention, e.g., by using defined cell banks. Currently, only a single center is routinely carrying out CHMI by infected red blood cells [16].

5 Ethical Considerations and Clinical Settings to Conduct CHMI Studies

Despite the inoculation of potentially life-threatening *P. falciparum* infections, CHMI has proven to be exceptionally safe and well tolerated. In fact, the procedure has now been carried out in thousands of study participants without a single case of severe malaria or death. This is a remarkable achievement and can be attributed to the implementation of stringent rules for conducting CHMI trials. Foremost, study participants must fully understand the risks inherent to exposure to a life-threatening pathogen. Full cooperation with all study procedures is required, lost to follow-up is *not* an option in CHMI studies, and should this occur, participants must accept the involvement of law enforcement. Secondly, starting on day 6 post-inoculation (day 0 is defined as day of inoculation), daily visits are mandated to detect emerging blood-stage infections and/or early signs of disease. Thirdly, upon detection of blood-stage infections, defined either by PCR or microscopy, supervised oral chemotherapy is initiated, and the regimen needs to reflect the chemosensitivity profile of the strain used in the CHMI protocol. Generally, the use of drug-resistant strains is discouraged, but the limited supply of gametocyte-producing strains puts limits on the practicality of this rule. All CHMI trials are conducted under the umbrella of good clinical practice (GCP), which is designed to safeguard the health of study participants and protect the quality of study data. This requires substantial investment in the training of dedicated study teams and in validating the clinical, laboratory, and data management infrastructure. Even if very small, the residual risk of life-threatening complications of CHMI in nonimmune individuals requires rapid access to intensive care departments in case of medical emergencies.

The difference in the immune status and, thus, the level of acquired protective immunity observed between residents of endemic areas and residents of malaria-free regions can dictate the selection of CHMI endpoints. For instance, in semi-immune individuals it should be possible to extend follow-up until a clinical endpoint is reached, i.e., low-grade fever in the presence of parasitemia, whereas in nonimmune participants early-as-possible detection of parasitemia, ideally before the onset of symptoms, is recommended.

6 Applications of CHMI Studies

The precise control of timing, dose, and genetic composition of exposure to malarial parasite transmission in CHMI studies offers unprecedented potential for both furthering our understanding of malaria and the development of novel interventions. Without such tight control of exposure, any study that examines protection—be it attributable to vaccines, host genetics, or immunology—requires enormous sample sizes to account for the randomness of highly heterogeneous natural transmission [17].

Primarily, CHMI is a tool for accelerating malaria vaccine development. Specifically, it is used with great success as challenge both in small cohorts of volunteers enrolled in proof-of-concept phase I-IIa vaccine trials and in larger cohorts in phase II vaccine trials. The use of defined doses at specific time points leads to a substantial reduction of sample sizes and heterologous challenges, which can potentially include local parasite isolates in the future, can also be included. Secondly, CHMI can serve as vehicle for delivering parasite antigens, as the core of whole-parasite vaccine strategies. These range from the inoculation of attenuated sporozoites to the inoculation of live sporozoites under chemoprophylaxis, both of which are promising vaccine strategies under active clinical development. Finally, CHMI is also used to interrogate stage-specific immunity toward identification of signatures of protective efficacy and to test new chemoprophylactic drug candidates.

7 Outlook

The firm and early placement of CHMI studies in the clinical development plan of virtually every novel malaria intervention strategy reflects the enormous value of CHMI for malaria research. Further improvements are desirable to better reflect the enormous strain and antigenic diversity of *Plasmodium* infections and to aim for a broader involvement of scientists, clinicians, and trial participants from malaria-endemic countries. Efforts are under way to (a) improve on the availability of heterologous strains from at least the major two human malarial parasites, *P. falciparum* and *P. vivax*, and (b) to gradually move away from CHMI centers in malaria-free, high-income countries to malaria-afflicted areas with distinct epidemiological patterns. Therefore, successful employment of CHMI trial centers in the tropics, particularly sub-Saharan Africa, will be one of the most critical advancements for translational malaria research.

Acknowledgments

K.M. is supported partly by the Alliance Berlin Canberra "Crossing Boundaries: Molecular Interactions in Malaria", which is co-funded by a grant from the Deutsche Forschungsgemeinschaft (DFG) for the International Research Training Group (IRTG) 2290 and the Australian National University. S.B. is investigator at the German Centre for Infection Research (DZIF) and a recipient of a DFG grant to study parasite-vector interactions. We acknowledge the many important contributions that have been made over the past 100 years in the field. For the purpose of this chapter, we selected a few seminal references and had to omit many equally important contributions. We apologize to our colleagues afflicted by this choice.

References

1. Sauerwein RW, Roestenberg M, Moorthy VS (2011) Experimental human challenge infections can accelerate clinical malaria vaccine development. Nat Rev Immunol 11:57–64
2. Payne RO, Griffin PM, McCarthy JS et al (2017) *Plasmodium vivax* controlled human malaria infection–progress and prospects. Trends Parasitol 33:141–150
3. Stanisic DI, McCarthy JS, Good MF (2018) Controlled human malaria infection: applications, advances and challenges. Infect Immun 86:e00479–e00417
4. Grassi B, Bignami A, Bastianelli G (1899) Ulteriore ricerche sul ciclo dei parassiti malarici umani sul corpo del zanzarone. Atti Reale Accad Lincei 8:21–28

5. Manson P (1900) Experimental proof of the mosquito-malaria theory. Br Med J 2:949–951
6. Clyde DF, Most H, McCarthy VC et al (1973) Immunization of man against sporozoite-induced falciparum malaria. Am J Med Sci 266:169–177
7. Trager W, Jensen JB (1976) Human malaria parasites in continuous culture. Science 193:673–675
8. Roestenberg M, Bijker EM, Sim BK et al (2013) Controlled human malaria infections by intradermal injection of cryopreserved *Plasmodium falciparum* sporozoites. Am J Trop Med Hyg 88:5–13
9. Teirlinck AC, Roestenberg M, van de Vegte-Bolmer M et al (2013) NF135.C10: a new *Plasmodium falciparum* clone for controlled human malaria infections. J Infect Dis 207:656–660
10. Walk J, Reuling IJ, Behet MC et al (2017) Modest heterologous protection after *Plasmodium falciparum* sporozoite immunization: a double-blind randomized controlled clinical trial. BMC Med 15:168
11. Hermsen CC, Telgt DS, Linders EH et al (2001) Detection of *Plasmodium falciparum* malaria parasites *in vivo* by real-time quantitative PCR. Mol Biochem Parasitol 118:247–251
12. Roestenberg M, McCall M, Hopman J et al (2009) Protection against malaria challenge by sporozoite inoculation. N Engl J Med 361:468–477
13. Coffeng LE, Hermsen CC, Sauerwein RW et al (2017) The power of malaria vaccine trials using controlled human malaria infection. PLoS Comput Biol 13:e1005255
14. Mordmüller B, Supan C, Sim KL et al (2015) Direct venous inoculation of *Plasmodium falciparum* sporozoites for controlled human malaria infection: a dose-finding trial in two centres. Malar J 14:117
15. Lell B, Mordmüller B, Dejon Agobe JC et al (2018) Impact of sickle cell trait and naturally acquired immunity on uncomplicated malaria after controlled human malaria infection in adults in Gabon. Am J Trop Med Hyg 98:508–515
16. Engwerda CR, Minigo G, Amante FH et al (2012) Experimentally induced blood stage malaria infection as a tool for clinical research. Trends Parasitol 28:515–521
17. Bejon P, Williams TN, Nyundo C et al (2014) A micro-epidemiological analysis of febrile malaria in Coastal Kenya showing hotspots within hotspots. elife 3:e02130s

Part III

Therapeutics

Chapter 8

In Vivo Assessments to Detect Antimalarial Resistance

Mehul J. Dhorda and Arjen M. Dondorp

Abstract

In vivo drug clinical trials are the gold standard for assessing the therapeutic efficacy of antimalarials. They must be conducted in a rigorous and standardized manner so that the resistance of antimalarial drugs can be compared both in time and in space. This chapter presents the methodology for conducting such clinical studies of antimalarials for the treatment of uncomplicated malaria and describes the logistical difficulties and limitations of this methodology. Finally it highlights the importance of such knowledge in preventing resistance, in prolonging the utility of existing antimalarial drugs, and in ensuring that all individuals and populations suffering from malaria get the right malaria treatment at the right time.

Key words Malaria, Therapeutic efficacy study, Resistance, Methodology

1 Introduction: Why Clinical Trials Are Important for Assessing Drug Efficacy

Naturally occurring infections of malaria in humans are caused by five species of Apicomplexan parasites of the genus *Plasmodium*—*P. falciparum*, *P. vivax*, *P. malariae*, *P. ovale*, and, in certain geographically limited zones, *P. knowlesi*. The disease caused by such infections and the outcomes following its treatment are affected by a complex interplay between a multitude of parasite and host-related factors [1]. This complexity, alongside the sociopolitical contexts in the places where it continues to be endemic, has meant that it has thus far been impossible to eradicate malaria despite the enormous scientific and operational advances made in improving its diagnosis, treatment, and prevention. The vast majority of cases and deaths due to malaria result from infections with *P. falciparum*, whereas a larger proportion of the global population is at risk of infections with *P. vivax* [2, 3]. Taken together, malaria infections caused over 216 million cases and 439,000 deaths leading to the loss of over 56 million DALYs (disability-adjusted life years) [4, 5]. Deployment of effective antimalarial drugs is a prerequisite for adequate malaria control and future elimination. Any evidence used to recommend deployment of new or changed

Frédéric Ariey et al. (eds.), *Malaria Control and Elimination*, Methods in Molecular Biology, vol. 2013,
https://doi.org/10.1007/978-1-4939-9550-9_8,

treatment regimens to improve treatment outcomes or to counter antimalarial drug resistance in the parasites would thus affect millions of lives and must be robust and of high quality. Generating such evidence necessitates the collection of data from standardized, controlled, repeatable, and repeated experiments to assess the efficacy of antimalarial drugs for the clearance of malaria infections. In the case of malaria and of all other infectious diseases, the gold standard for such experimental evidence is that generated from in vivo trials of drug efficacy conducted in multiple individuals and populations. Integration of drug efficacy assessment into routine surveillance is currently proposed, but these clinical assessments are labor-intensive and expensive. In areas of low transmission, which also tend to be the areas with antimalarial drug resistance, sufficiently rapid enrolment of patients into drug efficacy studies can be hard to achieve. Supplementing clinical efficacy data with in vitro susceptibility testing and assessment of molecular markers for drug resistance can also be valuable in monitoring and confirming resistance, as discussed in other chapters of this book.

An assessment of in vivo therapeutic efficacy requires the consistent implementation of clinical and laboratory procedures for all subjects in the study population. This ensures at a minimum that all subjects are selected, treated, and assessed in the same way and allows generalizable conclusions to be drawn from the trial. If the procedures and protocols are globally harmonized, the generated data or evidence is comparable over time and space, which further allows spatiotemporal trends in the spread or emergence of drug resistance to be discerned. Such standardization also aids the identification of genetic changes associated with drug resistance and the validation of in vitro drug susceptibility assays [6–9]. However, infections by parasites carrying resistance-conferring mutations and/or demonstrating a drug-resistant phenotype as detected by in vitro assays can sometimes still be cured effectively by the correspondent drug. Vice versa, treatment failures can occur due to host-related or other factors in infections caused by parasites susceptible to the antimalarials used. Thus, any signs of resistance detected through laboratory-based testing needs to be confirmed clinically through rigorous in vivo therapeutic efficacy assessments. We here describe in some detail the prerequisites for high-quality clinical studies on antimalarial drug efficacy.

2 Rationale for Methodologies

A simple definition of the efficacy of a drug therapy for an infectious disease is the proportion cured in a study population suffering from that disease following treatment with the drug or combination of drugs being tested. Measurement of drug efficacy thus requires that a case of the disease and the success or failure of the treatment be clearly defined and objectively verifiable. For antimalarial drug efficacy assessments, the most commonly used case definition of treatment failure is the presence of malaria parasites in the patient's peripheral blood along with clinical symptoms associated with malaria—usually febrile illness with or without other symptoms [10]. This implies that all cases must have parasite densities above the pyrogenic threshold, which varies with the malaria parasite species and the epidemiological context where the study is being conducted. Higher parasite densities may be needed to define a *Plasmodium falciparum* malaria case in zones with higher transmission of malaria, where microscopically patent but asymptomatic infections can be common, whereas presence of any parasitemia may be sufficient to confirm a case of *P. vivax* infection. Further, it is advisable to exclude subjects with low or very low initial parasite densities in studies aiming to detect parasite resistance to artemisinins. Artemisinins, unlike the other available antimalarials, have a broad stage specificity including on circulating ring-stage parasites. Initial parasite clearance dynamics are an important measure of drug efficacy. Measurement of parasite clearance rates is required in these instances which cannot be performed with accuracy and precision if the starting parasite densities are too low [11].

An episode of malaria is considered successfully treated when an adequate clinical and parasitological response (ACPR; *see* Table 1 for definitions) to the treatment is sustained over a pre-defined period following its administration. Confirming ACPR thus implies that the study subject needs to be monitored following treatment for the reappearance of parasitemia with or without associated symptoms. The duration of the follow-up is in part determined by the half-life of the drugs being tested, with longer follow-up periods required for drugs with slower in vivo elimination as they would suppress the recurrence of parasitemia until after the drug levels in the blood are below minimum inhibitory concentrations (MIC) (Fig. 1). Longer durations of follow-up, however, also increase the chances that the study subjects are reinfected following a fresh infective mosquito bite, which is in particular frequent in high transmission areas. Such events can only be differentiated from true recrudescence of the initial infection through genotyping of the parasites detected at baseline and upon follow-up given that the parasites will be morphologically indistinguishable by microscopy. Even if recrudescence is confirmed by molecular testing, the possibility that the infecting parasites were not exposed to inhibitory or lethal concentrations of the drugs due to sub-optimal dosing, poor absorption, altered host metabolism of the drug, or combinations thereof needs to be excluded by measuring the drug levels in the patients. Antimalarial treatment failures can thus be defined as genetically confirmed recrudescence of parasites despite appropriate dosing, absorption, and metabolism of the drugs. Treatment

Table 1
Recommended inclusion and exclusion criteria (adapted from WHO (2009))

Inclusion criteria
• Age, 6–59 months in areas of high transmission, all patients over 6 months of age in areas of low-to-moderate transmission
• Mono-infection with the species of interest detected by microscopy
• Asexual parasite density of 2000–200,000/μL in areas of high transmission, 1000–100,000/μL asexual forms in areas of low-to-moderate transmission (lower and upper limits can be modified depending on the epidemiological context and the drugs being assessed)
• Axillary or tympanic temperature 37.5 °C or oral or rectal temperature of 38 °C or history of fever during the past 24 h
• Ability to swallow oral medication
• Ability and willingness to comply with the study protocol for the duration of the study and to comply with the study visit schedule
• Informed consent from the patient or from a parent or guardian in the case of children
Exclusion criteria
• Presence of general danger signs in children aged under 5 years or signs of severe falciparum malaria according to the definitions of WHO
• Mixed or mono-infection with another *Plasmodium* species detected by microscopy
• Presence of severe malnutrition (defined as a child whose growth standard is below −3 z-score, who has symmetrical edema involving at least the feet, or who has a mid-upper arm circumference <110 mm)
• Presence of febrile conditions due to diseases other than malaria (e.g., measles, acute lower respiratory tract infection, severe diarrhea with dehydration) or other known underlying chronic or severe diseases (e.g., cardiac, renal, and hepatic diseases, HIV/AIDS)
• Regular medication, which may interfere with antimalarial pharmacokinetics
• History of hypersensitivity reactions or contraindications to any of the medicine(s) being tested or used as alternative treatment(s)
• A positive pregnancy test or breastfeeding (include this criterion only for adults)
• Unable to or unwilling to take contraceptives for the duration of the follow up (for women of childbearing age)
• Previous splenectomy (required for parasite clearance rate measurements only)

failure of 10% or more is used as a threshold for changing the first-line antimalarial treatment, as it is considered evidence of significant emerging resistance. Treatment failures are classified depending when parasites and symptoms recur or whether they are cleared in the first place. Emerging resistance is characterized by recrudescence detected 2–9 weeks after treatment, whereas parasitemia and symptoms may persist or indeed worsen despite adequate plasma drug concentrations in cases of high-level resistance. The distribution of treatment failures within these classifications provides useful

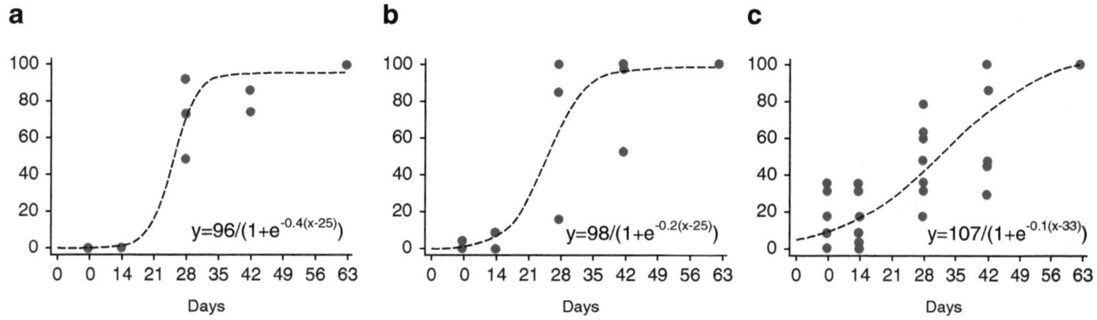

Fig. 1 Relationship between the proportion of antimalarial treatment failures detected and the duration of follow-up for (**a**) short half-life, (**b**) medium half-life, and (**c**) long half-life antimalarial drugs. PCR genotype-corrected results are shown [1]

information on the level of resistance in a given context and also requires repeated clinical and parasitological assessments to be performed over the duration of the follow-up of the patient, including daily assessments for a few days after start of treatment.

3 Confirming Disease and Detecting Recurrent Parasitemia

Infections with malaria parasites do not always result in illness. In high transmission zones, asymptomatic parasitemia is common, especially among partially immune older children and adults who may control or clear the infection without any antimalarial treatments. Symptomatic or clinical episodes are likely to occur in such populations only from an infection with a strain of the parasite to which the subject has not previously been exposed, resulting in higher parasite densities and a lower likelihood of clearing the infection without antimalarial treatment. However, febrile illnesses in such carriers may not only be caused by malaria, as it is often co-endemic with other fever-causing infectious diseases. Individuals in low transmission zones, on the other hand, are less likely to carry microscopically detectable parasitemia without concurrent febrile illness. The minimum criteria to define a case of malaria for monitoring of resistance must accordingly be the presence of microscopically detectable parasitemia in the peripheral blood associated with a febrile illness without signs of severity, along with other practical and ethical considerations (Table 2). In populations with “premunity,” identification of antimalarial drug resistance could be delayed in particular when subjects with lower initial parasitemia are included, because these parasites can be cleared by the human host even without full drug sensitivity [12]. The thresholds of parasite density for inclusion should hence be adjusted to account for the effect of transmission intensity as well as the drugs for which the assessment is being performed, as discussed later in

Table 2
Minimum requirements for microscopy

• Standardized blood volume, size, staining of films, microscopes
• 200 fields to declare slide negative
• Parasite density to be estimated using actual white blood cell or red blood cell counts
• 20–100% of slides rechecked locally and in reference lab depending on microscopist competency

this chapter. This increases the likelihood of recruiting adequate numbers of true cases of malaria while taking into consideration the intensity of malaria transmission where the study is being conducted. Finally, parasite densities also need to be assessed to exclude cases with very high parasitemia, which is one of the several forms of severe malaria characterized by altered clinical or laboratory findings or the presence of other underlying pathologies [13]. Such cases require parenteral treatment with artesunate and proper supportive management, which precludes their inclusion in routine assessments of the efficacy of antimalarials.

Confirming febrile illness is readily accomplished by measuring body temperature or by recording of the subject's medical history. The mode of measurement must nonetheless be recorded to allow for adjustments if needed, depending on whether the measurement was axillary, oral, temporal, or tympanic. Confirmation of malaria parasitemia to screen subjects for recruitment, however, is more involved as it requires detection, identification, and quantification of the parasites.

Lateral flow immunochromatographic rapid diagnostic tests (RDTs) detect circulating parasite antigens. In PfHRP2-based RDT, the antigen PfHRP2 can remain in the peripheral blood for weeks following an infection [14]. This can result in false-positive tests despite clearance of parasitemia and, even in cases of true infections, can only provide qualitative confirmation of parasitemia. Their utility in therapeutic efficacy assessments is thus limited to pre-screening of febrile cases for inclusion in efficacy trials, and not for patient follow-up. Polymerase chain reaction (PCR) assays to amplify genus- and species-specific segments of parasite genomes are increasingly used within the context of clinical trials, particularly in novel drug and vaccine trials involving controlled human malaria infections (CHMI). Such tests can be highly sensitive and specific with limits of detection far below those that can be achieved with other methodologies. Quantification of parasite density, however, can be complicated by the presence of multinucleate forms of the parasite (mostly for non-falciparum species), as well as the persistence of parasite genetic material after parasite clearance [15, 16], though the effect of such persistence may be minor and/or short-lived [17]. Methods using fluorescence-activated cell sorting

(FACS) or based on counting of differentially stained RBCs, alongside full blood counts with hematology analyzers, have recently been developed. These technologies look promising, but do not yet fully address the needs for malaria drug trials given their relatively high limits of detection and their inability to identify parasite species unequivocally. Further, as for PCR-based assays, the procedures, equipment, and materials required for such testing and its quality assurance are demanding, expensive, and difficult to standardize.

Microscopy is widely regarded as the gold standard for the diagnosis of malaria, especially in the research setting, and is the only accepted diagnostic test for malaria parasite detection, identification, and quantification in drug registration trials. It is likely to remain so for the medium to long term in the absence of alternative, validated, and standardized field-applicable methods, as discussed in the preceding paragraphs. Microscopy comes with its own challenges, however, as numerous factors can affect its quality. This includes the quality of the blood films and various parameters related to slide examination, in addition to stochastic variations in the detection of parasites, all of which must be controlled and standardized to ensure consistency and reliability of trial findings (Table 3) [18]. Nonetheless, given its wide acceptance and proven

Table 3
Classification of response to treatment (WHO 2009)

Early treatment failure (ETF)
• Danger signs or severe malaria on day 1, 2, or 3, in the presence of parasitemia
• Parasitemia on day 2 higher than on day 0, irrespective of axillary temperature
• Parasitemia on day 3 with axillary temperature 37.5°C
• Parasitemia on day 3 >25% of count on day 0
Late clinical failure (LCF)
• Danger signs or severe malaria in the presence of parasitemia on any day between day 4 and day 28 (day 42) in patients who did not previously meet any of the criteria of early treatment failure
• Presence of parasitemia on any day between day 4 and day 28 (day 42) with axillary temperature 37.5 °C in patients who did not previously meet any of the criteria of early treatment failure.
Late parasitological failure (LPF)
• Presence of parasitemia on any day between day 7 and day 28 (day 42 or day 63 for drugs with long $t_{½}$) with axillary temperature <37.5°C in patients who did not previously meet any of the criteria of early treatment failure or late clinical failure
Adequate clinical and parasitological response (ACPR)
• Absence of parasitemia on day 28 (day 42), irrespective of axillary temperature, in patients who did not previously meet any of the criteria of early treatment failure, late clinical failure, or late parasitological failure

feasibility, even in malaria endemic resource-limited settings, it remains the method of choice to identify subjects for recruitment and for their posttreatment follow-up in malaria drug trials.

4 Measuring Drug Efficacy

Drug efficacy, cure rate, or, more precisely, a point estimate of the probability of success of an antimalarial treatment is obtained by calculating the proportion of subjects who were successfully cured of malaria following treatment [19]. This definition, along with those of treatment success and failure, the procedures followed to determine those outcomes, and the interpretation of the generated results, have evolved over time starting with the early protocols developed in response to the emergence and spread of resistance to chloroquine and sulphadoxine-pyrimethamine [20–23]. At the time, it was rightly stressed that "... in assessment of the response of malaria parasites to treatment the strictest possible criteria should be applied" with respect to selection of subjects for the test, their treatment, and clinical and parasitological follow-up. The duration of follow-up was to be extended to 2 months in certain cases but was reduced to 28 days and/or to 14 days depending on the transmission intensity in subsequent versions of this protocol. A minimum follow-up period of 28 days is, however, now recommended, which may be extended to 42 or even 63 days depending on the plasma half-life of the drugs being assessed. Similarly, classifications of treatment responses initially took into account composite parasitological and clinical manifestations of disease, then only parasitological or clinical criteria, and back again to composite criteria. ACPR after a minimum follow-up period of 28 days irrespective of the epidemiological context is now the accepted standard, in keeping with evolutions in the understanding of the disease and its treatment thanks to a larger volume and diversity of available data [24–26]. Clinical and parasitological examinations of all included subjects must be performed at periodic (usually weekly) visits until completion of follow-up, with additional visits on days 1, 2, and 3 to detect early treatment failures (ETF), which usually result from high-grade resistance. An exeption is the evaluation of artemisinin resistance, where persistence of parasitemia at day 3 (72 hours) is not classified as ETF. If monitoring is systematically implemented, cases of ETF should be rare as treatments would be changed before high-grade resistance is prevalent.

In the simplest or most extreme cases where a single, fully resistant parasite is selected from the parasite population infecting a nonimmune adult host following treatment, parasites will become detectable by microscopy after they have gone through multiple life cycles. For *P. falciparum*, with a parasite muliplication factor of around 10 per 48-hour life cycle, recrudescent parasites would become microscopically patent in approximately 12 to 14 days. The time to recrudescence will be shorter when the resistant parasite population is larger at the time of treatment or in non-immune children, and longer in case of partial resistance in the parasite, immunity in the host, and longer elimination half-lives ($t_{½}$) of the drug [26, 27]. This has been confirmed in meta-analyses of *P. falciparum* antimalarial drug trials, wherein 14-day follow-up periods were clearly inadequate in detecting all except the highest levels of resistance; even a 42-day follow-up was less than 80% sensitive for confirmed recrudescence following antimalarial treatments with the longest elimination half-lives, suggesting a need for up to 63-day follow-up durations [24]. In the case of treatments for radical cure of *P. vivax*, follow-up for a few months to a year may be needed.

Sample sizes for single-arm studies such as those performed to assess the efficacy of already deployed drugs may differ depending on the goals of the trial. When no resistance is suspected, the lower limit of the confidence interval of the efficacy point estimate must be >90%, which is the prescribed threshold for changing first-line treatment. Conversely, if a trial is being conducted to verify early signals of emerging resistance, the upper limit of confidence interval of the estimate must be <90%. In practice, this translates to a minimum sample size of 76 if the expected efficacy is 95% and 204 if it is 85%, increasing to 91 and 245, respectively, if an attrition rate during patient follow-up of 20% is assumed [10, 25].

Strict "per protocol" (PP) assessments, wherein subjects experiencing any event that may interfere with, or confound the estimation of, efficacy are excluded from the analysis, are considered to be more accurate compared to "intention-to-treat" (ITT) analyses where all subjects are included in the analyses irrespective of outcomes. In PP analyses, all cases of protocol deviation, withdrawal, losses to follow-up, and recurrences of parasitemia due to new (PCR-confirmed) *P. falciparum* and/or non-falciparum parasites are excluded from the analyses, whereas in ITT analyses, all subjects with only partial protocol adherence are classified as treatment failures. Both these approaches are likely to underestimate efficacy, i.e., overestimate resistance or the risk of treatment failure, by excluding subjects who may have had an ACPR (PP analysis) or by counting them as treatment failures (ITT). Accordingly, Kaplan-Meier (K-M) "survival" analyses are currently recommended to derive the cumulative probability of treatment success or failure [25]. Such probability estimates take into account all data collected until a subject is censored following an event, which in PP or ITT analyses would lead to the subject being excluded or classified as treatment failure. This approach ensures that the maximum amount of available information is utilized and has the added benefit of reducing the impact of losses to follow-up, which tend to be larger with increasing duration of follow-up, on the final efficacy estimate

Table 4
Estimating drug efficacy (reproduced from Dahal et al. (2017))

Per protocol proportion
In a study, the proportion p of patients with treatment failure at time t can be computed as:
$$p = \frac{d}{n}$$
where d is the total number of recrudescence failures and n is the total number of patients who reach the end of the study who weren't lost to follow-up or didn't deviate from the protocol

Kaplan-Meier survival
Estimate of cumulative proportion of patients with cure is computed as:
$$K - M(t) = \prod_{k \leq t} \frac{n_k - d_k}{n_k}$$
where d_k is the number of recrudescences at time k and n_k is the total number of patients at risk of experiencing recrudescence just before time k, and the symbol Π presents the product over all distinct times when recrudescences or losses to follow-up were observed. The failure estimate is given by 1 minus the K-M

Cumulative incidence function
Cumulative incidence function at time t for event j is defined as:
$$\mathrm{CIF}_i(t) = \sum_{k \leq t} \frac{d_{ik}}{n_k} . \hat{S}(k-1)$$
where d_{ik} is the number of events of type i that occur at time k, n_k is the number at risk at time k, and $\hat{S}(k-1)$ is the K-M estimator of the survival probability of being free of any event type prior to time k

[28–30]. A refinement of this statistical approach, viz., cumulative incidence function, may provide an incremental improvement in the accuracy of the efficacy estimate but has not been widely used in antimalarial drug efficacy assessments (*see* Table 4 and supplementary information in [19] for a worked example).

Detecting resistance to artemisinins and their derivatives, which are extremely fast-acting but rapidly eliminated antimalarial drugs, constitutes a special case. These drugs are unique among antimalarials currently used to treat *Plasmodium falciparum* malaria in that they exert their parasiticidal effects on all parasite stages. For the treatment of uncomplicated malaria, they are only used in combination with a partner drug with longer plasma half-lives to clear the residual parasitemia [31]. Provided that the partner drug is effective, it follows that emerging resistance to artemisinins can be difficult to detect in vivo by assessing treatment outcomes in the weeks following treatment since those outcomes are a result of the cumulative effect of both drugs in the combination [32, 33]. Since artemisinins are the only class of drugs effectively killing circulating ring-stage parasites, the initial parasite clearance following treatment with ACTs is almost completely dependent on the artemisinin drug action. Hence, in vivo assessments of artemisinin resistance must necessarily involve measurement of the rates of parasite clearance, usually expressed as parasite clearance half-life or $PC_{1/2}$ obtained form the log-linear parasite clearance curve, following start of treatment [11]. Such measurements are cumbersome, as they require frequent sampling (up to three or more measurements per 24 h, *see* Table 5) to assess parasite densities over time, which are then log-transformed and plotted to

Table 5
Criteria for parasite clearance rate estimations [adapted from [34]; web-based tool for PCE estimations available here]

Minimum criteria
• Initial parasitemia ≥1000 parasites per microliter
• At least four non-zero parasite measurements (to detect lag phase at least three measurements in the first 24 h with <14 h between any two consecutive time points)
• Suggested sampling time points (acceptable window in brackets)
Hour 0 (0–2), 6 (4–8), 12 (10–14), 24 (22–26), 36 (34–36), and 48 (46–50). If parasitemia persists at hour 48 (46–50), sample at least once every 24 h until parasites are undetectable
Rejection criteria
• Last recorded non-zero parasitemia ≥1000 parasites per microliter
• Last recorded parasite density is ≥1000 parasites per microliter (and no subsequent measurement with a zero count)

determine the slope of the linear phase from which the $PC_{1/2}$ is derived [34, 35]. In settings where such assessments are not feasible, parasitological assessments must at a minimum be performed on all subjects at Day 3 (72 hours) following treatment. The proportion of subjects with Day 3 parasitemia detectable by light microscopy provides a proxy measure of parasite clearance rates—if this proportion is >10%, it should trigger more precise measurements of parasite clearance in that context with the corollary inclusion criteria of non-splenectomized subjects with a minimum starting parasite density of ≥1000/μL, preferably higher. A noteworthy caveat of such proxy measurements as parasite positivity at Day 3 is their dependence on the initial parasite density—infections of resistant parasites with initially low densities may not persist up to Day 3, and those with high densities may remain positive even with adequate parasite clearance [27, 36]. Further, Day 3 parasite positivity rates must be measured by light microscopy. Using much more sensitive detection methods such as PCR may be misleading as parasites, or their genetic material can usually be detected for longer than 3 days by such tests even in fully sensitive infections. Finally, a threshold proportion of 5% of patients remaining slide positive at Day 3 after ACT treatment may be more sensitive for the detection of emerging artemisinin resistance in high transmission contexts [27].

5 Confirming Resistance

As discussed earlier in this chapter, study subjects may need to be followed up for up to 9 weeks after they have been treated to ensure accurate estimation of drug efficacy, during which time they may be reinfected with malaria from a new mosquito bite, causing parasitemia to recur. Recurrent parasitemia during follow-up can also be caused by recrudesce of the infection, i.e., by parasites from the initial infection becoming microscopically detectable again after the drug levels in the blood drop below inhibitory levels. Recrudescent parasites are evidently more likely to be drug resistant. Reinfection or recrudescence cannot be distinguished morphologically by microscopy and thus requires additional testing before the recurrent infection can be categorized. Genetic polymorphisms within parasite populations are used to identify parasites for such categorization. Current recommendations for the identification of recrudescent infections are based on molecular genotyping assays targeting parasite genetic loci with length polymorphisms, with in P. falciparum the markers *glurp*, *msp1*, and *msp2* being the most commonly used [37]. Genetic segments of parasites detected before and after treatment are amplified followed by gene fragment electrophoresis to compare their lengths in base pairs. If the lengths of the amplified products are the same, the infection is deemed to be recrudescent (Fig. 2). While the principle of such determinations is straightforward, their practice and the interpretation of the results are complex, as it can be affected by malaria transmission in the context where the trial is conducted [38]. In low transmission settings where parasite populations tend to be more homogeneous, the chance of a recurrent infection being categorized as recrudescent is higher because parasite strains are more likely to carry the same genetic polymorphisms. Thus, in such contexts, the molecular assays have reduced specificity, i.e., they are more likely to result in false categorizations of recrudescence and hence an overestimation of drug resistance. High proportions of recrudescent infections (>10%) identified in such contexts must ideally be further examined by assessing the allele frequencies of the markers being used and selecting only the markers with the most diverse alleles. At the other end of the transmission spectrum, these assays may not be optimally sensitive nor specific for recrudescence. Patients in these high transmission settings are usually infected by multiple strains, and only one or a subset of these strains may be drug resistant. Unless the resistant strain or strains are predominant at the time of sample collection, the products from the amplification of the resistant parasites may be undetectable, leading to a false classification of the recurrent parasitemia as reinfection. On the other hand, if transmission and hence multiplicity of infection are extremely high, matching alleles may be detected for each of the markers by chance even if the infection is not recrudescent [38, 39]. Distinguishing recrudescence from reinfection in *P. vivax* infections is further complicated by recurrent episodes caused by relapses from the liver. If the relapsing parasites are homologous to those in the initially detected infection, as is often the case, they will be indistinguishable from those from the initial

INTERPRETATION OF GENOTYPING RESULTS WITH THREE MARKER GENES

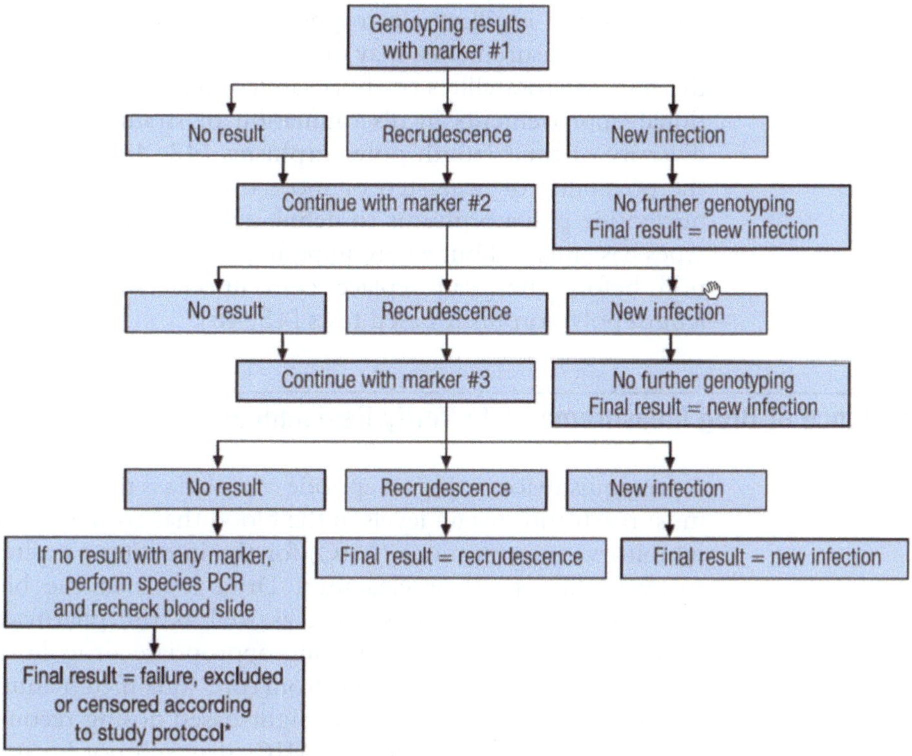

Fig. 2 Decision tree for confirming recrudescence. Assessments of length polymorphisms at three loci are recommended. For *P. falciparum*, sequential testing with *msp2*, *msp1*, and *glurp* is usually performed per the decision tree above. If there is at least one common allele for all three markers, the recurrent parasitemia is classified as recrudescence. In all other cases, the infection is classified as a new infection or reinfection. (WHO 2007)

infection, resulting in an erroneous interpretation of treatment failure. Relapses due to heterologous parasites originating from liver hypnozoites from a previous infection will also, confound assessments of anti-vivax drug efficacy. The latter will be more common in high P. vivax transmission settings, but can also occur in low transmission areas. Despite these limitations, molecular testing importantly improves the qualiy of drug efficacy assessments, provided it is performed correctly with robust quality assurance measures to ensure standardization and consistency. Results must be interpreted along with the biology of malaria parasites, the epidemiological context of the trial site, and the pharmacokinetics of the drugs being tested [40–42].

The ability of molecular assays to distinguish recrudescent infections from reinfections can be improved by using optimized or more advanced methods to determine the genotypes or simply by adding more markers to the comparisons. For example, using labelled primers in PCR amplifications to improve detection of poorly amplified products, along with restriction digests of the products and capillary electrophoresis to improve the resolution of length measurements, may improve the discriminatory power of the test. Microsatellites or short tandem repeats can provide additional improvements in discrimination of strains due the higher diversity of their length polymorphisms [43, 44]. More recently, the possibility of using ten or more of highly determinant single nucleotide polymorphisms to define genome-wide parasite haplotypes has emerged but will require further development and validation before they can replace conventional amplified fragment length polymorphism-based tests [45, 46].

6 Importance of Drug Measurements to Verify Resistance

A prerequisite for curing an episode of malaria is that the drugs used must reach and sustain levels in the blood that are above minimum inhibitory concentrations (MIC) for the infecting parasites, eventually leading to their clearance. Drug levels in the blood are affected by the treatment dose, as well as the pharmacokinetic properties of the drugs. Ensuring appropriate drug levels starts with using only approved drugs from (pre-)qualified manufacturers and following up-to-date bodyweight-based dosing recommendations. Despite adequate dosing, MICs may still not be attained in some patients due to poor absorption and/or incomplete metabolism of the drug, thus increasing the chances of recrudescence in that patient. To correctly categorise cases as true resistance, it is advisable to include drug concentration measurements in studies to verify whether recrudescence occurred in the presence of drug concentrations that would be parasiticidal or at least inhibitory in susceptible parasite infections. Current techniques only require a few drops of blood for measuring drug concentrations; for an increasing number of antimalarial drugs, blood dried on absorbent paper is sufficient to assess drug concentrations [47, 48].

7 Data Management

The strength of evidence generated by drug efficacy studies is improved if they are corroborated by other standardized studies conducted at the same location over time, at different locations at the same time, or both [32, 49]. In recognition of the value of standardization of drug efficacy studies, the World Health

Organization supports a global network of sentinel sites for therapeutic efficacy studies following a common protocol [10]. Harmonization is further aided by using common tools for data collection, management, and analysis [50, 51]. A significant added benefit of the systematic implementation of harmonized protocols and procedures is that the data generated through the studies can be pooled for individual patient-level analyses. Pooling data collected across different populations, locations, and time periods enables analyses to detect emerging trends or risks that are not always evident from individual studies [52, 53]. Such knowledge is critical in preventing resistance, in prolonging the utility of existing antimalarial drugs, and in ensuring that all individuals and populations suffering from malaria get the right malaria treatment at the right time.

Acknowledgments

We thank Dr. Mavuto Mukaka for the advice and assistance in providing the sample size calculations.

References

1. Miller LH, Baruch DI, Marsh K et al (2002) The pathogenic basis of malaria. Nature 415:673–679
2. Guerra CA, Howes RE, Patil AP et al (2010) The international limits and population at risk of *Plasmodium vivax* transmission in 2009. PLoS Negl Trop Dis 4:e774
3. Hay SI, Guerra CA, Gething PW et al (2009) A world malaria map: *Plasmodium falciparum* endemicity in 2007. PLoS Med 6:e1000048
4. World Health Organization (2017) World malaria report 2017. World Health Organization, Geneva
5. DALYs GBD, Collaborators H (2017) Global, regional, and national disability-adjusted life-years (DALYs) for 333 diseases and injuries and healthy life expectancy (HALE) for 195 countries and territories, 1990-2016: a systematic analysis for the Global Burden of Disease Study 2016. Lancet 390:1260–1344
6. Ariey F, Witkowski B, Amaratunga C et al (2014) A molecular marker of artemisinin-resistant *Plasmodium falciparum* malaria. Nature 505:50–55
7. Witkowski B, Amaratunga C, Khim N et al (2013) Novel phenotypic assays for the detection of artemisinin-resistant *Plasmodium falciparum* malaria in Cambodia: in-vitro and ex-vivo drug-response studies. Lancet Infect Dis 13:1043–1049
8. Witkowski B, Duru V, Khim N et al (2017) A surrogate marker of piperaquine-resistant *Plasmodium falciparum* malaria: a phenotype-genotype association study. Lancet Infect Dis 17:174–183
9. Duru V, Khim N, Leang R et al (2015) *Plasmodium falciparum* dihydroartemisinin-piperaquine failures in Cambodia are associated with mutant K13 parasites presenting high survival rates in novel piperaquine in vitro assays: retrospective and prospective investigations. BMC Med 13:305
10. World Health Organization (2009) Methods for surveillance of antimalarial drug efficacy. World Health Organization, Geneva
11. White NJ (2011) The parasite clearance curve. Malar J 10:278
12. O'Flaherty K, Maguire J, Simpson JA et al (2017) Immunity as a predictor of anti-malarial treatment failure: a systematic review. Malar J 16:158
13. World Health Organization (2014) Severe malaria. Tropical Med Int Health 19:7–131
14. Dalrymple U, Arambepola R, Gething PW et al (2018) How long do rapid diagnostic tests

remain positive after anti-malarial treatment? Malar J 17:228

15. Vafa Homann M, Emami SN, Yman V et al (2017) Detection of malaria parasites after treatment in travelers: A 12-months longitudinal study and statistical modelling analysis. EBioMedicine 25:66–72
16. Imwong M, Stepniewska K, Tripura R et al (2016) Numerical distributions of parasite densities during asymptomatic malaria. J Infect Dis 213:1322–1329
17. Imwong M, Woodrow CJ, Hendriksen IC et al (2015) Plasma concentration of parasite DNA as a measure of disease severity in falciparum malaria. J Infect Dis 211:1128–1133
18. World Health Organization (2015) Microscopy for the detection, identification and quantification of malaria parasites on stained thick and thin blood films in research settings (version 1.0); procedure: methods manual. World Health Organization, Geneva
19. Dahal P, Simpson JA, Dorsey G et al (2017) Statistical methods to derive efficacy estimates of anti-malarials for uncomplicated *Plasmodium falciparum* malaria: pitfalls and challenges. Malar J 16:430
20. World Health Organization (1996) Assessment of therapeutic efficacy of antimalarial drugs for uncomplicated falciparum malaria in areas with intense transmission. World Health Organization, Geneva
21. World Health Organization (2003) Assessment and monitoring of antimalarial drug efficacy for the treatment of uncomplicated falciparum malaria. World Health Organization, Geneva
22. World Health Organization (1965) Resistance of malaria parasites to drugs. Report of a WHO scientific group. World Health Organization, Geneva
23. World Health Organization (1967) Chemotherapy of malaria. Report of a WHO sientific group. World Health Organization, Geneva
24. Stepniewska K, Taylor WR, Mayxay M et al (2004) *In vivo* assessment of drug efficacy against *Plasmodium falciparum* malaria: duration of follow-up. Antimicrob Agents Chemother 48:4271–4280
25. Stepniewska K, White NJ (2006) Some considerations in the design and interpretation of antimalarial drug trials in uncomplicated falciparum malaria. Malar J 5:127
26. White NJ (2002) The assessment of antimalarial drug efficacy. Trends Parasitol 18:458–464
27. PCSG WWARN (2015) Baseline data of parasite clearance in patients with falciparum malaria treated with an artemisinin derivative: an individual patient data meta-analysis. Malar J 14:359
28. Ashley EA, Pinoges L, Turyakira E et al (2008) Different methodological approaches to the assessment of *in vivo* efficacy of three artemisinin-based combination antimalarial treatments for the treatment of uncomplicated falciparum malaria in African children. Malar J 7:154
29. Verret WJ, Dorsey G, Nosten F et al (2009) The effect of varying analytical methods on estimates of anti-malarial clinical efficacy. Malar J 8:77
30. Guthmann JP, Pinoges L, Checchi F et al (2006) Methodological issues in the assessment of antimalarial drug treatment: analysis of 13 studies in eight African countries from 2001 to 2004. Antimicrob Agents Chemother 50:3734–3739
31. Nosten F, White NJ (2007) Artemisinin-based combination treatment of falciparum malaria. Am J Trop Med Hyg 77:181–192
32. Ashley EA, Dhorda M, Fairhurst RM et al (2014) Spread of artemisinin resistance in *Plasmodium falciparum* malaria. N Engl J Med 371:411–423
33. Dondorp AM, Nosten F, Yi P et al (2009) Artemisinin resistance in *Plasmodium falciparum* malaria. N Engl J Med 361:455–467
34. Flegg JA, Guerin PJ, Nosten F et al (2013) Optimal sampling designs for estimation of *Plasmodium falciparum* clearance rates in patients treated with artemisinin derivatives. Malar J 12:411
35. Flegg JA, Guerin PJ, White NJ et al (2011) Standardizing the measurement of parasite clearance in falciparum malaria: the parasite clearance estimator. Malar J 10:339
36. WWARN AbCTABSG (2015) Clinical determinants of early parasitological response to ACTs in African patients with uncomplicated falciparum malaria: a literature review and meta-analysis of individual patient data. BMC Med 13:212
37. World Health Organization (2008) Methods and techniques for clinical trials on antimalarial drug efficacy–genotyping to identify parasite populations: informal consultation organized by the Medicines for Malaria Venture and cosponsored by the World Health Organization, 29–31 May 2007, Amsterdam, The Netherlands. World Health Organization, Geneva
38. Juliano JJ, Taylor SM, Meshnick SR (2009) Polymerase chain reaction adjustment in antimalarial trials: molecular malarkey? J Infect Dis 200:5–7

39. Messerli C, Hofmann NE, Beck HP et al (2017) Critical evaluation of molecular monitoring in malaria drug efficacy trials and pitfalls of length-polymorphic markers. Antimicrob Agents Chemother 61. https://doi.org/10.1128/AAC.01500-16
40. Snounou G, Beck HP (1998) The use of PCR genotyping in the assessment of recrudescence or reinfection after antimalarial drug treatment. Parasitol Today 14:462–467
41. Juliano JJ, Gadalla N, Sutherland CJ et al (2010) The perils of PCR: can we accurately 'correct' antimalarial trials? Trends Parasitol 26:119–124
42. White MT, Karl S, Koepfli C et al (2018) *Plasmodium vivax* and *Plasmodium falciparum* infection dynamics: re-infections, recrudescences and relapses. Malar J 17:170
43. Greenhouse B, Myrick A, Dokomajilar C et al (2006) Validation of microsatellite markers for use in genotyping polyclonal *Plasmodium falciparum* infections. Am J Trop Med Hyg 75:836–842
44. Thanapongpichat S, McGready R, Luxemburger C et al (2013) Microsatellite genotyping of *Plasmodium vivax* infections and their relapses in pregnant and non-pregnant patients on the Thai-Myanmar border. Malar J 12:275
45. Daniels R, Volkman SK, Milner DA et al (2008) A general SNP-based molecular barcode for *Plasmodium falciparum* identification and tracking. Malar J 7:223
46. Lerch A, Koepfli C, Hofmann NE et al (2017) Development of amplicon deep sequencing markers and data analysis pipeline for genotyping multi-clonal malaria infections. BMC Genomics 18:864
47. White NJ, Stepniewska K, Barnes K et al (2008) Simplified antimalarial therapeutic monitoring: using the day-7 drug level? Trends Parasitol 24:159–163
48. World Health Organization (2011) Methods and techniques for assessing exposure to antimalarial drugs in clinical field studies. World Health Organization, Geneva
49. Phyo AP, Ashley EA, Anderson TJC et al (2016) Declining efficacy of Artemisinin combination therapy against *P. falciparum* malaria on the Thai-Myanmar border (2003-2013): The role of parasite genetic factors. Clin Infect Dis 63:784–791
50. Tools for monitoring antimalarial drug efficacy [http://www.who.int/malaria/areas/drug_resistance/efficacy-monitoring-tools/en/]
51. Malaria Clinical Trials Toolkit [http://www.wwarn.org/tools-resources/malaria-clinical-trials-toolkit]
52. Adjuik MA, Allan R, WorldWide Antimalarial Resistance Network ASAQSG et al (2015) The effect of dosing strategies on the therapeutic efficacy of artesunate-amodiaquine for uncomplicated malaria: a meta-analysis of individual patient data. BMC Med 13:66
53. WorldWide Antimalarial Resistance Network (2013) The effect of dosing regimens on the antimalarial efficacy of dihydroartemisinin-piperaquine: a pooled analysis of individual patient data. PLoS Med 10:e1001564

Chapter 9

Plasmodium falciparum In Vitro Drug Resistance Selections and Gene Editing

Caroline L. Ng and David A. Fidock

Abstract

Malaria continues to be a global health burden, threatening over 40% of the world's population. Drug resistance in *Plasmodium falciparum*, the etiological agent of the majority of human malaria cases, is compromising elimination efforts. New approaches to treating drug-resistant malaria benefit from defining resistance liabilities of known antimalarial agents and compounds in development and defining genetic changes that mediate loss of parasite susceptibility. Here, we present protocols for in vitro selection of drug-resistant parasites and for site-directed gene editing of candidate resistance mediators to test for causality.

Key words Malaria, *Plasmodium falciparum*, Drug resistance, Selections, Gene editing, ZFN, CRISPR/Cas9

1 Introduction

In 2017, there were an estimated 219 million reported cases of malaria, resulting in 435,000 deaths, the majority due to *Plasmodium falciparum* [1]. The World Health Organization recommends artemisinin-based combination therapies (ACTs) as first-line treatments for malaria [1]. Alarmingly, resistance has emerged to artemisinin—the cornerstone of ACTs [2–5]—as well as to several partner drugs and earlier first-line therapies. Detailed analyses of genetic determinants of antimalarial resistance benefit molecular surveillance campaigns to monitor the appearance and spread of drug resistance and inform therapeutic strategies to overcome resistance. Important insights in drug development are also gained by subjecting compounds in the antimalarial pipeline to in vitro drug selections, in order to assess the resistance liabilities and search for their resistance mechanisms that in some instances correspond to the actual drug targets.

To simulate the evolution of parasites that happens in clinical settings, several groups including ours have pressured parasites with sublethal concentrations of drugs, enriching for parasites that have

Frédéric Ariey et al. (eds.), *Malaria Control and Elimination*, Methods in Molecular Biology, vol. 2013,
https://doi.org/10.1007/978-1-4939-9550-9_9,

mutated as a means to survive drug pressure [6–8]. In vitro drug resistance selections can be performed in a single-step, stepwise, or pulse manner. Briefly, single-step selections involve large numbers of parasites pressured at one drug concentration, often 3–5× IC_{50} values, where the IC_{50} is calculated as the concentration that produces half-maximal growth inhibition of parasites exposed to drug for 48 or 72 hr. The benefit of this method is that drug-resistant parasites are obtained relatively quickly, typically within 1–2 months. However, this requires handling large amounts of culture (often multiple flasks of 100–200 mL each) and also necessitates large quantities of red blood cells and culture media. Stepwise selections are easier to handle, as these can be performed using parasite cultures of only 5 mL. Parasites are incubated with drug media starting at 1× IC_{50}, and the concentration of drug exposure is slowly increased over time. Parasites must be monitored carefully, and this selection method can result in a lengthy selection period (requiring several months of continuous culture). In situations where drug-resistant parasites cannot be obtained with either of the methods described, an alternative method is to briefly pulse parasites with drug. Here, parasites are exposed to drug for 1–2 days, then drug is washed off, and parasites are allowed to recover. To obtain drug-resistant parasites that stably maintain their phenotype, we prefer single-step selections.

Once drug-resistant mutants are obtained, these are typically cloned by limiting dilution, and resistance is verified by observing a shift in IC_{50} values. Genetic mutations are then identified by whole-genome sequencing or, in the case of known candidates, Sanger sequencing. To confirm that these mutations confer drug resistance, the mutation is reintroduced into drug-sensitive parasites, or the mutation in drug-resistant parasites is reverted to the wild-type sequence to confer drug sensitivity. Genetic manipulation of *P. falciparum* has historically been challenging. With the newfound ability to precisely introduce double-strand breaks in the genome, as opposed to earlier methods of single or double crossover-based recombination methods [9, 10], researchers no longer need to wait for stochastic breaks in the DNA in order to achieve homologous recombination. Site-directed gene editing via zinc-finger nucleases (ZFN) or clustered regularly interspaced short palindromic repeats (CRISPR)/CRISPR-associated gene 9 (Cas9) has revolutionized our ability to efficiently edit parasite genomes [11–13]. While ZFNs were developed first for *Plasmodium*, CRISPR/Cas9 has become a more widely used tool and thus is first discussed below.

The CRISPR/Cas9 system widely used in gene-editing technologies relies on the type II endonuclease Cas9 [14–16], which cleaves double-stranded DNA three nucleotides upstream of the protospacer-adjacent motif (PAM) via its RuvC and HNH nuclease domains. Cas9 is directed to cleavage sites by complementary base pairing with the guide RNA, which is composed of two distinct components: the CRISPR RNA (crRNA) and the trans-activating CRISPR RNA (tracrRNA). In a landmark discovery, Jinek et al. demonstrated that a single-guide RNA (sgRNA) can be engineered to act in place of the crRNA and tracrRNA [14]. Thus, to mediate a particular site-directed break, one only needs to replace the sgRNA targeting sequence in vectors that express sgRNA and Cas9. A break in the integrity of the genome is potentially catastrophic and must be repaired. *P. falciparum* do not possess components of the nonhomologous end-joining (NHEJ) pathway. Instead, these parasites rely primarily on homologous recombination to repair DNA breaks [17, 18]. Thus, *P. falciparum* gene editing can be mediated by supplying three elements: (1) a Cas9 endonuclease, (2) a sgRNA, and (3) a donor template with homology regions upstream and downstream of the cleavage site. An important consideration is that donor templates must include silent mutations at the Cas9 recognition sites to prevent cleavage of either the supplied donor template or the template that has been integrated into the genome. Nucleotide mutations within the PAM or in the seed region, which is the 12 nucleotide sequence directly upstream of the PAM motif, are most effective in disrupting Cas9 binding [14]. The ability to direct double-stranded breaks rather than waiting for a break to occur stochastically has dramatically reduced the amount of time needed to genetically manipulate parasites. In addition, the relatively low cost of performing CRISPR/Cas9 has led to its adoption in many laboratories.

The pioneering studies of CRISPR/Cas9 in *P. falciparum*, published within months of each other in *Nature Biotechnology* and *Nature Methods*, employed two-plasmid approaches to express Cas9, sgRNA, and a donor template [12, 13]. At the same time, studies in *P. yoelii* employed a one-plasmid approach [19]. These studies utilize *Streptococcus pyogenes* Cas9 (SpCas9), which has a PAM recognition motif of 5′-NGG-3′ downstream of the protospacer element [14]. Ghorbal et al. delivered SpCas9 on the pUF1 plasmid, which also contains a yeast dihydroorotate dehydrogenase (y*dhodh*) expression cassette that confers resistance to PfDHODH inhibitors such as DSM1 [20]. The second plasmid, pL7, delivered a sgRNA expressed under the *P. falciparum* U6 snRNA polymerase III promoter and a donor template. pL7 also expresses human dihydrofolate reductase (h*dhfr*) and y*fcu* (yeast cytosine deaminase and uridyl phosphoribosyl transferase), allowing positive selection with WR99210 and negative selection with 5-fluorocytosine, respectively [21, 22]. Gene knockouts were successfully obtained with transfection of pL7 as an intact or a linearized plasmid. Using CRISPR/Cas9, Ghorbal et al. engineered gene knockouts and marker-free point mutations. Successful editing was observed within 3 weeks of transfection of ring-stage parasites and in as little as 8 days with nucleofection of schizont stages [13].

Because the *P. falciparum* U6 snRNA polymerase III promoter had not been well defined, Wagner et al. chose instead to use promoter and terminator sequences from T7 RNA polymerase to express sgRNA. pCas9-sgRNA-T, which contains a blasticidin S-deaminase (*bsd*) selectable marker, was used to deliver SpCas9 and the sgRNA [12]. The second plasmid, pT7-RNAP-HR, delivers T7 RNA polymerase and the donor template. This group selected only for the Cas9-expressing plasmid and obtained successful marker-free gene disruption within 4–6 weeks.

For similar reasons, Marcus Lee (group leader at the Wellcome Sanger Institute in Hinxton, UK, formerly in the Fidock lab at Columbia University in New York, USA) also decided on a two-plasmid approach in which sgRNA transcription was driven by a T7 RNA polymerase promoter sequence. The first plasmid, named pDC2-Cas9-sgRNA-h*dhfr*, delivers SpCas9 driven by the calmodulin promoter and a sgRNA driven by the T7 RNA polymerase promoter, and also contains the selectable marker h*dhfr*. The second plasmid, pDC2-T7Pol-donor-*bsd*, expresses a calmodulin-driven T7 RNA polymerase and a *bsd* selectable marker. These plasmids have been used to mediate point mutations in three genes, and successful editing was observed within 3–4 weeks [23–25]. By replacing the T7 promoter with a U6 snRNA polymerase III promoter (pDC2-cam-Cas9-U6-sgRNA-h*dhfr*), he obviated the need to express T7 RNA polymerase, and thus the second plasmid was simplified to only express the donor template and *bsd* (pDC2-donor-*bsd*). Using these plasmids, successful editing was obtained within 2–8 weeks of transfection [6, 24].

An alternative plasmid-free approach is to deliver SpCas9 protein, a dual guide RNA (dgRNA) comprising of both tracrRNA and crRNA, and a single-strand template DNA for repair. Parasites were selected using a compound that confers resistance to parasites that incorporate the mutation of interest, and editing was obtained within 4–5 weeks post-electroporation [26].

Multiple groups have used original or modified pUF1 and pL7 plasmids [13] to introduce point mutations [27], generate reporter lines [28], tag proteins of interest [29, 30], or produce gene knockouts [31, 32]. Importantly, this technology can now be used to demonstrate the nonessentiality of conserved genetic elements [33] and genes [30, 34–36], a subset of which had earlier been proposed to be essential due to previous unsuccessful knockout attempts. Variations of these plasmids have been used to achieve particular goals. In a conditional knockdown study, three plasmids were used, one each for SpCas9, sgRNA, and the donor template, respectively [36]. The pDC2-cam-Cas9-U6-sgRNA-h*dhfr* vector [6, 24] was modified to pDC2-Cas9-hDHFRyFCU, in which hDHFR is fused with yFCU and used in combination with a markerless plasmid encoding the dimerization-competent Cre (DiCre) recombinase and flanked with sequences to insert the recombinase into p230p or pfs47. Marker-free parasite clones were successfully obtained 7 weeks post-transfection in this study, thereby establishing the benefit of using CRISPR/Cas9 to rapidly generate parasite lines expressing dimerization-competent Cre (DiCre)-recombinase [37]. *P. falciparum* parasites constitutively expressing Cas9 have also been generated. These parasites, when paired with a tetracycline-controlled conditional knockdown system, have been used to investigate the essentiality of several genes [38–40].

In the rodent malaria parasite *P. yoelii,* CRISPR/Cas9 has been used for gene deletion, gene insertion, and the introduction of point mutations [19]. Here, SpCas9, sgRNA, and the donor template were delivered on a single plasmid. sgRNA was driven by a *P. yoelii* U6 snRNA promoter, while SpCas9 was driven by the *P. berghei* eef1α promoter. Also encoded in this pYC vector was the donor template that included regions for homologous recombination and a h*dhfr* cassette that mediate resistance to the selection agent pyrimethamine. *P. yoelii* transfected with these constructs were then intravenously injected into mice for parasite propagation, and pyrimethamine was supplied in the drinking water 1 day after parasite injection. Edited parasites were observed in as little as 5 days postinjection [19]. This strategy was also used to investigate the functions of the PyApiP2 gene family using knockout studies, in which 12 out of 24 genes were successfully targeted [41]. Zhang et al. then modified pYC such that h*dhfr* was replaced with a h*dhfr-yfcu* cassette to allow positive and subsequent negative selection, which as described earlier permits sequential genetic modification of parasites. This strategy was used to tag an ookinete surface protein and to confirm using knockout studies that genes shown to be involved in ookinete motility in *P. berghei* have similar functions in *P. yoelii* [42].

Precise gene editing can also be mediated by ZFNs, whose use in *P. falciparum* predated CRISPR/Cas9. This technology relies on a pair of zinc fingers that each recognize unique 15–18 nucleotide DNA sequences located several nucleotides apart on either strand of the DNA helix. Each zinc-finger sequence is fused to separate halves of the FokI restriction endonuclease, such that the enzyme can refold as an obligate heterodimer upon binding of the two DNA-binding zinc-finger proteins. This results in the introduction of a double-stranded break [43, 44]. ZFN-mediated gene editing in *P. falciparum* has proven to be efficient [11, 45–47] but requires custom design of ZFNs and can be cost-prohibitive.

Here we describe a method for single-step in vitro resistance selections, followed by gene editing via a two-plasmid U6 expression-based CRISPR/Cas9 strategy or ZFNs in *P. falciparum*.

2 Materials

2.1 Parasite Cultures

1. Dd2, NF54, 3D7, Cam3.II, and V1/S parasite lines, available from the Malaria Research and Reference Reagent Resource Center (MR4, Manassas, VA—http://www.malaria.mr4.org), are routinely used for in vitro drug resistance selections and gene editing. The procedures described here are not restricted to these particular parasites.
2. RPMI 1640 with L-glutamine (Invitrogen, Carlsbad, CA), 25 mM *N*-2-hydroxyethylpiperazine-*N′*-2-ethanesulfonic (HEPES; CalBiochem, San Diego, CA), 50 mg/L hypoxanthine (Sigma-Aldrich, St. Louis, MO), 0.25% sodium bicarbonate ($NaHCO_3$; Sigma-Aldrich) and 0.01 mg/mL gentamicin (Invitrogen) medium is supplemented with 0.5% Albumax II (Invitrogen) to constitute complete medium. Store at 4 °C. Media used in this protocol are always complete media.
3. Human red blood cells (RBCs) are obtained from Interstate Blood Bank (Memphis, TN). RBC must be fresh and no more than 2 weeks old when used.

2.2 In Vitro Drug Resistance Selections

1. Drug compound to be examined.
2. SYBR Green I (Invitrogen by Thermo Fisher Scientific, Waltham, MA), supplied at 10,000× in DMSO. It detects parasite DNA and is used at 1×. Store at −20 °C, avoid repeat freeze-thaw cycles, and keep away from light.
3. Mitotracker Deep Red FM (Molecular Probes, Eugene, OR) supplied at 50 μg and reconstituted in DMSO to 500 μM. It detects mitochondria-active parasites and is used at 100 nM. Store at −20 °C, avoid repeat freeze-thaw cycles, and keep away from light.
4. BD Accuri C6 Plus Flow Cytometer to measure drug inhibition of parasite growth (*see* **Note 1**).
5. Softwares FlowJo (Becton Dickinson) and Prism (GraphPad).

2.3 Site-Specific Editing Using CRISPR/Cas9 or ZFN

1. Plasmids for CRISPR/Cas9-mediated editing express Cas9, sgRNA sequence that targets the endonuclease to its cleavage site, and a donor template containing silent mutations at the Cas9 binding site.
2. Plasmids for ZFN-mediated editing express a pair of ZFNs (custom-ordered from Sigma-Aldrich, St. Louis, MO) and a donor repair template that contains silent mutations at the ZFN binding site. Several customized ZFNs, specific for *pfcrt*, *eef1a*, *pfmdr1*, *k13*, *lipoic acid ligase (lipB)*, *elongase1*, or *pfs47*, have already been published or obtained by the Fidock lab and are available upon request to that lab.

3. For both types of site-directed gene editing, we use a two-plasmid approach in which one plasmid encodes a *bsd* selectable marker, while the other encodes a h*dhfr* expression cassette, thus allowing plasmid selection using blasticidin and the antifolate drug WR99210 [21, 24, 25, 48].

2.4 Parasite Transfection and Selection of Recombinant Lines

1. Cytomix (1×): 120 mM KCl, 0.2 mM $CaCl_2$, 2 mM EGTA, 10 mM $MgCl_2$, 25 mM HEPES, 5 mM K_2HPO_4, 5 mM KH_2PO_4; pH 7.6. Store at room temperature.
2. An electroporator, e.g., Gene Pulser XCell (BioRad, Hercules, CA) and 0.2-cm cuvettes (BioRad).
3. Blasticidin HCl (Invitrogen) is dissolved in tissue culture-grade water at 10 mg/mL, sterile-filtered, and stored in aliquots at −80 °C. Parasites are exposed to a concentration of 2.5 μg/mL.
4. WR99210 (Jacobus Pharmaceuticals, Princeton, NJ; molecular weight 394.35) is dissolved in tissue culture-grade water, and working stocks of sterile-filtered, 25 μM WR99210 are stored in aliquots at −80 °C. Parasites are exposed to a concentration of 2.5 nM.

3 Methods

3.1 In Vitro Drug Resistance Selections

1. Thaw parasite of choice, and grow under standard hypoxic conditions (5% O_2, 5% CO_2, 90% N_2; [48]). Recently cloned parasites are preferred to minimize genetic drift.
2. Determine the concentration at which drug compound inhibits 50% growth (IC_{50}). Parasites predominantly in the ring stages (*see* **Note 2**) seeded at 0.2% parasitemia and 1% hematocrit in a 96-well plate are exposed to serially increasing concentrations of drug compound. After incubation for 72 h at 37 °C in a hypoxic environment (5% O_2, 5% CO_2, 90% N_2), samples are resuspended, and 5 μL of each well is removed and mixed with 40 μL of stain (1× SYBR Green I and 100 nM MitoTracker Deep Red, diluted in 1× phosphate-buffered saline (PBS)). Assays are read on a BD Accuri C6 Flow Cytometer and analyzed using FlowJo®. IC_{50} values are determined by nonlinear regression analysis using the Prism software. At least three biological repeats are performed to accurately determine IC_{50} values [25, 49].
3. For single-step selections, large numbers of parasites (2×10^9) are pressured at 3–5× IC_{50}, and the experiment is performed in triplicate. Grow parasites to the appropriate volume, ensuring that cultures are always healthy and maintained at a parasitemia between 1% and 5%. Prior to beginning the selection, it is

preferable to start with a culture with lower volume and higher parasitemia rather than higher volume and lower parasitemia (even though this gives the same number of parasites) to ensure that the parasites are actively growing. A 100 mL culture at 5% parasitemia and 4% hematocrit corresponds to 2×10^9 parasites (*see* **Note 3**). Since this experiment is performed in triplicate, you will need >300 mL of culture in total before starting. These cultures will then be diluted from 5% to ~2–2.5%, so each of the triplicate flasks will eventually hold ~200–250 mL. When beginning the selections, cultures should be predominantly ring stages. If culturing in multiple vessels, combine all cultures together. Remove 10 mL cultures to freeze in Glycerolyte 57 (Fenwal) as a preselection comparative line. Add the appropriate amount of drug (5× IC_{50}) and RBC to achieve ~2–2.5% parasitemia and 4% hematocrit (*see* **Note 4**). Divide into three flasks, and incubate at 37 °C in hypoxic conditions.

4. Early the next day, remove the supernatant and supply cultures with fresh medium containing the selection concentration of drug. Parasitemia is monitored by Giemsa staining a thin blood smear. Continue this procedure for 6 days, ensuring that the parasitemia is sufficiently reduced. By day 6, parasitemia should be close to zero.
5. On day 7, refresh drug medium and add fresh red blood cells, equivalent to an additional 0.5% hematocrit.
6. Refresh drug medium every other day. Once parasites are no longer detected, monitoring can be reduced from every other day to once a week.
7. On day 14, and every week thereafter, fresh RBC is added, and total culture volume is reduced. The new total culture volume will be 75% of the current total volume. To achieve this, culture medium is aspirated, and a thin blood smear is made to check parasitemia. Measure or estimate the remaining volume and discard 50% of this culture. Add fresh RBC to achieve 4% hematocrit for ¼ of the total new volume. Add fresh drug media to achieve the new reduced total volume (*see* **Note 5** for sample calculation). Culture volume is repeatedly diminished in this way every 7 days until cultures are 50 mL, a volume that we find easy to handle and maintain. At this point, when it's time to refresh RBC, ¼ of resuspended culture is removed, 1 mL of fresh RBC (from the 50% hematocrit stock) is added, and volume is brought up to 50 mL with fresh drug media. Throughout this process, continue to refresh drug medium every 2–3 days (three times per week is a useful schedule).
8. The experiment is carried out to until parasites are visually detected by microscopy. Cultures are discarded if no parasites are visible by day 60 (*see* **Note 6**).

3.2 Site-Specific Editing Using CRISPR/Cas9: Design of Plasmids

1. This strategy outlines a two-plasmid approach using the U6 promoter to drive sgRNA expression. The first plasmid encodes a *P. falciparum* calmodulin-driven SpCas9, a *P. falciparum* U6 promoter-driven sgRNA, and a h*dhfr* selectable marker. The second plasmid encodes the region to be replaced, and homology arms on either side, plus a *bsd* selectable marker (Fig. 1) [6].
2. Identify suitable guide RNAs that will bind to 20 nucleotides upstream of a 5′-NGG-3′ PAM motif (*see* **Note 7**). The study by Ghorbal et al. demonstrated that unlike its counterpart in mammalian cells, *P. falciparum* RNA polymerase III does not have a strict requirement for a G nucleotide at the 5′ end to initiate transcription. PAMs and sgRNA can be on either strand of DNA. The cleavage site, which occurs three nucleotides upstream of the PAM sequence, should be as close as possible to sequences to be modified to facilitate efficacy, although we have had success with cleavage sites up to 750 bp away from the modified site [25]. In addition, ensure that the sgRNA binds to a sequence that is unique within the genome. This can be done using a variety of tools, including https://chopchop.rc.fas.harvard.edu/, E-CRISP, or downloading Protospacer Workbench [50] from http://www.protospacer.com/. Select the best two guides by proximity to site of interest or the Doench score. Be sure to select guide sequences with G or C nucleotides interspersed along the sequence, and avoid sequences that contain long tracts of only A or T nucleotides.
3. Custom synthesize these sequences with BbsI restriction site overhangs, which allows insertion behind the U6 promoter in pDC2-Cas9-U6-sgRNA-h*dhfr* [6]. To do so, order phosphorylated primers with 5′-ATAGN_{20} as the forward primer and 3′-AAACN_{20} as the reverse primer, where N_{20} is the sgRNA identified above. Note that only the protospacer, and not the PAM sequences, are included in these N_{20}. Anneal primer pairs to generate dsDNA, and insert into BbsI-digested pDC2-Cas9-U6-sgRNA-h*dhfr* (Fig. 1a, b).
4. Select a donor that contains the region of interest, with homology arms on either side of ~750 bp each (*see* **Note 8**). PCR amplify this region using primers with ApaI and BamHI restriction sites at the 5′ and 3′ ends, respectively. Clone into pGEM-T for further modification of nucleotides at sites of interest to achieve desired mutations/insertions/deletions. Mutate at least one nucleotide at the PAM site (Fig. 1a, red box, c, red arrow) or two nucleotides in the seed region (the first 12 nucleotides upstream of the PAM site) closest to the PAM (Fig. 1a, purple box, c, purple arrows) to prevent Cas9-mediated cleavage of the donor plasmid or integrated DNA. Sequence both strands of the donor template in full to avoid plasmids with unwanted mutations. Insert fragment into ApaI- and BamHI-digested pDC2-donor-*bsd* plasmid [6] (Fig. 1c).

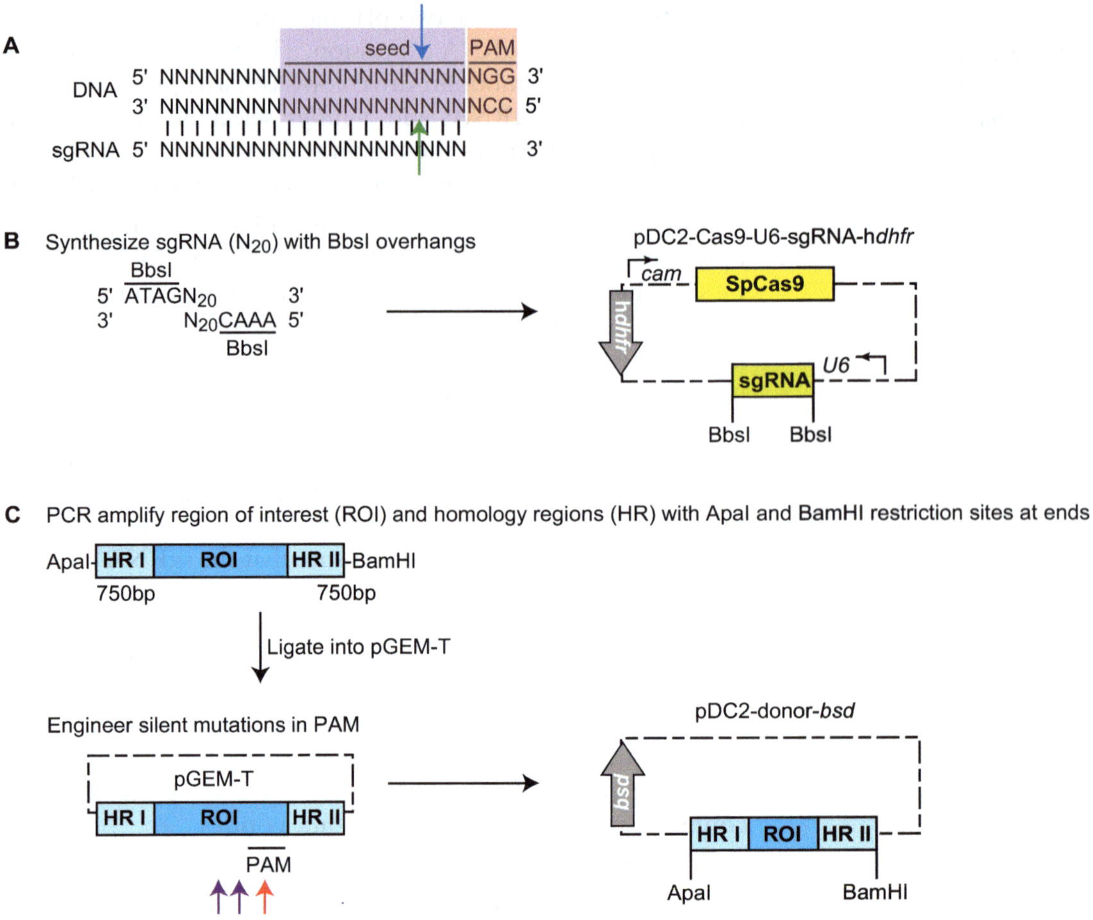

Fig. 1 CRISPR/Cas9-mediated editing using a two-plasmid approach. (**a**) This diagram shows the sgRNA binding via complementary base pairing to the 20 nucleotides of DNA upstream of the PAM sequence (red box). When custom ordering primers to engineer double-stranded sgRNAs, do not include the PAM sequence. When brought to the DNA sequence by sgRNA, Cas9 mediates a blunt double-stranded break via its RuvH nuclease domain, which cleaves three nucleotides upstream of the PAM in the sequence that is complementary to the recognized DNA strand (blue arrow), and its HNH nuclease domain, which cleaves the strand that is recognized (green arrow). The seed region (purple box) is the 12 nucleotides immediately upstream of the PAM. Mutations within the PAM will be most effective in blocking Cas9 recognition and binding to DNA (and thus cleavage). If it is not possible to introduce silent mutations within the PAM, mutate two nucleotides within the seed region, preferably close to the PAM. (**b**) pDC2-Cas9-U6-sgRNA-h*dhfr* delivers SpCas9 and a U6-driven sgRNA and contains a h*dhfr* selectable marker. Custom synthesize the sgRNA with BbsI overhangs, and then insert into BbsI-digested pDC2-Cas9-h*dhfr* to generate pDC2-Cas9-U6-sgRNA-h*dhfr*. (**c**) pDC2-donor-*bsd* delivers the donor repair template and contains a *bsd* selectable marker. PCR amplify a fragment containing the region of interest (ROI) flanked by ~750 bp homology region (HR), with ApaI and BamHI restriction sites at the ends. Clone the fragment into pGEM-T to engineer silent mutations at the Cas9 binding site. Ideally, one nucleotide within the PAM is mutated (red arrow). If this is not possible, two nucleotides within the seed region and close to the PAM site are mutated (purple arrows). Insert this fragment into ApaI- and BamHI-digested pDC2-*bsd* to generate pDC2-donor-*bsd*

This general protocol can also be followed if using other pairs of plasmids. For cloning strategies using pUF1-Cas9 and pL7 plasmids [13] (*see* **Note 9**). For cloning into pCas9-sgRNA-T and pT7-RNAP-HR plasmids [12] (*see* **Note 10**). To clone into pDC2-Cas9-sgRNA-h*dhfr* and pDC2-T7pol-donor-*bsd* plasmids [24, 25] (*see* **Note 11**). Lastly, a one-plasmid approach can also be employed to deliver SpCas9, sgRNA, and a donor template (*see* **Note 12**).

3.3 Site-Specific Editing Using ZFN: Design of Plasmids

1. Pairs of ZFNs can be ordered through Sigma-Aldrich (CompoZr ZFNs, Product No. CSTZFN-1KT). Specify the target region of interest, and ensure that the cleavage site is close to the site of the desired modification. Select the two most active pairs based on the yeast proxy cleavage assays, results of which are provided by the company.
2. The ZFN pair is cloned into a pDC2 vector expressing a *bsd* selectable marker (pZFN-*bsd*), downstream of a calmodulin promoter and upstream of a *hsp86* 3′ untranslated region (UTR) [11]. The ZFN described here can be excised with AvrII and XhoI restriction enzymes to be replaced with custom ZFNs of interest that have been digested with NheI and XhoI (Fig. 2a). The ZFN pair is expressed from the same promoter

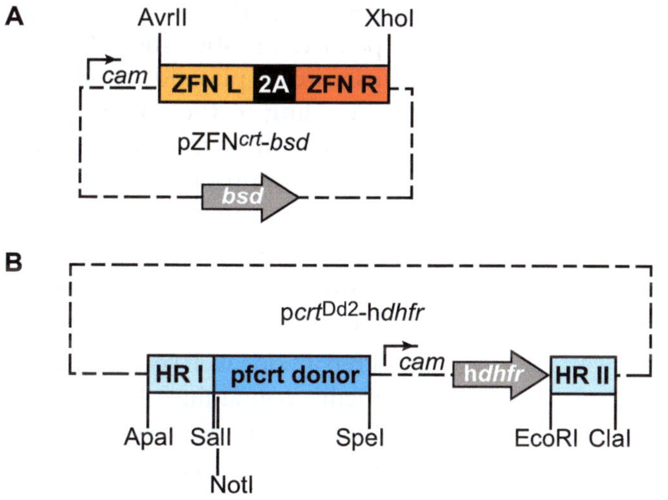

Fig. 2 ZFN-mediated editing using a two-plasmid approach. (**a**) pZFN^{crt}-*bsd* delivers two zinc-finger sequences fused to separate halves of the FokI restriction endonuclease and contains a *bsd* selectable cassette. This particular pair of ZFNs can be excised with AvrII and XhoI restriction enzymes to be replaced with custom ZFNs digested with NheI and XhoI. (**b**) p*crt*^{Dd2}-h*dhfr* delivers the donor repair template. This vector and the restriction enzyme sites that can be used to clone in donor regions are shown as described in [11]. Note that donor templates can be made on any standard *P. falciparum* expression plasmid

and is separated by a "2A ribosome skip peptide" sequence that yields two separate proteins translated from one combined transcript.

3. Select a donor that contains the region of interest, with homology arms on either side of about 750 bp each (*see* **Note 8**). Amplify this region by PCR, cloning into pGEM-T for further modifications including gene mutations and silent binding site mutations. To prevent FokI-mediated cleavage of the donor plasmid or the integrated plasmid, engineer silent mutations at the binding sites. This is then cloned into a pDC2 vector encoding the h*dhfr* cassette [11] (Fig. 2b).

3.4 Parasite Transfection and Selection of Recombinant Lines

1. 50 μg of each plasmid is required for transfection. In the case of ZFN, these are the plasmids encoding ZFN and that of the donor. In the case of CRISPR/Cas9, these plasmids encode Cas9 and sgRNA and the donor. When preparing the plasmids, directly resuspend these plasmids in 1× Cytomix.
2. When ready to transfect, parasites should be at ~5% parasitemia and consist predominantly of ring stages. 2.5 mL of culture should be used per transfection. Parasite cultures are harvested, pelleted at 500 × *g* for 3 min, supernatant removed, and resuspended in an equal volume of 1× Cytomix. This resuspension is then spun again at 500 × *g* for 3 min and resuspended in 300–400 μL of 1× Cytomix. Total volume of parasites + plasmids should be ~450 μL, so add 1× Cytomix according to the volume of plasmid DNA. Be sure to keep a stock of frozen parasites made the day of electroporation to have an appropriate control for future comparisons with transfected parasites.
3. Put the plasmids in a 1.5 mL centrifuge tube. Mix in the resuspended parasite culture. Transfer to an electroporation cuvette.
4. Prepare one well (per transfection) of a six-well plate with 4 mL media containing 4% hematocrit. Aliquot 1 mL media per transfection into a conical tube.
5. Settings for electroporation of infected red blood cells are voltage of 0.31 kV and capacitance of 950 μF. Electric resistance is infinite, and cuvette gap is 2 mm.
6. Immediately after electroporation, add 1 mL of complete media to the cuvette.
7. Transfer the contents of the cuvette to the six-well plate, and place at 37 °C. Once the RBC have settled, tilt the plate at a 45° angle, remove the supernatant, and add fresh culture medium. Incubate at 37 °C.

8. The next day, transfected parasites are exposed to culture medium with 2.5 nM WR99210 and 2.5 μg/mL blasticidin for 6 days. 1.5 nM WR99210 is sufficient if parasites express wild-type *P. falciparum dhfr*. If preferred, drug selection can be kept on until edited parasites are detected. Parasitemia is monitored to ensure it does not exceed 10%. Parasites should be undetectable 6–7 days post-transfection. Evidence of abundant gametocytes on day 6 is a sign of culture stress and reduces the likelihood of successful transfections.
9. When parasites are detectable by microscopy, usually 14–21 days post-electroporation, culture them to ~5% parasitemia, harvest the gDNA, and verify by PCR whether parasites now harbor the desired changes. It is important to verify that binding site mutations are present to be certain that mutations were incorporated by CRISPR/Cas9- and/or ZFN-mediated gene editing. CRISPR/Cas9-mediated editing often edits close to 100% and may obviate further parasite cloning. If mixed cultures prevail, clone out bulk cultures by limiting dilution to obtain pure populations.

4 Notes

1. Parasitemia can also be assayed via other means, e.g., hypoxanthine incorporation, determination of SYBR Green I staining (only) with a plate reader, or DAPI (Molecular Probes, Eugene, OR)-stained parasites on a high-content imager such as the Operetta CLS (Perkin Elmer, Waltham, MA). We note that parasite inhibition assays with only SYBR Green I may yield skewed IC_{50} values [49].
2. We have found that there is generally no necessity to tightly synchronize parasites. A culture with 70–90% rings produces good IC_{50} growth curves. If the drug compound is particularly sensitive to parasite stage, parasites can be synchronized using 5% sorbitol [51].
3. Assuming one parasite per infected red blood cell (iRBC), parasite numbers can be approximated by the following formula: iRBC/mL = $(1 \times 10^{10}) \times$ (% parasitemia) $\times$ (% hematocrit).
4. It is imperative to start with no more than 3% parasitemia; we find 2% parasitemia is ideal. Cultures with a high starting parasitemia will crash before the drug has a chance to take effect. Slow-acting drugs, or drugs that act on different stages of the lifecycle, may allow parasitemia to increase before killing.
5. When reducing culture volumes, if at day 14 the current flask volume is 200 mL, then the new total volume will be 150 mL.

If after aspirating the supernatant you are left with 100 mL, discard 50 mL. To this, add 3 mL fresh RBC (washed and stored at 50% hematocrit). The calculation for this is that ¼ of 150 mL is 37.5 mL, and to achieve a 4% hematocrit, it takes 1.5 mL packed RBC (at 100% hematocrit). Since our RBC is washed and stored at 50% hematocrit, we will need to add 3 mL of washed RBC.

6. If selection with 5× IC_{50} yields no parasite-positive flasks after 60 days, the experiment can be repeated at a lower drug concentration (e.g., 3× IC_{50}). Alternatively, stepwise selections where a single 6-well culture is pressured at 1× IC_{50} can also be performed. A yet milder selection strategy is pulsing parasites with drug for a day, then removing drug and allowing them to recover, and repeating the process until resistant parasites emerge.
7. The method described is for *Streptococcus pyogenes* Cas9 (SpCas9)-mediated editing, which is most commonly used in *P. falciparum* and was used in pioneering studies [12, 13, 19]. SpCas9 recognizes the PAM motif 5′-NGG-3′ [14, 15]. If space on a vector is limiting, the smaller *Staphylococcus aureus* Cas9 (SaCas9) is an attractive alternative. SaCas9 recognizes the motif 5′-NNGRRT-3′ where R represents A or G [52].
8. Longer homology arms lead to higher recombination efficiency. If the region of interest to be inserted is large, this will generate large plasmids that might be unstable and scramble in *Escherichia coli* or provide very low yields. In this case, homology arms can be reduced to as little as 250 bp.
9. The strategy described in Ghorbal et al. [13] employs a two-plasmid approach and a U6-expressed sgRNA. No modification is necessary to pUF1-Cas9, which delivers SpCas9 and has a y*dhodh* selection marker. pL7 delivers U6-expressed sgRNA, donor template, and h*dhfr* and y*fcu* selectable markers. The donor template is constructed by PCR amplification of the region of interest and homology arms on either side from parasite of interest and subsequent modification at the PAM or seed regions (Fig. 1a). Alternatively, the donor is custom synthesized. In both instances, the donor template is cloned into pL7 using AflII/SpeI and NcoI/EcoRI restriction sites. The pL7 containing donor template is then digested with BtGZI, and sgRNA is inserted using the In-Fusion HD Cloning Kit. Parasites harboring pUF1-Cas9 are selected with DSM1, and parasites transformed with pL7 are selected with WR99210, which can be followed with 5-fluorocytosine for negative selection [13].

10. The strategy described in Wagner et al. [12] employs a two-plasmid approach and a T7 polymerase-expressed sgRNA. PCR amplify the region of interest and left and right homology arms, introduce silent mutations in the PAM or seed regions (Fig. 1a), and then assemble into SalI-digested pT7-RNAP in a Gibson reaction to produce pT7-RNAP-HR. This plasmid also delivers T7 RNA polymerase. To insert a T7 polymerase-driven sgRNA into pCas9, order custom primers to synthesize the double-stranded sgRNA, and then PCR amplify this product using the T7 promoter adaptor and T7 terminator adaptor primers as described in [12]. This is then inserted into pCas9 using SalI restriction sites to generate pCas9-sgRNA-T. This plasmid will deliver SpCas9 and sgRNA and has a *bsd* selectable marker. Transfections should be selected with *bsd*.
11. The strategy described in Ng et al. [25] employs a two-plasmid approach and a T7 polymerase-expressed sgRNA. Custom synthesize sgRNA with BbsI overhangs, which allows insertion behind the T7 promoter in pDC2-Cas9-h*dhfr* to produce pDC2-Cas9-sgRNA-h*dhfr*. This plasmid delivers SpCas9, a T7 promoter-driven sgRNA, and a h*dhfr* selectable marker. To generate the donor plasmid, PCR amplify the region of interest with SacI and AatII restriction sites at the 5′ and 3′ ends, respectively. Introduce silent mutations at the PAM or seed regions (Fig. 1a), and then insert fragment into SacI- and AatII-digested pDC2-T7pol-*bsd* to generate pDC2-T7pol-donor-bsd. This plasmid expresses a T7 RNA polymerase and a *bsd* selectable marker. Select transfections with WR99210 and *bsd* [25].
12. A one-plasmid approach for *P. falciparum* CRISPR/Cas9 editing has also been developed by Marcus Lee (Fig. 3). pDC2-cam-coSpCas9-U6sgRNA-donor-h*dhfr* delivers SpCas9 codon-optimized for *P. falciparum* (coSpCas9), U6-expressed sgRNA, a donor template, and contains a h*dhfr* selectable marker. Insert sgRNA generated using the methods described in Subheading3.2 into a BbsI-digested pDC2-cam-coSpCas9-U6-h*dhfr* to generate pDC2-cam-coSpCas9-U6sgRNA-h*dhfr* (Fig. 3a). PCR amplify the region of interest and homology arms with EcoRI and AatII restriction sites at the 5′ and 3′ ends, respectively, and engineer silent mutations in the PAM or seed regions (Fig. 1a). Then insert this fragment into EcoRI- and AatII-digested pDC2-cam-coSpCas9-U6sgRNA-h*dhfr* to generate pDC2-cam-coSpCas9-U6sgRNA-donor-h*dhfr* (Fig. 3b). Select transfections with WR99210.

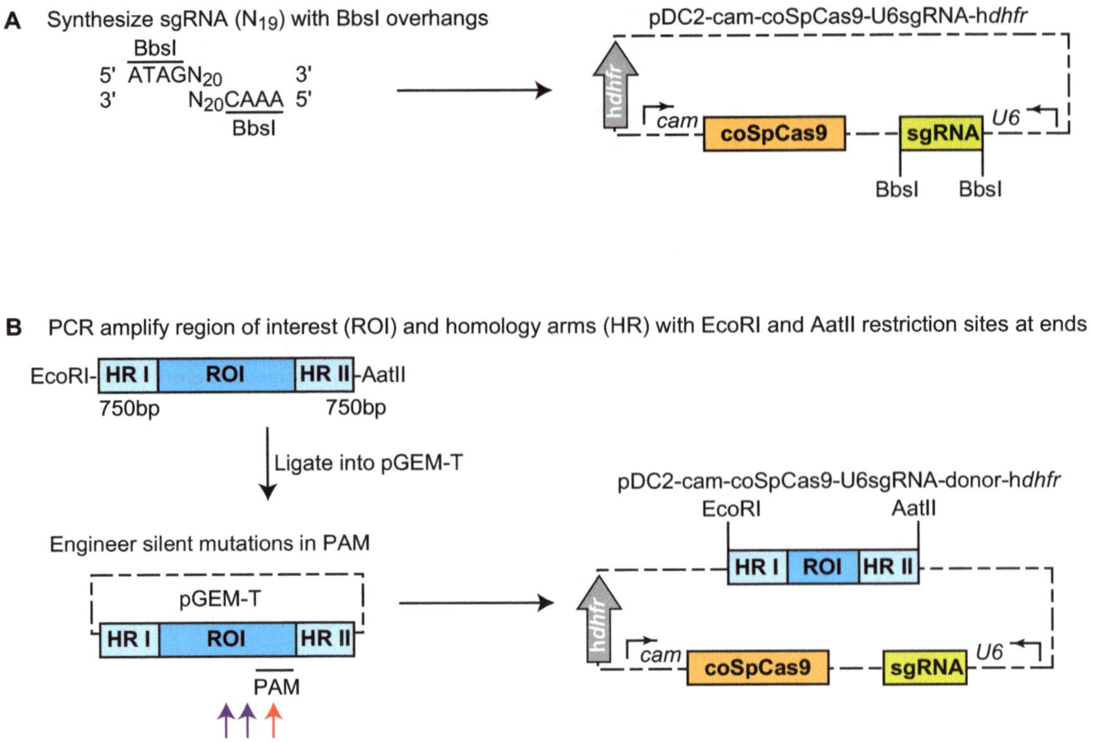

Fig. 3 CRISPR/Cas9-mediated editing using a one-plasmid approach. The final vector, pDC2-cam-coSpCas9-U6sgRNA-donor-h*dhfr*, delivers SpCas9 codon-optimized for *P. falciparum*, a U6-driven sgRNA, and the donor template and contains a h*dhfr* selectable marker. (**a**) Custom synthesize sgRNA with BbsI overhangs, and then insert into BbsI-digested pDC2-cam-coSpCas9-U6-h*dhfr* to generate pDC2-cam-coSpCas9-U6sgRNA-h*dhfr*. (**b**) PCR amplify a fragment containing the region of interest (ROI) flanked by ~750 bp homology region (HR), with EcoRI and AatII restriction sites at the ends. Clone the fragment into pGEM-T to engineer silent mutations within the PAM or seed region. Ideally, one nucleotide at the PAM site is mutated (red arrow). If this is not possible, two nucleotides in the seed region and close to the PAM are mutated (purple arrows). Insert this fragment into EcoRI- and AatII-digested pDC2-cam-coSpCas9-U6sgRNA-h*dhfr* to generate pDC2-cam-coSpCas9-U6sgRNA-donor-h*dhfr*

Acknowledgments

We thank Marcus Lee for his development of several T7- and U6-based editing systems that are discussed herein.

References

1. World Health Organization (2018) World malaria report 2018. https://www.who.int/malaria/publications/world-malaria-report-2018/report/en
2. Dondorp AM, Nosten F, Yi P et al (2009) Artemisinin resistance in *Plasmodium falciparum* malaria. N Engl J Med 361:455–467
3. Ashley EA, Dhorda M, Fairhurst RM et al (2014) Spread of artemisinin resistance in *Plasmodium falciparum* malaria. N Engl J Med 371:411–423
4. Takala-Harrison S, Jacob CG, Arze C et al (2015) Independent emergence of artemisinin resistance mutations among *Plasmodium*

falciparum in Southeast Asia. J Infect Dis 211:670–679

5. Tun KM, Imwong M, Lwin KM et al (2015) Spread of artemisinin-resistant *Plasmodium falciparum* in Myanmar: a cross-sectional survey of the K13 molecular marker. Lancet Infect Dis 15:415–421
6. Sonoiki E, Ng CL, Lee MC et al (2017) A potent antimalarial benzoxaborole targets a *Plasmodium falciparum* cleavage and polyadenylation specificity factor homologue. Nat Commun 8:14574
7. Vanaerschot M, Lucantoni L, Tao L et al (2017) Hexahydroquinolines are antimalarial candidates with potent blood stage and transmission-blocking activity. Nat Microbiol 2:1403–1414
8. Cowell AN, Istvan ES, Lukens AK et al (2018) Mapping the malaria parasite druggable genome by using *in vitro* evolution and chemogenomics. Science 359:191–199
9. Sidhu AB, Verdier-Pinard D, Fidock DA (2002) Chloroquine resistance in *Plasmodium falciparum* malaria parasites conferred by *pfcrt* mutations. Science 298:210–213
10. de Koning-Ward TF, Gilson PR, Crabb BS (2015) Advances in molecular genetic systems in malaria. Nat Rev Microbiol 13:373–387
11. Straimer J, Lee MC, Lee AH et al (2012) Site-specific genome editing in *Plasmodium falciparum* using engineered zinc-finger nucleases. Nat Methods 9:993–998
12. Wagner JC, Platt RJ, Goldfless SJ et al (2014) Efficient CRISPR-Cas9-mediated genome editing in *Plasmodium falciparum*. Nat Methods 11:915–918
13. Ghorbal M, Gorman M, Macpherson CR et al (2014) Genome editing in the human malaria parasite *Plasmodium falciparum* using the CRISPR-Cas9 system. Nat Biotechnol 32:819–821
14. Jinek M, Chylinski K, Fonfara I et al (2012) A programmable dual-RNA-guided DNA endonuclease in adaptive bacterial immunity. Science 337:816–821
15. Mali P, Yang L, Esvelt KM et al (2013) RNA-guided human genome engineering via Cas9. Science 339:823–826
16. Cong L, Ran FA, Cox D et al (2013) Multiplex genome engineering using CRISPR/Cas systems. Science 339:819–823
17. Lee AH, Symington LS, Fidock DA (2014) DNA repair mechanisms and their biological roles in the malaria parasite *Plasmodium falciparum*. Microbiol Mol Biol Rev 78:469–486
18. Kirkman LA, Lawrence EA, Deitsch KW (2014) Malaria parasites utilize both homologous recombination and alternative end joining pathways to maintain genome integrity. Nucleic Acids Res 42:370–379
19. Zhang C, Xiao B, Jiang Y et al (2014) Efficient editing of malaria parasite genome using the CRISPR/Cas9 system. MBio 5: e01414–e01414
20. Ganesan SM, Morrisey JM, Ke H et al (2011) Yeast dihydroorotate dehydrogenase as a new selectable marker for *Plasmodium falciparum* transfection. Mol Biochem Parasitol 177:29–34
21. Fidock DA, Wellems TE (1997) Transformation with human dihydrofolate reductase renders malaria parasites insensitive to WR99210 but does not affect the intrinsic activity of proguanil. Proc Natl Acad Sci U S A 94:10931–10936
22. Duraisingh MT, Triglia T, Cowman AF (2002) Negative selection of *Plasmodium falciparum* reveals targeted gene deletion by double crossover recombination. Int J Parasitol 32:81–89
23. LaMonte G, Lim MY, Wree M et al (2016) Mutations in the *Plasmodium falciparum* cyclic amine resistance locus (PfCARL) confer multidrug resistance. MBio 7:e00696–e00616
24. Lim MY, LaMonte G, Lee MC et al (2016) UDP-galactose and acetyl-CoA transporters as *Plasmodium* multidrug resistance genes. Nat Microbiol 1:16166
25. Ng CL, Siciliano G, Lee MC et al (2016) CRISPR-Cas9-modified *pfmdr1* protects *Plasmodium falciparum* asexual blood stages and gametocytes against a class of piperazine-containing compounds but potentiates artemisinin-based combination therapy partner drugs. Mol Microbiol 101:381–393
26. Crawford ED, Quan J, Horst JA et al (2017) Plasmid-free CRISPR/Cas9 genome editing in *Plasmodium falciparum* confirms mutations conferring resistance to the dihydroisoquinolone clinical candidate SJ733. PLoS One 12: e0178163
27. Bansal A, Ojo KK, Mu J et al (2016) Reduced activity of mutant calcium-dependent protein kinase 1 is compensated in *Plasmodium falciparum* through the action of protein kinase G. MBio 7:e02011–e02016
28. Mogollon CM, van Pul FJ, Imai T et al (2016) Rapid generation of marker-free *P. falciparum* fluorescent reporter lines using modified CRISPR/Cas9 constructs and selection protocol. PLoS One 11:e0168362

29. Kuang D, Qiao J, Li Z et al (2017) Tagging to endogenous genes of *Plasmodium falciparum* using CRISPR/Cas9. Parasit Vectors 10:595
30. Miliu A, Lebrun M, Braun-Breton C et al (2017) Shelph2, a bacterial-like phosphatase of the malaria parasite *Plasmodium falciparum*, is dispensable during asexual blood stage. PLoS One 12:e0187073
31. Nacer A, Claes A, Roberts A et al (2015) Discovery of a novel and conserved *Plasmodium falciparum* exported protein that is important for adhesion of PfEMP1 at the surface of infected erythrocytes. Cell Microbiol 17:1205–1216
32. Bansal A, Molina-Cruz A, Brzostowski J et al (2018) PfCDPK1 is critical for malaria parasite gametogenesis and mosquito infection. Proc Natl Acad Sci U S A 115:774–779
33. Bryant JM, Regnault C, Scheidig-Benatar C et al (2017) CRISPR/Cas9 genome editing reveals that the intron is not essential for *var2csa* gene activation or silencing in *Plasmodium falciparum*. MBio 8:e00729–e00717
34. Wezena CA, Alisch R, Golzmann A et al (2017) The cytosolic glyoxalases of *Plasmodium falciparum* are dispensable during asexual blood-stage development. Microb Cell 5:32–41
35. Bansal A, Molina-Cruz A, Brzostowski J et al (2017) *Plasmodium falciparum* calcium-dependent protein kinase 2 is critical for male gametocyte exflagellation but not essential for asexual proliferation. MBio 8:e01656-17
36. Cobb DW, Florentin A, Fierro MA et al (2017) The exported chaperone PfHsp70x is dispensable for the *Plasmodium falciparum* intraerythrocytic life cycle. mSphere 2:e00363–e00317
37. Knuepfer E, Napiorkowska M, van Ooij C et al (2017) Generating conditional gene knockouts in *Plasmodium* - a toolkit to produce stable DiCre recombinase-expressing parasite lines using CRISPR/Cas9. Sci Rep 7:3881
38. Walczak M, Ganesan SM, Niles JC et al (2018) ATG8 is essential specifically for an autophagy-independent function in apicoplast biogenesis in blood-stage malaria parasites. MBio 9: e02021–e02017
39. Nasamu AS, Glushakova S, Russo I et al (2017) Plasmepsins IX and X are essential and druggable mediators of malaria parasite egress and invasion. Science 358:518–522
40. Sidik SM, Huet D, Ganesan SM et al (2016) A genome-wide CRISPR screen in *Toxoplasma* identifies essential apicomplexan genes. Cell 166:1423–1435
41. Zhang C, Li Z, Cui H et al (2017) Systematic CRISPR-Cas9-mediated modifications of *Plasmodium yoelii* ApiAP2 genes reveal functional insights into parasite development. MBio 8: e01986–e01917
42. Zhang C, Gao H, Yang Z et al (2017) CRISPR/Cas9 mediated sequential editing of genes critical for ookinete motility in *Plasmodium yoelii*. Mol Biochem Parasitol 212:1–8
43. Doyon Y, Vo TD, Mendel MC et al (2011) Enhancing zinc-finger-nuclease activity with improved obligate heterodimeric architectures. Nat Methods 8:74–79
44. Miller JC, Holmes MC, Wang J et al (2007) An improved zinc-finger nuclease architecture for highly specific genome editing. Nat Biotechnol 25:778–785
45. McNamara CW, Lee MC, Lim CS et al (2013) Targeting *Plasmodium* PI(4)K to eliminate malaria. Nature 504:248–253
46. Straimer J, Gnadig NF, Witkowski B et al (2015) K13-propeller mutations confer artemisinin resistance in *Plasmodium falciparum* clinical isolates. Science 347:428–431
47. Gabryszewski SJ, Modchang C, Musset L et al (2016) Combinatorial genetic modeling of *pfcrt*-mediated drug resistance evolution in *Plasmodium falciparum*. Mol Biol Evol 33:1554–1570
48. Fidock DA, Nomura T, Wellems TE (1998) Cycloguanil and its parent compound proguanil demonstrate distinct activities against *Plasmodium falciparum* malaria parasites transformed with human dihydrofolate reductase. Mol Pharmacol 54:1140–1147
49. Ekland EH, Schneider J, Fidock DA (2011) Identifying apicoplast-targeting antimalarials using high-throughput compatible approaches. FASEB J 25:3583–3593
50. MacPherson CR, Scherf A (2015) Flexible guide-RNA design for CRISPR applications using Protospacer Workbench. Nat Biotechnol 33:805–806
51. Lambros C, Vanderberg JP (1979) Synchronization of *Plasmodium falciparum* erythrocytic stages in culture. J Parasitol 65:418–420
52. Ran FA, Cong L, Yan WX et al (2015) *In vivo* genome editing using *Staphylococcus aureus* Cas9. Nature 520:186–191

Chapter 10

An Update on Artemisinin Resistance

Frédéric Ariey and Didier Ménard

Abstract

While the precise mode of action of artemisinin (ART) derivatives remains obscure, it is nonetheless commonly accepted that ART generates reactive oxygen intermediates that contribute to cell death. Also, numerous studies confirm that point mutations in the propeller domain of K13 protein play a key role in resistance to ART derivatives. Because of its homology with the KEAP1 protein, it is thought that this protein may have a role in the polyubiquitination of proteins and that its alteration may cause resistance of young parasite stages to the drug. In this chapter, we present our current knowledge of K13-related resistance to ART and its spread in Southeast Asia and discuss its possible emergence and/or diffusion in Africa.

Key words Artemisinin derivatives, Resistance, K13 protein, Southeast Asia, Africa

1 Introduction

Malaria is a potentially fatal disease caused by protozoan parasites from the genus *Plasmodium* and widespread in tropical regions. The most dangerous malaria species is *Plasmodium falciparum*, which is especially frequent in sub-Saharan Africa where most clinical cases and deaths occur. According to the World Health Organization (WHO), 216 million clinical cases of malaria have been reported worldwide in 2016, giving rise to 445,000 deaths: this represents a 45% decrease in mortality since 2000. These spectacular statistics are partly due to the massive use of artemisinin (ART)-based combination therapies (ACTs) as first-line treatments, which lead to the recent award of the Nobel Prize in Physiology or Medicine 2015 to Youyou Tu for the discovery of ART. Because of these recent advances, the WHO announced its support for a more ambitious goal, i.e., progressive malaria elimination in endemic countries leading to its complete eradication. Unfortunately, since 2008 there has been a worrying decrease in the efficacy of ACT treatments in Southeast Asia (SEA), due to the emergence and spread of drug-resistant *Plasmodium falciparum* parasites

Frédéric Ariey et al. (eds.), *Malaria Control and Elimination*, Methods in Molecular Biology, vol. 2013,
https://doi.org/10.1007/978-1-4939-9550-9_10,

[1, 2]. Indeed, ART-resistant *P. falciparum* might threaten malaria control and elimination efforts in case they spread to, or emerge in, sub-Saharan Africa. In the 1980s, the spread of chloroquine-resistant *P. falciparum* isolates from SEA to sub-Saharan Africa was accompanied by a major increase in malaria-related mortality, due to the lack of a readily available alternative as first-line treatment.

ART resistance (ARTr) is clinically defined as a reduced parasite clearance rate, expressed as an increased parasite clearance half-life [2]. However, clinical studies are very expensive, labor-intensive, and difficult to apply to national/regional scales. Molecular markers of drug resistance are therefore key tools to monitor in time and space the evolution of drug resistance [3]. A few years ago, non-synonymous mutations in the *P. falciparum k13* (*pfk13*) gene were identified as marker [4] and determinant [5] of ARTr (only one *pfk13* mutation is sufficient to confer ARTr). This ground-breaking discovery led to major biological insights into parasite biology [6] and to real-time survey of ARTr evolution [7].

2 Artemisinin Mechanism of Action

While the precise mode of action of ART remains obscure, it is nonetheless commonly accepted that ART (or its bioactive derivative dihydroartemisinin—DHA) treatment of *P. falciparum*-infected red blood cells (iRBC) generates reactive oxygen intermediates (ROS) and that ROS production contributes to cell death [8–10]. It has long been known that upon aging of normal RBC, the oxidative stress stemming from metHb production generates oxidized erythrocyte plasma membrane lipids via a calcium-activated lipoxygenase activity [11]. As DHA treatment of iRBC promotes ROS production, it follows that this could lead to the generation of oxidant metabolites and oxidized lipids [12, 13].

The oxidative stress caused by ART is not only acting on lipids but also involves widespread damage to parasite proteins in different cellular compartments [14]. This causes polyubiquitination of the damaged proteins, which are then degraded by the proteasome. In 2018, Bridgford and collaborators identified the proteasome as a key target of DHA and pinpointed the buildup of polyubiquitinated proteins and endoplasmic reticulum (ER) stress response as the key toxic events during artemisinin treatment [15].

3 K13-Propeller Mutations Are Linked to ART Resistance

ARTr *P. falciparum* parasites were shown to harbor a mutated *pfk13* allele. Mutations segregated in a specific region of the corresponding parasite protein, which contains a domain composed of 6 Kelch-like motifs (Fig. 1), and their presence were

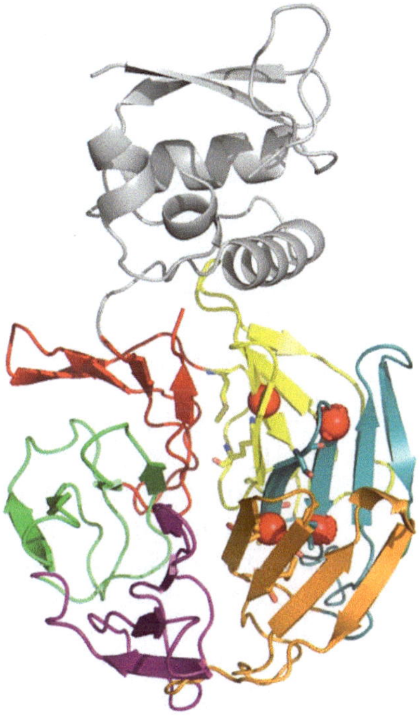

Fig. 1 Three-dimensional structure of PfK13 (provided by Ray Hui)

predictive of the Cambodian *P. falciparum* ARTr phenotype for both in vitro culture and clinical cases [4]. Using reverse genetic approaches, the introduction of the most frequent ARTr-related *pfk13* mutations (encoding C580Y, R539T, I543T, and Y493Y) into a *P. falciparum* ART-sensitive (ARTs) clone resulted in ARTr recombinant parasites. In addition, the reversion of the *pfk13* mutant alleles to the wild-type allele led to the recovery of the ARTs phenotype [5]. Taken together, the abovementioned reports not only confirmed that *pfk13* is the first parasite gene clearly linked to ARTr but also defined *pfk13* as a key upstream player that undergoes several independent and/or synergetic mutations that induce the *P. falciparum* ARTr phenotype.

The K13-propeller shows homology with human KLHL12 and KLHL2, involved in ubiquitin-based protein degradation, and Keap1, involved in cell adaptation to oxidative stress. Keap1 (*see* **Note 1**) is involved via its interaction with the transcription factor Nrf2 (nuclear factor erythroid 2-related factor 2) in the control of the antioxidant response in mammalian cells, through transcription of genes possessing antioxidant-responsive and electrophile-responsive elements (ARE and EpRE, respectively) [16]. Keap1 is a conserved protein composed of two main domains, separated by an intervening region: the BTB/POZ (broad complex, tramtrack, and bric-a-brac/poxvirus and zinc finger) domain, which is involved in Keap1 homodimerization to facilitate Cullin

3-binding and subsequent ubiquitylation, and the DGR (double glycine region) Kelch-containing domain, which is composed of six Kelch-like motifs that form a 6-bladed propeller structure binding to Nrf2.

Since most Kelch-containing modules are involved in protein-protein interactions, the hypothesis that the *Plasmodium* K13 Kelch domain plays a similar function and that ARTr-associated mutations alter the binding of K13 to its partners has recently been confirmed by Mbengue and collaborators [6]. The binding of *P. falciparum* PfPI3K to the PfKelch13-C580Y mutant is reduced compared to the wild-type PfK13. As a consequence, the polyubiquitination-mediated proteolysis of PfPI3K is decreased in ring stages, leading to an accumulation of the PfPI3K lipid product PI3P, the level of which correlates with the ARTr phenotype.

However, different observations suggest that the ARTr phenotype might not be explained only by the modified level of PfPI3K. The proposed hypothesis that K13 could interact with several proteins is supported by transcriptomic analyses, which showed that the expression level of several genes belonging to different metabolic pathways in different intraerythrocytic stages of *P. falciparum* was modified in ARTr parasites [17]. Additionally, special attention should be given to K13 partners predicted to be involved in the ubiquitination pathway, since a recent report claims that the *P. falciparum* ARTr phenotype is associated with an upregulation of the ubiquitin/proteasome system and that inhibition of polyubiquitination proteins helps parasites resist DHA-mediated killing [15, 18]. Altogether, K13 is likely to be an upstream master player that regulates several pathways, like Keap1-Nrf2 that initiates the complex ARE-EpRE responses, even if no Nrf2 homologue has been identified in the *Plasmodium* genome.

4 ART-Induced Dormancy

Another type of escape from ART treatment is represented by parasite recrudescence after treatment [19]. In this case, as documented by in vitro studies, treatment with dihydroartemisinin (DHA) leads to the developmental arrest of some ring-stage parasites, for up to 20 days. These "dormant rings," induced by and somewhat protected from ART exposure, are likely responsible for the recrudescence of infections that are sometimes observed after ART monotherapy, remerging as ARTs parasites when ART has been cleared. In 2010, two papers reported an ART-induced falciparum dormancy phenotype that could be linked to resistance. Teuscher and collaborators [20] argued that the temporary growth arrest of ring-stage parasites (dormancy) they observed after cultured parasites were exposed to ART drugs provides a plausible explanation for this phenomenon. Witkowski and collaborators

[21], through long-term ART in vitro pressure, obtained an ART-tolerant strain that can survive extremely high doses of ART. They showed that drug pressure could induce the developmental arrest of a subpopulation of ring stages, which could explain the ART tolerance in *P. falciparum* found in Cambodian isolates. Based on this phenotype, Witkowsky and collaborators [22, 23] developed a new in vitro test dedicated to ARTr determination, called the ring-stage survival assay (RSA), which corresponds to the percentage of parasites that survive a pulse of 700 nM ART. This new phenotype led to the identification of the K13 molecular marker and paved the way for the understanding of the mechanism of resistance to ART.

In 2011, Mok and collaborators [24] used DNA microarrays to profile the physiological gene expression pattern of Cambodian falciparum ARTr isolates. They observed reduced expression of many basic metabolic and cellular pathways, which suggests a slower growth and maturation of these parasites during the first half of the asexual intraerythrocytic developmental cycle. This has been confirmed through a large transcriptomic analysis performed with more than 1000 field isolates cultivated in vitro under ART exposure. Resistant parasites entered a quiescence-like phase, with an apparent drop in their metabolism. The authors identified an increased expression of genes involved in the unfolded protein response (UPR) pathways, which correlates with a decelerated progression of ARTr parasites through the first part of the asexual intraerythrocytic development cycle, i.e., ring stages [17]. It has been recently proposed that an early signal is PK4-mediated phosphorylation of eIF2α, followed by a global protein translational shutdown [25].

5 Emergence and Spread of Antimalarial Drug Resistance

With regard to malaria control, it is feared that the emergence of ARTr will resemble the historical diffusion of chloroquine resistance, which also emerged in Cambodia in the late 1950s before spreading only later to Africa where it resulted in millions of malaria deaths [26]. The discovery that K13-propeller mutations are the major determinants of resistance has provided opportunities for monitoring such resistance on a global scale. The analysis of the K13-propeller sequence polymorphism, performed in 14,037 samples collected between 2012 and 2014 in 59 countries in which malaria is endemic, showed no evidence of ARTr outside Southeast Asia and China [7].

Over the last decade, there has been a complete replacement of the wild-type K13 by the K13 C580Y mutant in Cambodia. Moreover, recent results suggest that the dominant ARTr C580Y lineage probably arose in western Cambodia and then spread to Thailand

and Laos, outcompeting other parasites and acquiring piperaquine resistance [27, 28]. The emergence and spread across the Greater Mekong Subregion of fitter ARTr *P. falciparum* parasite lineages, which then acquired partner drug resistance, suggests that these successful lineages carry some specific advantageous traits. Furthermore, Amato et al. [28] showed that K13 mutations have multiple independent origins, so that two samples with the same mutation might not be epidemiologically related (i.e., their alleles are identical by state, but they might not have common descent). By analyzing the haplotype structure of K13 and its flanking regions and using statistical chromosome painting to estimate the level of shared ancestry between samples, they were able to assign each sample to a K13 haplogroup. This approach identified 38 K13 haplogroups, each of which was presumed to represent a distinct lineage of ARTr. The C580Y signature was found in six different K13 haplogroups in 2007, of which one invaded the whole Cambodian parasite population. Unfortunately, the authors could not determine if a specific genetic background, unrelated to the *pfk13* mutation, was associated with the invasion process, but highlighted the fact that K13-related ARTr was a highly frequent event.

Recent reports from SEA showed that ARTr is also linked to a decrease in efficacy of partner drugs. In Cambodia, since 2008 dihydroartemisinin-piperaquine (DHA-PPQ) has replaced treatment with artesunate-mefloquine (ASMQ) that was showing reduced efficacy due to increasing resistance to mefloquine [29]. However, in recent years there has been a significant decrease in the efficacy of DHA-PPQ, which has been linked to the emergence of resistance to piperaquine [30]. These observations not only strengthen the need to finely follow and contain the dissemination of ARTr parasites but also pose the question of the best partner drugs to be associated in the future with ART to optimize the killing of recrudescent ARTr parasites days after the end of the treatment. Anyway, it is now well established that resistance to ART combination therapy (ACT) arose in SEA.

In Africa, resistance to antimalarials (chloroquine, pyrimethamine, sulfadoxine) is widespread and has consistently arisen after emerging in SEA [26, 31, 32]. Parasite resistance in Africa occurred through importation or arose locally [33]. In addition to the risk of importation, which is likely to increase with the augmentation of human migrations between malaria-endemic areas [34], reduced malaria transmission in parts of Africa could be a new risk factor for the local emergence of ACT-resistant parasites and its rapid spread [35, 36]. The efficacy of ACTs remains high in Africa [37], although some case reports of ACT treatment failure warrant intensive investigation and surveillance [38]. As mentioned, robust molecular markers of resistance to ART derivatives and piperaquine have been identified in parasites from SEA [4, 30]. However, the molecular basis of resistance to lumefantrine and amodiaquine—

the two main ACT partner drugs used in Africa—remains poorly understood, and no molecular marker of clinical resistance has yet been validated. Further, whether ARTr in Africa will proceed through the same genetic events than in SEA remains an open question; recent cross-sectional surveys in Uganda and a probable Chinese imported case from Equatorial Guinea showed that parasites carrying K13 mutations exhibited high survival rate [39, 40]. Anyhow, in vitro studies have clearly demonstrated that high levels of ARTr can be generated through different selection schemes and can be expressed as different in vitro phenotypes [20, 21, 41].

6 Conclusion

ACT-resistant parasites are now spreading from western Cambodia to the Greater Mekong Subregion, and there is a real risk that these parasites will invade Africa. This is extremely worrisome and could lead to a public health threat due to the loss of efficacy of the front-line malaria treatment. These observations not only strengthen the need to closely follow and contain the dissemination of ACT-resistant parasites in SEA but also require the implementation of proactive monitoring and surveillance of antimalarial drug resistance in Africa, in order to be able to rapidly respond and prevent a potentially uncontrollable invasion of antimalarial-resistant parasites. Constant access to genomics tools will help us keep our eyes open.

7 Note

1. Keap1 stands for **K**elch-like **E**CH-**a**ssociated **p**rotein 1, where ECH stands for erythroid cell-derived protein with CNC homology and CNC for cap "n" collar proteins. Kelch (goblet in German) is the name of a *Drosophila* mutant whose phenotype corresponds to abnormal eggs, their anterior shell remaining open, forming cup shape.

References

1. Noedl H, Se Y, Schaecher K et al (2008) Evidence of artemisinin-resistant malaria in western Cambodia. N Engl J Med 359:2619–2620
2. Dondorp AM, Nosten F, Yi P et al (2009) Artemisinin resistance in *Plasmodium falciparum* malaria. N Engl J Med 361:455–467
3. Mita T, Tanabe K, Kita K (2009) Spread and evolution of *Plasmodium falciparum* drug resistance. Parasitol Int 58:201–209
4. Ariey F, Witkowski B, Amaratunga C et al (2014) A molecular marker of artemisinin-resistant *Plasmodium falciparum* malaria. Nature 505:50–55
5. Straimer J, Gnädig NF, Witkowski B et al (2015) Drug resistance. K13-propeller mutations confer artemisinin resistance in *Plasmodium falciparum* clinical isolates. Science 347:428–431

6. Mbengue A, Bhattacharjee S, Pandharkar T et al (2015) A molecular mechanism of artemisinin resistance in *Plasmodium falciparum* malaria. Nature 520:683–687
7. Ménard D, Khim N, Beghain J et al (2016) A worldwide map of *Plasmodium falciparum* K13-propeller polymorphisms. N Engl J Med 374:2453–2464
8. Antoine T, Fisher N, Amewu R et al (2014) Rapid kill of malaria parasites by artemisinin and semi-synthetic endoperoxides involves ROS-dependent depolarization of the membrane potential. J Antimicrob Chemother 69:1005–1016
9. Hu W, Chen SS, Zhang JL et al (2014) Dihydroartemisinin induces autophagy by suppressing NF-κB activation. Cancer Lett 343:239–248
10. Efferth T, Giaisi M, Merling A et al (2007) Artesunate induces ROS-mediated apoptosis in doxorubicin-resistant T leukemia cells. PLoS One 2:e693
11. Kiefer CR, Snyder LM (2000) Oxidation and erythrocyte senescence. Curr Opin Hematol 7:113–116
12. O'Neill PM, Gary HP (2004) A medicinal chemistry perspective on artemisinin and related endoperoxides. J Med Chem 47:2945–2964
13. Kumura N, Furukawa H, Onyango AN et al (2009) Different behavior of artemisinin and tetraoxane in the oxidative degradation of phospholipid. Chem Phys Lipids 160:114–120
14. Wang J, Zhang CJ, Chia WN et al (2015) Haem-activated promiscuous targeting of artemisinin in *Plasmodium falciparum*. Nat Commun 6:10111
15. Bridgford JL, Xie SC, Cobbold SA et al (2018) Artemisinin kills malaria parasites by damaging proteins and inhibiting the proteasome. Nat Commun 9:3801
16. Itoh K, Wakabayashi N, Katoh Y et al (1999) Keap1 represses nuclear activation of antioxidant responsive elements by Nrf2 through binding to the amino-terminal Neh2 domain. Genes Dev 13:76–86
17. Mok S, Ashley EA, Ferreira PE et al (2015) Drug resistance. Population transcriptomics of human malaria parasites reveals the mechanism of artemisinin resistance. Science 347:431–435
18. Dogovski C, Xie SC, Burgio G et al (2015) Targeting the cell stress response of *Plasmodium falciparum* to overcome artemisinin resistance. PLoS Biol 13:e1002132
19. Kyle DE, Webster HK (1996) Postantibiotic effect of quinine and dihydroartemisinin on *Plasmodium falciparum* in vitro: implications for a mechanism of recrudescence. In: XIVth International Congress for Tropical Medicine and Malaria
20. Teuscher F, Gatton ML, Chen N et al (2010) Artemisinin-induced dormancy in *Plasmodium falciparum*: duration, recovery rates, and implications in treatment failure. J Infect Dis 202:1362–1368
21. Witkowski B, Lelièvre J, Barragán MJ et al (2010) Increased tolerance to artemisinin in *Plasmodium falciparum* is mediated by a quiescence mechanism. Antimicrob Agents Chemother 54:1872–1877
22. Witkowski B, Amaratunga C, Khim N et al (2013) Novel phenotypic assays for the detection of artemisinin-resistant *Plasmodium falciparum* malaria in Cambodia: in-vitro and ex-vivo drug-response studies. Lancet Infect Dis 13:1043–1049
23. Witkowski B, Khim N, Chim P et al (2013) Reduced artemisinin susceptibility of *Plasmodium falciparum* ring stages in western Cambodia. Antimicrob Agents Chemother 57:914–923
24. Mok S, Imwong M, Mackinnon MJ et al (2011) Artemisinin resistance in *Plasmodium falciparum* is associated with an altered temporal pattern of transcription. BMC Genomics 12:391
25. Zhang M, Gallego-Delgado J, Fernandez-Arias C et al (2017) Inhibiting the *Plasmodium* eIF2a kinase PK4 prevents artemisinin-induced latency. Cell Host Microbe 22:766–776
26. Wootton JC, Feng X, Ferdig MT et al (2002) Genetic diversity and chloroquine selective sweeps in *Plasmodium falciparum*. Nature 418:320–323
27. Imwong M, Suwannasin K, Kunasol C et al (2017) The spread of artemisinin-resistant *Plasmodium falciparum* in the Greater Mekong subregion: a molecular epidemiology observational study. Lancet Infect Dis 17:491–497
28. Amato R, Pearson RD, Almagro-Garcia J et al (2018) Origins of the current outbreak of multidrug-resistant malaria in southeast Asia: a retrospective genetic study. Lancet Infect Dis 18:337–345
29. Phyo AP, Ashley EA, Anderson TJC et al (2016) Declining efficacy of artemisinin combination therapy against *P. falciparum* malaria on the Thai-Myanmar border (2003-2013): the role of parasite genetic factors. Clin Infect Dis 63:784–791
30. Witkowski B, Duru V, Khim N et al (2017) A surrogate marker of piperaquine-resistant *Plasmodium falciparum* malaria: a phenotype-genotype association study. Lancet Infect Dis 17:174–183

31. Ariey F, Fandeur T, Durand R et al (2006) Invasion of Africa by a single *pfcrt* allele of South East Asian type. Malar J 5:34
32. Maïga O, Djimdé AA, Hubert V et al (2007) A shared Asian origin of the triple-mutant *dhfr* allele in *Plasmodium falciparum* from sites across Africa. J Infect Dis 196:165–172
33. Vinayak S, Alam MT, Mixson-Hayden T et al (2010) Origin and evolution of sulfadoxine resistant *Plasmodium falciparum*. PLoS Pathog 6:e1000830
34. Tatem AJ, Smith DL (2010) International population movements and regional *Plasmodium falciparum* malaria elimination strategies. Proc Natl Acad Sci U S A 107:12222–12227
35. Ariey F, Robert V (2003) The puzzling links between malaria transmission and drug resistance. Trends Parasitol 19:158–160
36. Scott N, Ataide R, Wilson DP et al (2018) Implications of population-level immunity for the emergence of artemisinin-resistant malaria: a mathematical model. Malar J 17:279
37. Zani B, Gathu M, Donegan S et al (2014) Dihydroartemisinin-piperaquine for treating uncomplicated *Plasmodium falciparum* malaria. Cochrane Database Syst Rev (1): CD010927
38. Sutherland CJ, Lansdell P, Sanders M et al (2017) pfk13-independent treatment failure in four imported cases of *Plasmodium falciparum* malaria treated with artemether-lumefantrine in the United Kingdom. Antimicrob Agents Chemother 61. https://doi.org/10.1128/AAC.02382-16
39. Ikeda M, Kaneko M, Tachibana SI et al (2018) Artemisinin-resistant *Plasmodium falciparum* with high survival rates, Uganda, 2014-2016. Emerg Infect Dis 24:718–726
40. Lu F, Culleton R, Zhang M et al (2017) Emergence of indigenous artemisinin-resistant *Plasmodium falciparum* in Africa. N Engl J Med 376:991–993
41. Rocamora F, Zhu L, Liong KY et al (2018) Oxidative stress and protein damage responses mediate artemisinin resistance in malaria parasites. PLoS Pathog 14:e1006930

Chapter 11

Antimalarial Drugs for Malaria Elimination

Jerome Clain, Abderaouf Hamza, and Frédéric Ariey

Abstract

The diversity of *Anopheles* species and the environmental issues posed by the large-scale use of insecticides make it unlikely that malaria elimination will be achieved by fighting mosquitoes only. Malaria elimination necessitates targeting the parasite itself. For this, in the absence of efficient vaccines against the disease, antimalarial drugs remain the primary tool. We present here the limitations of currently available antimalarials and the different implementation strategies of these drugs, which ultimately depends on the epidemiological context of the disease.

Key words Malaria, Elimination, Antimalarials, Strategy

1 Introduction: WHO Eradication Campaign

From 1955 to 1969, the WHO launched a malaria eradication campaign consisting of "mass drug administration," or MDA, combined with vector control [1]. The idea was to combine wide and systematic treatment of local populations in endemic areas with chloroquine, along with massive DDT spraying. This highly interventional procedure proved to be effective until the early 1970s in Europe, some Asian countries, and the USA, greatly reducing morbidity. But this strategy has found its limits in sub-Saharan Africa [2, 3]. For example, the Garki project, a quasi-military application of that protocol in a Nigerian province, failed to eradicate the disease, with prevalence rates even returning to numbers equivalent to those prior to the campaign [4]. At that time, ecological considerations also became prominent, like the potential negative effects of massive DDT spraying on flora and fauna [5], all the while resistance to major antimalarial drugs started to emerge [6].

Thus, in the early 1980s, the WHO malaria eradication strategy was halted and, in large part due to the spread of chloroquine resistance, the burden of the disease even significantly increased in Africa [7, 8]. At the beginning of the 2000s, the WHO, with the financial support of global funds [9], reviewed its strategy, and the

Frédéric Ariey et al. (eds.), *Malaria Control and Elimination*, Methods in Molecular Biology, vol. 2013,
https://doi.org/10.1007/978-1-4939-9550-9_11,

fight against malaria was reoriented around three main axes: (1) vector control with insecticide treatment in endemic areas and the use of long-lasting impregnated nets (LLINs); (2) the use of rapid diagnostic tests (RDT) to better target malaria patients; and (3) ACT (artemisinin-based combination therapy) as a first-line treatment. The promising results observed in the years following the application of this strategy revived the possibility of eradicating the disease: in 2009, the WHO, supported by the Gates Foundation, the UNICEF, the World Bank, and the United Nations Development Programme (UNDP), proposed a new malaria elimination program [10].

2 Drugs and Elimination

The WHO has defined three progressive stages on the path to malaria eradication, depending on the endemicity of the parasite in the area. When the number of cases of fever attributed to malaria is greater than 5%, the program continues the standard malaria control strategy (combination of rapid diagnosis, prompt treatment, and mass distribution of LLINs). When the rate falls below 5%, the program goes into the pre-elimination phase. Finally, the elimination phase is defined by malaria incidence in the high-risk population less than 0.1% [11]. It is within the framework of these two epidemiological conditions—pre-elimination and elimination—that we discuss below possible treatment strategies depending on the micro-epidemiological context of the endemic zone.

3 Available Drugs

Several types of antimalarial drugs can play a key role in achieving malaria elimination.

3.1 The Alpha and Omega of Antimalarials: Artemisinin Combination Therapies (ACTs)

Artemisinin originates from the Chinese traditional pharmacopoeia. For centuries Chinese authorities have described malaria as a major public health issue, from ancient Chinese writings to modern WHO reports, and have invested immense effort in controlling the disease. The annual incidence of malaria decreased from 24 million at the beginning of the 1970s to tens of thousands by the end of the 1990s. In 2010, the Chinese government even launched an ambitious campaign with the explicit aim of eliminating the disease within its border by 2020. In the context of a vast plant screening research program initiated by Chairman Mao Zedong to find new cures for malaria, ART was isolated from *Artemisia annua* (named qinghaosu in Chinese), a common herb used by Chinese herbalists for more than 2000 years for the treatment of fever. Tu Youyou, one of the lead scientists among the hundreds behind that research, received the Nobel Prize in Physiology or Medicine in 2015 [12].

Studies on artemisinin derivatives conducted in many different countries demonstrated both their effectiveness and their ease of administration, with injectable or daily dose oral forms available. They eliminate the parasites present in the blood more quickly than any other antimalarial drug [13], especially when administered in combination with another molecule with a longer elimination half-life (e.g., sulfadoxine-pyrimethamine, amodiaquine, mefloquine, lumefantrine, pyronaridine or piperaquine). Artemisinin derivatives having a relatively short half-life, the residual parasitemia remaining in the patient's body is eliminated by the second (or partner) antimalarial drug [14, 15]. These combined drugs, which have the added effect of delaying the emergence of resistance, are called artemisinin-based combination therapies (ACTs).

In the mid-1990s, because of the high frequency of resistance to commonly used drugs (chloroquine, sulfadoxine-pyrimethamine) in the border areas of Thailand, the first-line treatment was changed to mefloquine followed by 3 days of artesunate (MQA3) [16]. This restored the cure rates to 90–95% and resulted in a substantial decrease in disease incidence. The discussion then moved to whether the use of ACTs could be expanded to first-line malaria treatment in Africa, mainly because of the large difference in malaria prevalence and transmission between these two endemic areas. Yet today, due to the high mortality associated with resistance to chloroquine and sulfadoxine-pyrimethamine, and the successful rollout ACT in Africa, ACTs are now the only medical malaria treatment recommended by the WHO [17].

3.2 Transmission-Blocking Drugs

In the absence of newly available antimalarials, ACTs have become the alpha and omega of any uncomplicated malaria treatment strategy. However, although it appears that artemisinin derivatives have an effect on immature gametocytes, ACTs alone have not demonstrated a significant effect on transmission [18], a property that would be paramount in the context of disease elimination. The only molecule used today as a transmission-blocking agent is primaquine, but new strategies are exploring the benefit of endectocide molecules such as ivermectin.

3.2.1 Single Low Dose of Primaquine to Facilitate Elimination

Plasmoquine (pamaquine), the forerunner of primaquine, was the first of many compounds derived from aniline dye methylene blue, in 1925. Wilhelm Roehl, Paul Ehrlich's pupil, developed a standardized test system in canaries infected with *Plasmodium relictum*, in which plasmoquine showed efficacy [19]. Although the results of human trials were disappointing, the drug still exhibited two novel properties, prevention of relapses from *Plasmodium vivax* and gametocide activity [20, 21], making it the first drug of the

8-aminoquinoline class to potentially block the parasite infectious cycle. Primaquine and tafenoquine are analogs of pamaquine.

Remarkably, primaquine is the only drug lethal to *P. vivax* and *P. ovale* dormant liver stages (hypnozoites). It also displays potency at the low micromolar range during the replicative blood stage. Its exact mechanism of action is not fully understood but could depend on cell damage by oxidative stress [22]. Primaquine is well-absorbed in the gut, extensively distributes in the body without accumulating in red blood cells, and is quickly metabolized by liver enzymes; its primary metabolite is carboxyprimaquine (which is devoid of antimalarial activity) along with a myriad of other hydroxylated metabolites that bear some of the antimalarial activities of primaquine [23].

The most serious adverse effect of primaquine is observed in patients with glucose-6-phosphate dehydrogenase deficiency (G6PD), which is unfortunately very common in malaria-endemic areas. In those patients, a high-dose regimen over several days (necessary for the elimination of *P. ovale* and *P. vivax* hypnozoites) can induce hemolytic anemia, which can be fatal, even though the number of published cases is small [24].

In addition to its activity against hypnozoite forms of *P. vivax* or *P. ovale*, primaquine is interesting for its activity on *P. falciparum* mature gametocytes even at low doses. Numerous studies have shown that the combination of a single dose of primaquine along with standard malaria treatment leads to a large decrease of human-to-mosquito parasite transmission rates [25, 26]. It has recently been shown that the short-lived exposition to low circulating levels of primaquine following a single-dose administration does not put subjects at risk of severe hemolytic anemia, even in G6PD-deficient people [27]. In areas of low transmission, the WHO advocates for a single-dose regimen of 0.25–0.75 mg/kg primaquine with ACT in patients with *P. falciparum* malaria (except pregnant women, infants aged <6 months, and breastfeeding women of infants aged <6 months) to reduce transmission, without requiring to test G6PD deficiency status. Conversely, tafenoquine should not be associated with ACT for *P. falciparum* elimination strategy, since its long half-life (2–3 weeks) prohibits its use among people suffering from G6PD deficiency.

3.2.2 Ivermectin: A New Concept

Ivermectin is the most widely used and efficient endectocide developed in the last 30 years [28, 29]. Its use in veterinary settings has massively increased animal husbandry productivity [30]. In 2015, William C. Campbell and Satoshi Ōmura (along with the above-mentioned Youyou Tu) were awarded the Nobel Prize in Physiology or Medicine for the discovery of ivermectin: its medical use has indeed revolutionized the treatment of many parasitic diseases, primarily onchocerciasis and filariasis, and was even extended in recent years to the treatment of ectoparasites such as scabies or lice [31].

Ivermectin, a macrocyclic lactone, is a derivative of avermectins, a compound isolated from the fermentation of *Streptomyces avermitilis*. It can be administered either orally or parenterally and its digestive resorption is quick, with a peak plasma concentration reached within 4 h and a plasmatic half-life of 12 h [32]. Although its mechanism of action is not yet fully established, it is known that ivermectin exerts its effect via action on the parasite nervous system and muscle function, disrupting neurotransmission. Notably, it has a significant affinity for glutamate-dependent chloride channels present in the nerves and muscle cells of invertebrates [33], and the resistances described during its massive use in veterinary practice have been explained by the selection of mutations on chloride channels [34]. Because of its high efficacy against insects, even at very low doses, ivermectin has been recently suggested for use as a transmission-blocking adjunct to antimalarial treatment campaigns; the "theoretical" rationale was that mosquitoes having fed on people treated with ivermectin would die and thus break the parasite infectious cycle. The first obvious factor this strategy depends on is the feasibility of achieving efficient ivermectin blood levels. Recent studies conducted to evaluate the LC50 (blood concentration able to kill 50% of feeding mosquitoes) after standard treatment with ivermectin [35] showed that an effect was observed up to 2 weeks after treatment. A field study in Senegal showed a significant decrease in the number of *Anopheles gambiae* (ss) infected with *Plasmodium falciparum* in the villages following MDA campaigns of ivermectin carried out to fight onchocerciasis and lymphatic filariasis [36]. Extended and delayed release forms currently under preclinical development could prolong the diffusion of the drug over a dozen days [37]. However, the side effects of long-term treatment with ivermectin have not yet been fully explored.

The relatively limited side effects of ivermectin reported during MDA campaigns, mostly related to increased mortality in hyperparasitemic *Loa loa* patients, could be explained by the absence of glutamate-dependent chloride channels in mammals. However, ivermectin also interacts with ligand-dependent chloride channels involving the neuro-mediator GABA (gamma-aminobutyric acid) [38]. Even if it does not appear to easily cross the blood-brain barrier in mammals, a recent study on multiday administration of ivermectin reducing alcohol intake in mice suggest that ivermectin action on the mammalian central nervous system does exist [39]. In 2001, a study conducted in Collie dogs, which have a natural mutation on the *mdr1* gene (leading to the absence of protein), shows that there is indeed a significant intracerebral passage of ivermectin, resulting in heavy neurological complications [40]. In addition, abamectin, a molecule related to ivermectin, has been classified as a Class II compound by the EPA (i.e., moderately toxic) so large-scale, long-term prophylactic use of ivermectin must be approached with caution [41]. Moreover, we must not neglect the effects of active product dissemination in the environment via feces, which can be extremely toxic for insects and aquatic organism ecosystems, thus posing more general problems of ecotoxicology [42].

In a 2017 article, Carlos Chaccour and N. Regina Rabinovich proposed scenarios and strategies for the use of ivermectin in the fight against malaria and agreed that the use of ivermectin as a transmission blocker in the context of an elimination campaign of malaria should be first tested by field studies to identify possible side effects [43]. As of today, ivermectin does not yet seem to be an immediately operational option.

4 Strategies for Implementing Drugs for Malaria Elimination

There is currently only a single safe pharmacological option recommended by the WHO for the elimination of malaria in the short term (i.e., before new drugs and new drug combinations eventually become available): the association of ACT and SLDP (single low dose of primaquine). However, strategies for implementing this regimen are still a subject of debate, crystalizing in two opposing approaches: (1) mass drug administration where everyone, whether infected or not, in a given area is treated [MDA and intermittent preventive therapy or treatment (IPT)] and (2) the test, treat, and track strategy [TTT or focal screening and treatment (FSAT)] where parasite carriers are identified before treatment. Diagnosis before treatment is where those two approaches fundamentally differ.

4.1 MDA vs. FSAT Strategy

MDA is undoubtedly an efficient strategy to reduce malaria burden. A large MDA campaign (with and without SLDP) was carried out in Anjouan in 2012–2013, with a high coverage of the population (above 80%). Results were excellent, with an average monthly malaria hospitalization rate per 100,000 people falling from 310.8 to 2.1 in the artemisinin-piperaquine (AP) with low-dose primaquine population and from 412.1 to 2.60 in the AP-treated population, although falling short of achieving elimination [44]. A 2013 Cochrane review based on 32 MDA studies concluded that MDA appears to reduce the initial risk of malaria parasitemia [45]. However, few studies showed a sustained impact beyond 6 months post-MDA, and those that did were conducted on small islands or in highland settings.

One major problem revolves around population participation. In a recent study conducted in Myanmar, the authors reported a maximum of participation to three MDA courses of the two thirds of the population, even going down to only one third in larger villages [46]. Another point is ethical considerations related to the iatrogenic risks of this type of intervention and the massively increased risk of emergence of drug resistance due to selective pressure. Contrary to MDA, a TTT/FSAT strategy designed to treat only people who carry parasites would expose fewer people to the drug and give less opportunities for malaria parasites to encounter residual, sub-therapeutic drug concentrations when infecting recently treated people.

The principle of FSAT is to carry out massive diagnosis campaigns and treat only people infected by the parasite, which requires very sensitive diagnosis techniques. Thanks to molecular diagnosis, we now have powerful tools capable of identifying patients with less than one parasite per microliter of blood, with a lab report ready within 48 h. But while this method allows to appropriately target treatments, the logistics of carrying out these diagnosis campaigns are expensive and time-consuming: they require delocalized technical equipment available within the villages and a trained and competent team to carry out sample analysis [47].

Initiated by the WHO, a group of experts met in April 2015 to review recent evidence on the use of MDA, mass screening and treatment (MSAT), and focal screening and treatment (FSAT) in specific epidemiological settings. They concluded that MDA was safe and feasible and could accelerate the elimination of *P. falciparum* when combined to other measures. But it has to be implemented with a real knowledge of local preferences for community mobilization, delivery, and timing. On the other hand, they buried the FSAT strategy, arguing that using current diagnostic tests, MSAT and FSAT are not suitable methods to reduce malaria transmission (Table 1, *see* recommendation 6).

4.2 Elimination Strategies and Malaria Epidemiology

Recently, a new strategic approach has been proposed: the SERCaP (Single Exposure Radical Cure and Prophylaxis) [48]. SERCaP has a double action. First, a fast-acting medical treatment clears the parasite from the blood of those infected. Second, prophylaxis is administered to prevent reinfection. If this approach seems interesting theoretically, it is essential to identify the epidemiological settings in which this strategy can work.

Infectious disease epidemiology shows that the average number of individuals that can be contaminated by an infected person, over the course of the infectious period, is related to the stability of the disease. This number, defined in an ideal, otherwise non-infected population, is called the basic reproduction ratio and is denoted R_0. If $R_0 < 1$, then an individual will contaminate less than one individual, which means that the disease will eventually disappear from the population.

Levins [49] defined a metapopulation as a set of small populations living in patches, in a balance between extinction and

Table 1
Recommendations proposed by the WHO evidence review group, for consideration by the WHO Malaria Policy Advisory Committee

Proposed recommendations
1. Use of MDA to interrupt transmission of *falciparum* malaria can be considered in endemic island communities and in low-endemic non-island settings approaching elimination, where there is minimal risk of reintroduction of infection, good access to treatment, and implementation of vector control and surveillance
2. In view of the growing threat of multidrug resistance and the need to use extreme measures, MDA can be considered as a component of malaria elimination efforts in the Greater Mekong Subregion, in areas with good access to treatment, vector control, and good surveillance
3. Use of MDA to rapidly reduce malaria morbidity and mortality can be considered for epidemic control as part of the immediate response, while other interventions are put in place
4. Use of MDA to reduce malaria morbidity and mortality can be considered during exceptional circumstances, where the health system is overwhelmed and unable to serve the affected communities
5. There is insufficient evidence to provide guidance on use of MDA in settings with moderate or high transmission; more research is required to inform future recommendations
6. Using current diagnostic tests, MSAT and FSAT are not suitable as interventions to reduce malaria transmission

colonization, i.e., as a "population of populations." A metapopulation is stable if the colonization rate of a patch (unitary population) is equal or superior to its extinction rate or, in other words, if a patch colonizes at least one other patch before becoming extinct ($R_0 > 1$). The minimum viable metapopulation size was defined by Hanski as the minimum number of interacting local populations necessary for long-term persistence. The main objective of this theory is to formalize the dynamics of ecological systems, such as island colonization or deforestation processes, and to define the critical number of connected populations leading to species extinction.

In malaria infection, if we consider a human host as a patch and the parasites infecting one host as a population, we can regard a malaria transmission unit (MTU) as a typical metapopulation. In that case, knowing the size of the minimum viable metapopulation (MTU size above which malaria remains stable) would help in estimating the malaria stability in an endemic area. Hanski defined the T_M/T_L ratio as the ratio between time before extinction in the metapopulation compared to the mean time before extinction in the population (which could be interpreted as the duration of parasite carriage before treatment) [50]: $T_M = T_L$ exp. $[HP^2/2(1 - P)]$, where T_L is the expected time to local extinction (parasite carriage), H the number of suitable habitat patches (MTU size), and P the fraction of occupied patches at a stochastic steady state (prevalence). This ratio depends on the size of the metapopulation,

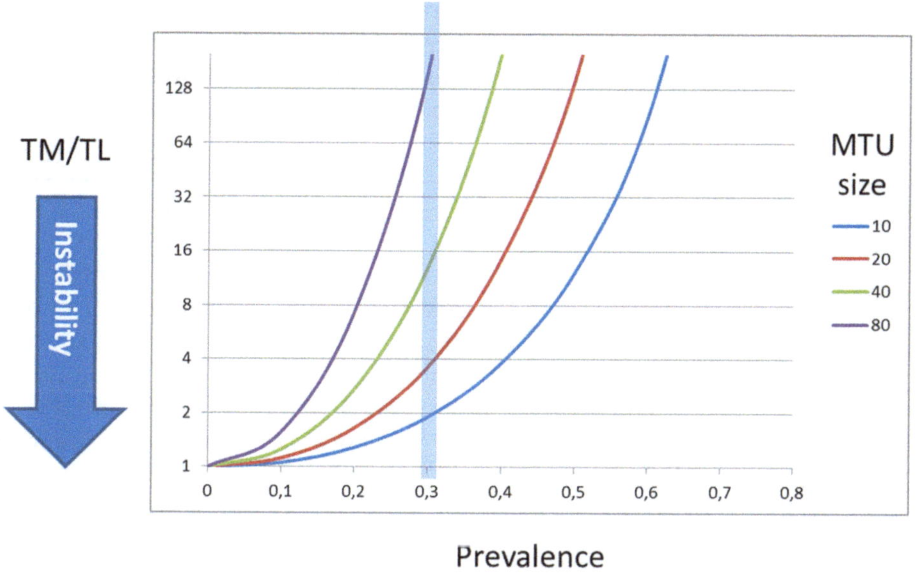

Fig. 1 The figure shows the theoretical stability (T_M/T_L) of malaria transmission unit (MTU) as a function of the prevalence and the MTU size (number of people susceptible to malaria infection in the endemic area). If we consider 2 weeks (T_L) as the average parasitic carriage, we can consider that the MTU will be stable if T_M is ten times larger (i.e., less than half year). The blue line indicates a prevalence of ~30%, usually found in populations at risk; the decrease in the number of people susceptible to infection (as a consequence of using chemoprophylaxis and/or vaccine) begins to act on the probability of elimination when the size of the MTU is less than 40 with an exponential effect of the decrease in the number of susceptible persons on the probability of sterilization of the endemic area

i.e., the number of susceptible members within the MTU. As expected, when the number of potential targets for the parasite is small, the prevalence of the disease must be high for the infection to become perennial and not go extinct.

In the case of SERCaP, chemoprophylaxis makes a fraction of the MTU unsusceptible to infection, thus decreasing its size and increasing the probability of parasite extinction. Figure 1 shows the theoretical stability (T_M/T_L) of MTU as a function of the prevalence and the MTU size (number of people susceptible to malaria infection in the endemic area). In areas of very low transmission, the SERCaP strategy could be very efficient even with basic logistics. This highlights the crucial importance of understanding parasite microcirculation to estimate the infection stability, especially in low or very low prevalence areas.

As incidence decreases, two opposite epidemiological situations can arise: overall homogenous reduction in transmission (large panmictic MTU) or epidemiological heterogeneity with pockets of high infectious risk (small, highly structured MTU). Examples of the latter are Southeast Asia and the Amazonian forest, where a small proportion of the population suffers from malaria while the vast majority of inhabitants live in disease-free areas. Elimination strategies must therefore be adapted to epidemiological conditions by using presumptive treatment and MDA in situations where the risk is homogeneous and adopting a targeted SERCAP-type strategy where targeting small, at-risk populations is necessary.

5 Conclusion

It is therefore essential to map the risks and identify pockets of transmission and at-risk populations. The stratification of national malaria maps should be revised regularly to guide a strategy that is rational, up-to-date, and adapted to the epidemiological context.

The main pitfall of malaria eradication is the number of drugs available, as we are now living in a therapeutic stalemate with a great risk that resistance will make elimination even more complex. It is necessary to make the most out of the current mobilization to achieve elimination at least in the most unstable endemic areas and where the incidence is low while limiting the risk of resistance emergence as much as possible. As we anticipate the arrival of new drugs, we must do our best to manage those available now, controlling their use and reinforcing resistance monitoring, especially within transmission pockets, which are proven to be breeding grounds for drug resistance [51].

References

1. Mayo CW, Brady FJ (1955) The eighth World Health Assembly. Public Health Rep 70:1057–1060
2. Bruce-Chwatt LJ (1969) Malaria eradication at the crossroads. Bull N Y Acad Med 45:999–1012
3. Bruce-Chwatt LJ (1987) Malaria and its control: present situation and future prospects. Annu Rev Public Health 8:75–110
4. Molineaux L, Gramiccia G (1980) The Garki project: research on the epidemiology and control of malaria in the Sudan savanna of West Africa. World Health Organization, Geneva. ISBN 9241560614
5. Carson R (1962) Silent spring. Houghton Mifflin, Boston, MA
6. Palacios Fraire S (1975) Analysis of the principal problems impeding normal development of malaria eradication programs. Bull Pan Am Health Organ 9:283–294
7. Trape JF, Pison G, Preziosi MP et al (1998) Impact of chloroquine resistance on malaria mortality. C R Acad Sci III 321:689–697
8. Trape JF (2001) The public health impact of chloroquine resistance in Africa. Am J Trop Med Hyg 64:12–17
9. Nordstrom A (2002) Global fund for AIDS, tuberculosis and malaria. Lancet 359:1621–1622
10. Alonso PL, Brown G, Arevalo-Herrera M et al (2011) A research agenda to underpin malaria eradication. PLoS Med 25:e1000406
11. World Health Organization (2009) Chapter 5: Elimination of malaria. World Health Organization, Geneva
12. Tu Y (2011) The discovery of artemisinin (qinghaosu) and gifts from Chinese medicine. Nat Med 11:1217–1220
13. Qinghaosu Antimalarial Coordinating Research Group (1979) Antimalarial studies on qinghaosu. Chin Med J 92:811–816
14. Li GQ, Arnold K, Guo XB et al (1984) Randomised comparative study of mefloquine, qinghaosu, and pyrimethamine-sulfadoxine in patients with falciparum malaria. Lancet 15:1360–1361

15. White NJ (1999) Delaying antimalarial drug resistance with combination chemotherapy. Parassitologia 41:301–308
16. Nosten F, Luxemburger C, ter Kuile FO et al (1994) Treatment of multidrug-resistant *Plasmodium falciparum* malaria with 3-day artesunate-mefloquine combination. J Infect Dis 170:971–977
17. Attaran A, Barnes K, Curtis C et al (2004) WHO, the Global Fund, and medical malpractice in malaria treatment. Lancet 363:237–240
18. Targett G, Drakeley C, Jawara M et al (2001) Artesunate reduces but does not prevent posttreatment transmission of *Plasmodium falciparum* to *Anopheles gambiae*. J Infect Dis 183:1254–1259
19. Roehl W (1926) Die Wirkung of Plasmochins auf die Vogelmalaria. Arch Schiffs Tropenhyg 30:311–318
20. Manifold J (1931) Report on a trial of plasmoquine and quinine in the treatment of benign tertian malaria. J R Army Med Corps LVI:321–338; 410–423
21. Dick GW, Bowles RV (1947) The value of plasmoquine as a gametocide in sub-tertian malaria. Trans R Soc Trop Med Hyg 40:447–450
22. Guerra F (1977) The introduction of cinchona in the treatment of malaria. Part II. J Trop Med Hyg 80:135–140
23. Marcsisin SR, Reichard G, Pybus BS (2016) Primaquine pharmacology in the context of CYP 2D6 pharmacogenomics: current state of the art. Pharmacol Ther 161:1–10
24. Ashley EA, Recht J, White NJ (2014) Primaquine: the risks and the benefits. Malar J 13:418
25. Eziefula AC, Bousema T, Yeung S et al (2014) Single dose primaquine for clearance of *Plasmodium falciparum* gametocytes in children with uncomplicated malaria in Uganda: a randomised, controlled, double-blind, dose-ranging trial. Lancet Infect Dis 14:130–139
26. Steketee RW, ter Kuile F (2014) Single low-dose primaquine to reduce malaria transmission. Lancet Infect Dis 14:91–92
27. Recht J, Ashley EA, White NJ (2018) Use of primaquine and glucose-6-phosphate dehydrogenase deficiency testing: divergent policies and practices in malaria endemic countries. PLoS Negl Trop Dis 12:e0006230
28. Chabala JC, Mrozik H, Tolman RL et al (1980) Ivermectin, a new broad-spectrum antiparasitic agent. J Med Chem 23:1134–1136
29. Campbell WC, Fisher MH, Stapley EO et al (1983) Ivermectin: a potent new antiparasitic agent. Science 221:823–828
30. Omura S (2008) Ivermectin: 25 years and still going strong. Int J Antimicrob Agents 31:91–98
31. Roos TC, Alam M, Roos S et al (2001) Pharmacotherapy of ectoparasitic infections. Drugs 61:1067–1088
32. Fisher MH, Mrozik H (1992) The chemistry and pharmacology of avermectins. Annu Rev Pharmacol Toxicol 32:537–553
33. Vassilatis DK, Arena JP, Plasterk RH et al (1997) Genetic and biochemical evidence for a novel avermectin-sensitive chloride channel in *Caenorhabditis elegans*. Isolation and characterization. J Biol Chem 272:33167–33174
34. R G, Andersen EC, Shapiro JA et al (2012) Natural variation in a chloride channel subunit confers avermectin resistance in *C. elegans*. Science 335:574–578
35. Smit MR, Ochomo EO, Aljayyoussi G et al (2018) Safety and mosquitocidal efficacy of high-dose ivermectin when co-administered with dihydroartemisinin-piperaquine in Kenyan adults with uncomplicated malaria (IVERMAL): a randomised, double-blind, placebo-controlled trial. Lancet Infect Dis 18:615–626
36. Kobylinski KC, Sylla M, Chapman PL et al (2011) Ivermectin mass drug administration to humans disrupts malaria parasite transmission in Senegalese villages. Am J Trop Med Hyg 85:3–5
37. Bellinger AM, Jafari M, Grant TM et al (2016) Oral, ultra-long-lasting drug delivery: application toward malaria elimination goals. Sci Transl Med 8:365ra157
38. Hernando G, Bouzat C (2014) *Caenorhabditis elegans* neuromuscular junction: GABA receptors and ivermectin action. PLoS One 9: e95072
39. Yardley MM, Neely M, Huynh N et al (2014) Multiday administration of ivermectin is effective in reducing alcohol intake in mice at doses shown to be safe in humans. Neuroreport 25:1018–1023
40. Mealey KL, Bentjen SA, Gay JM et al (2001) Ivermectin sensitivity in collies is associated with a deletion mutation of the *mdr1* gene. Pharmacogenetics 11:727–733
41. Molinari G, Soloneski S, Larramendy ML (2010) New ventures in the genotoxic and cytotoxic effects of macrocyclic lactones, abamectin and ivermectin. Cytogenet Genome Res 128:37–45
42. Verdú JR, Lobo JM, Sánchez-Piñero F et al (2018) Ivermectin residues disrupt dung beetle diversity, soil properties and ecosystem functioning: an interdisciplinary field study. Sci Total Environ 618:219–228

43. Chaccour C, Rabinovich NR (2017) Ivermectin to reduce malaria transmission II. Considerations regarding clinical development pathway. Malar J 16:166

44. Deng C, Huang B, Wang Q et al (2018) Large-scale artemisinin-piperaquine mass drug administration with or without primaquine dramatically reduces malaria in a highly endemic region of Africa. Clin Infect Dis 67 (11):1670–1676. https://doi.org/10.1093/cid/ciy364

45. Poirot E, Skarbinski J, Sinclair D et al (2013) Mass drug administration for malaria. Cochrane Database Syst Rev (12):CD008846

46. Landier J, Kajeechiwa L, Thwin MM et al (2017) Safety and effectiveness of mass drug administration to accelerate elimination of artemisinin-resistant falciparum malaria: A pilot trial in four villages of Eastern Myanmar. Wellcome Open Res 2:81

47. Hoyer S, Nguon S, Kim S et al (2012) Focused screening and treatment (FSAT): a PCR-based strategy to detect malaria parasite carriers and contain drug resistant *P. falciparum*, Pailin, Cambodia. PLoS One 7:e45797

48. malERA Consultative Group on Integration Strategies (2011) A research agenda for malaria eradication: cross-cutting issues for eradication. PLoS Med 8:e1000404

49. Levins R (1969) Some demographic and genetic consequences of environmental heterogeneity for biological control. Bull Entomol Soc Am 15:237–240

50. Hanski I (1999) Metapopulation ecology. Oxford University Press, Oxford

51. Scott N, Ataide R, Wilson DP et al (2018) Implications of population-level immunity for the emergence of artemisinin-resistant malaria: a mathematical model. Malar J 17:279

Part IV

Vaccinology

Chapter 12

Vaccine Development: From Preclinical Studies to Phase 1/2 Clinical Trials

Cécile Artaud, Leila Kara, and Odile Launay

Abstract

Vaccines are biological pharmaceutical products prescribed as prevention of a hypothetical infection. Development of a new vaccine is the result of a long process involving several stages. During all developmental phases, priority is the safety of the new product, which is often used in young infants. The initial research phase lasts 1–5 years and is followed by a clinical and pharmaceutical development phase (preclinical and clinical phases), which can last from 15 to 20 years on average before licensure is obtained. There are, however, exceptions, like the malaria vaccine for which research has been going on for more than 30 years and at least 30 candidate vaccines have been assessed. This chapter summarizes the different phases of vaccine candidate development from preclinical studies to phase 2 vaccine trials.

Key words Vaccine development, Clinical trial, Challenge, Safety

1 Introduction

Developing a vaccine, unlike other medicinal products, is a challenge. Vaccines are unique pharmaceutical products. Their major characteristics are related to their mechanism of action (inducing a long-lasting immune response), production process (biological products), indication (especially regarding preventative vaccines given to healthy subjects, often children), and impact. Development of a new vaccine is the result of a long process involving several stages. The initial research phase lasts 1–5 years and is followed by a clinical and pharmaceutical development phase (preclinical and clinical phases), which can last from 15 to 20 years on average before licensure can be obtained (Fig. 1).

Several basic steps compose the manufacturing process. The first step is to generate the antigen that will be used to induce an immune response, which mainly consists in the culture of the pathogen itself (pathogens may be grown on cells, yeast, bacteria, etc.). The next step is to release, isolate, and purify the antigen. The formulation of the vaccine consists of combining all components

Frédéric Ariey et al. (eds.), *Malaria Control and Elimination*, Methods in Molecular Biology, vol. 2013, https://doi.org/10.1007/978-1-4939-9550-9_12, © Springer Science+Business Media, LLC, part of Springer Nature 2019

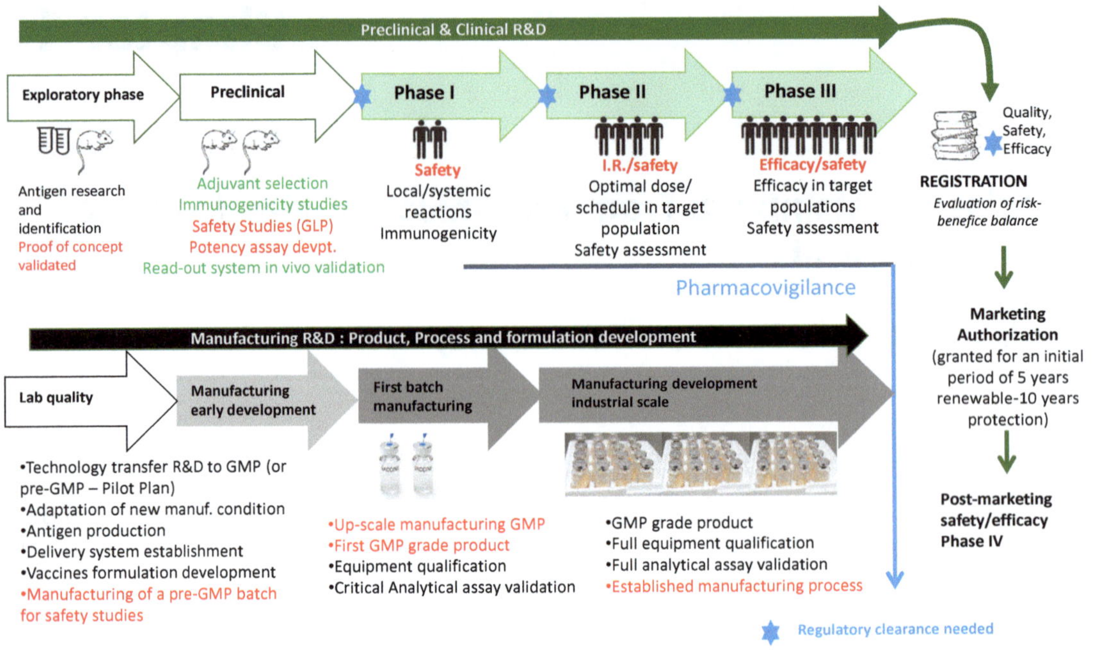

Fig. 1 Pre-clinical and clinical phases of drug development

that constitute the final vaccine: it may include an adjuvant to enhance the immune response, stabilizers to prolong the vaccine shelf life, and preservatives to allow multidose vials to be delivered. During this phase, containers are filled with vaccine and sealed with sterile stoppers or plungers. Quality control testing consists of safety, potency, purity, sterility, and other assays that may be specific to the product. As vaccines are biological products, they are produced through living systems. As a consequence, there is a high variability of the seeds and yields, which differ from a simple chemical product. Their production requires high technology levels, is very complex, and is strictly regulated. Any modification in the manufacturing process can modify the final product in terms of stability or efficacy.

To accomplish this, the vaccine developer must establish a multidisciplinary team including expert scientists, established manufacturers, medical doctors, and legal and regulatory experts. Regular communication with competent authorities throughout the entire vaccine development process is also necessary, starting during the proof of concept and continuing through the preclinical and clinical development stages.

Clinical evaluation of new vaccines aims at gathering information on a candidate vaccine in terms of safety, immunogenicity, efficacy, and administration conditions in order to obtain a licensure. As for other drugs, the vaccine developer will conduct a series of clinical trials in a predefined order.

2 Preclinical Vaccine Development: From Proof-of-Concept to Regulatory Submission for Phase 1 Clinical Trial

Vaccines represent the most diverse class of product candidates in the pharmaceutical industry (e.g., live attenuated or inactivated pathogens, purified or recombinant proteins, polysaccharide and conjugated vaccines, DNA vaccines, therapeutic vaccines, adjuvants). Hence, the types of product characterization, quality assessment, and safety evaluation involved in the preclinical development of new vaccines are numerous and complex [1]. Preclinical testing is a prerequisite to move a candidate vaccine from the laboratory to the clinic and includes all aspects of testing, product characterization, proof-of-concept/immunogenicity studies, and safety testing in animals conducted prior to introducing the product into humans [2].

2.1 First Step: Defining a Quality Control System for Vaccine Production for Clinical Trial

Once the proof of concept has been demonstrated and decisions have been made to move forward into vaccine development, the vaccine developer identifies an established manufacturer that will be able to provide information to demonstrate compliance with the principals of Good Manufacturing Practices (GMP).

GMPs are essential to ensure that products are consistently produced and controlled to the quality standards appropriate to their intended use and required by the marketing authorization [2]. GMPs have evolved and improved throughout the twentieth century, as quite a number of errors or accidents were made during the manufacture or testing of pharmaceutical products that resulted in health problems or deaths (Table 1).

Thus, the manufacturer has to constitute a quality control testing program for the candidate vaccine in compliance with the cGMP and to follow the technical guidelines established by national or international authorities or professional societies to preserve human safety. This includes identification and control of raw materials used to manufacture the vaccine and establishment of a panel of release assays that include identity, purity, potency, and stability. Specification and analytical methods are defined, qualified, and validated before being approved by regulatory authorities [3] (Table 2).

Once the vaccine has been characterized and its specification validated by a qualified person (QP), i.e., a licensed pharmacist, biologist or chemist with several years of experience working in pharmaceutical manufacturing operations, a certificate of analysis (CoA) is edited—the vaccine is termed "released" for preclinical or clinical testing. This document, which contains all specifications and analytical descriptions of the product, shows that the product is in compliance with company standards and all applicable legal and regulatory requirements.

Table 1
Key timelines for the evolution of GMP

YEAR	COUNTRY	GMP EVOLUTION
1902	USA	*Biologics control Act:* to improve the assurance of safety and purity of sera, vaccines, and other biological products
1938	USA	Revised Food, Drug, and Cosmetic Act
1962	USA	The "thalidomide tragedy" leads the US Congress to add GMP to the Food, Drugs, and Cosmetic Act. The FDA publishes their first Regulation on Good Manufacturing Practices"
1969	WHO	The World Health Organization publishes the first universal guideline "Basic Rules for the Manufacture of Pharmaceuticals and the Assurance of their Quality"
1978	USA	cGMP Final Rules for Drugs (21 CFR Parts 210–211)
1978–1994	FRANCE	The EU and the FDA open negotiations on the mutual recognition of GMP inspections (Agreement was finally reached and a DRAFT was signed)
2001	ICH	ICH Q7A API Guidance ICH's "Good Manufacturing Practice Guidance for Active Pharmaceutical Ingredients (APIs)"

2.2 Second Step: Establishing the Safety Profile of the Vaccine Before Testing in Humans

The purpose of a preclinical safety study in animals is to assess pharmacological and toxicological effects of a new vaccine before, and in parallel to, the clinical development. This assessment includes in vitro and in vivo studies. However, regulators encourage vaccine developers and manufacturers to further develop in vitro assays to minimize as much as possible the use of animals in research. For ethical reasons, it is asked to apply the 3Rs concept of "Replace, Reduce, Refine" when designing the preclinical studies [4].

Safety concerns for vaccine may include the potential inherent/intrinsic toxicities of the vaccine component such as the antigen, adjuvant, excipient in the final formulation, or any contaminant toxicity that may not have been identified during QC. Additionally, the pharmacodynamic activity of the vaccine may also lead to undesired toxic side effects due to a potential elicited immune-modulator and/or inflammatory response. Thus, a panel of toxicity studies is required by the regulatory agency such as single-dose toxicity, repeated-dose toxicity, and safety pharmacology to address these questions (Table 3). The goals of these studies are to: (a) provide information on systemic toxicity and local tolerance; (b) identify potential target organs for toxicity and assess whether such toxicity is reversible; (c) identify safety parameters for clinical monitoring and help plan protocols for subsequent clinical studies in human subjects; and (d) identify an initial safe dose and subsequent dose escalation schemes in humans [2, 5].

Table 2
Establishment of vaccine specification

RELEASE ASSAY	OBJECTIVES	EXAMPLE OF ANALYTICAL METHODS
Identity (*ICH Q6B*)	To show that the vaccine contains the intended immunogenic component	Mass spectrophotometry, peptide mapping, Western blot (protein, peptide vaccine), quantitative PCR (DNA, viral, inactivated vaccine), nuclear magnetic resonance (polysaccharide-protein conjugate)
Purity/Impurity (*ICH Q3A*) *R2*	To identify and characterize any component present in the product that is not the desired product. An impurity may be either process- or product-related	Levels of residual nucleic acid and protein from cell substrate; polyacrylamide gel electrophoresis (PAGE); chromatographic methods (HPLC); qPCR methods
Potency (*ICH Q6B*)	To estimate the biological activity and immunological strength of a vaccine	In vitro (e.g., transfection efficiency, viral infectivity in cell culture systems) or in vivo (e.g., immunogenicity studies)
Stability (*ICH Q5C*)	To demonstrate that the product vaccine is stable in the final container and to set a shelf life under appropriate storage condition	Methods for content identification and measurement, impurity profile, potency assay. Real-time study or accelerated study in stress condition (e.g., pH, temperature variation)
Viral safety testing (*ICH Q5A*)	To identify and control viral contamination of the cell banks, virus seeds, or vaccine bulk that may arise from the original source of the cell lines or from adventitious introduction of virus during production processes	Transmission electron microscopy (TEM) for retrovirus detection; infectivity assay; PCR-based assay
Transmissible Spongiform Encephalopathy agent (*EMA/410/0 1 rev3 2011/ C 73/01*)	To minimize the risk of transmitting animal spongiform encephalopathy agents via human and veterinary medicinal products.	Establishment of a *risk assessment* taking into consideration several factors as identified in the note for guidance: note for guidance on minimizing the risk of transmitting animal spongiform encephalopathy agents via human and veterinary medicinal products (EMA/410/01 rev.3)

Table 3
Regulatory toxicology requirement

PRECLINICAL SAFETY STUDIES	REGULATORY REQUIREMENT
Single dose toxicity	Yes[a]
Repeated dose toxicity	Yes[a]
Safety pharmacology	Yes
Genotoxicology	Generally not needed for vaccine but recommended for new chemical entities (adjuvant)
Pharmacokinetics and biodistribution study	Generally not needed but should be considered in case of alternative routes of administration or for genetically modified organism and concern about tropism and shedding
Reproductive toxicity	Should be considered to support the use of vaccine in special population (pregnant woman or childbearing potential females)

[a]One pivotal toxicology study may respond to these critical questions

2.3 Preclinical Safety Assessment Study Design

Toxicity studies should be designed to mimic the intended use in the clinic. Thus, the relevant animal species/strain, dosing schedule, and method of vaccine administration as well as timing of evaluation of endpoints (e.g., sampling for clinical chemistry, antibody evaluation, necropsy, etc.) should all mimic the intended clinical use. Special consideration should also be given to the quality of the lots of antigen to be used in preclinical studies, as they must be representative of the final vaccine formulation. Although there is no regulatory obligation to use a full GMP grade material for these studies, the manufacturer should ensure strict comparability of the vaccine used in the preclinical study and the clinical material, to justify the extrapolation of any finding.

The choice of the relevant animal species is a complicated question, as the selected species should fulfill several criteria. The selected species should in particular be able to develop an immune response to the vaccine that is similar to the expected response in humans after vaccination [5] and should be susceptible to infection by the wild-type organism. However, most of the time, no animal model meets all these criteria. In this case, purely practical factors should be considered, such as the feasibility of the route of administration and volume to be given, as well as the availability of reagents for immunological analyses [5]. Rodents and rabbits are often used for vaccine safety studies, although monkeys are sometimes the most appropriate choice. In all cases, the 3R rule should apply. However, animal models are not always indicative of the effect in humans since pathogenesis and immune responses are frequently species-specific. Nevertheless, any signal observed in preclinical toxicity studies must be carefully addressed in human clinical trials and may require additional preclinical testing.

Traditional routes of administration for vaccination are intramuscular, subcutaneous, or intradermal; however, alternative routes are used for specific vaccines, e.g., mucosal (nasal, rectal or vaginal) or oral routes or topical administration. The choice of the administration route should correspond to that intended for use in the clinic. If toxic effects are observed using a particular route of administration, a different route should be used to help in understanding the full spectrum of the product toxicity [2].

Although the administration of a full human dose (HD) is recommended by regulatory agencies, there might be cases when the limited animal size might prevent dosing the full HD. Nonetheless, this can be overcome by using several sites of administration.

The schedule of vaccine administrations should mimic the clinical protocol. However, regulatory agencies recommend using the $R + 1$ rule, which means that the animal should receive one more dose compared to what is to be administered in the clinic. Also, intervals between doses may be reduced in preclinical studies to 2–3 weeks compared to longer intervals in clinical studies. This interval may be defined based on the kinetics of the immune response observed in animals.

As previously mentioned, there are several types of safety assessment studies, which should address the potential for local inflammatory reaction, systemic toxicity, and effect on the immune system. Generally, one pivot repeat-dose toxicity study is sufficient in one species. During this study, in-life parameters should be monitored, for example, by daily clinical observation, weekly body weights, and weekly food consumption. Hematology and serum chemistry analyses should also be collected during the treatment period and treatment free phase. At study termination, blood samples should be collected for hematology and serum chemistry counts but also for the evaluation of the immune response induced by the vaccine. A complete gross necropsy and tissue collection and preservation should also be conducted through histopathological examination of the tissues. Special attention should be paid to immune organs (lymph nodes, thymus, spleen, etc.), pivotal organs (brain, kidney, liver, etc.), and the site of vaccine injection. Regulatory agencies have established the list of organs to be analyzed during a preclinical study [2].

2.4 Third Step: Preparation of the Regulatory Dossier for First-in-Human Trial

Once the manufacturing process is developed and toxicity studies are performed, the sponsor can submit a regulatory dossier to the competent national authority for approval. This dossier must include the description of manufacturing and testing processes and a summary of the results of toxicity studies and should describe the proposed clinical study. Once approved, the sponsor can start the clinical trial.

3 Clinical Evaluation of Vaccines

The goal of the clinical development plan is to demonstrate vaccine safety, immunogenicity, and efficacy. There are generally three separate phases in the clinical evaluation of a new vaccine at the pre-marketing stage. These phases may overlap, and multiple phase 1 or 2 trials may be performed as new data are obtained. Phase 1 trials are intended to provide a preliminary evaluation of safety and immunogenicity. These trials are conducted in a small number of closely monitored adult volunteers (20 to 80 subjects). Phase 2 studies may involve several hundred participants (usually 100 to 300). They are often randomized and well controlled. They provide further information on safety and immunogenicity and data on the doses and schedule that will be used in phase 3. Phase 3 studies are large-scale trials that need to provide a definite assessment of efficacy and a more thorough assessment of safety. They usually involve thousands of subjects and sometimes tens of thousands when they are designed to evaluate rare adverse events (e.g., 70,000 subjects for rotavirus vaccine phase 3 trial to assess the risk of intussusception). When the disease is rare, the measurement of the immune response to the vaccine could be an alternative approach (e.g., meningococcal vaccines). In some cases, a proof of concept of efficacy is tested in a phase 2b trial that allows showing efficacy trends in a high-risk population or in challenge studies, before embarking on a large phase 3 study. Finally, phase 4, post-marketing studies are designed to provide additional assessments of rare adverse events and assess effectiveness of the new vaccine in "real life" and duration of vaccine-induced immunity. In addition, during the post-marketing phase, there is continued surveillance of the product and of the manufacturer's production activities. Vaccine manufacturers have to develop data before and after licensing that demonstrate the stability of their vaccine under recommended storage conditions for claimed shelf life.

Several guidelines on various aspects of clinical trials of vaccines are available from WHO (http://www.who.int/biologicals/vaccines/clinical_evaluation/en/), FDA (https://www.fda.gov/BiologicsBloodVaccines/GuidanceComplianceRegulatoryInformation/Guidances/Vaccines/default.htm), and EMA (http://www.ema.europa.eu/ema/index.jsp?curl=pages/regulation/general/general_content_000407.jsp&mid=WC0b01ac058002958b). Below, we address phase 1 and phase 2 studies.

3.1 Phase 1 Vaccine Trials (Dose-Escalating Studies)

Phase 1 trials are intended to provide a preliminary evaluation on safety and immunogenicity of the vaccine candidate in a small number of closely monitored adult volunteers. Phase 1 trials are principally designed to assess the safety and tolerability of multiple dose levels of the vaccine candidate to select the doses to use for further development. The objective is to gather information on safety and to observe the immune response after vaccine candidate administration. Usually, only two or three doses are tested as the doses have already been assessed during the preclinical phases in animal models. The best dose is the lowest dose that gives the appropriate immune response with an acceptable safety profile. Usually, these phase 1 studies are blinded, dose-ranging placebo-controlled studies, involving 20–80 subjects, and they may last up to 1 year. Of note, even if the target population for the vaccine is infants or young children, the first administration of vaccine candidate in humans is always done in adults.

During phase 1 studies, various compositions/formulations of the vaccine candidate may be tested (e.g., monovalent versus multivalent vaccines such as dengue serotype 2 or dengue serotypes 1, 2, 3, 4 together). The necessity of adjuvants and various antigen dosages are also tested.

3.2 Phase 2 Vaccine Trials

Phase 2 trials aim to provide further information on safety and immunogenicity and data on the doses and schedule of the vaccine candidate that will be used in the phase 3 study. Phase 2 studies are larger than phase 1 studies and involve several hundred participants (usually 100 to 300). They evaluate the immunogenicity of the vaccine and provide preliminary estimates of common adverse events. They are usually randomized, controlled studies. Phase 2a studies focus on immunogenicity, dose, and schedule finding, whereas phase 2b studies are designed as proof-of-concept efficacy trials.

3.2.1 Phase 2a Studies

The objectives of phase 2a studies are to find out:

1. The optimum vaccine dose if not determined from phase 1 studies, for example comparing two doses.
2. The number of vaccine doses needed to elicit a proper immune response (antibodies active with regard to clinical endpoints), i.e., the administration schedule.
3. The need for an adjuvant and choice of the adjuvant.
4. The need for booster doses (study of antibody persistence through the follow-up of vaccinated subject cohorts for several months or years). The recommendation for boosting may have to be based on long-term follow-up and data that are obtained during the post-authorization period.
5. The administration route: injectable (intramuscular/subcutaneous/intradermal) or mucosal (oral, intranasal).
6. The induction of an immune memory and the reactivation kinetics of memory-B cells.

Phase 2a studies aim to characterize the immunological response, i.e., the kinetics of the specific antibody response (IgG, IgM, IgA) after each dose (percentage of participants with seroconversion, seroprotection above a given threshold (not always known in general and never known for a new vaccine) and GMT (geometric mean titers). The exploration of cellular responses is also an important tool for phase 2 studies to better explore the immune response.

Phase 2 studies can also assess the influence of maternal antibodies for infants or other preexisting immunity (dengue, malaria, etc.) acquired from natural disease or vaccination. Furthermore, if the vaccine has to be given together with other vaccines (generally pediatric vaccines), phase 2 clinical development should include immunogenicity and preliminary safety data on the concurrent administration of the vaccine.

3.2.2 Phase 2b Studies

Phase 2b studies are early proof-of-concept efficacy trials (POC studies). The objective is to evaluate the preliminary efficacy of the vaccine candidate before the initiation of a pivotal phase 3 trial, which is expensive and complex. Phase 2b trials require sample sizes of hundreds to thousands of volunteers and long follow-up periods. Prior to starting such a trial, "Go/No-Go" criteria should be established, on which the decision to proceed further will be based. In certain situations, they can be considered as pivotal studies. The efficacy of the vaccine candidate is measured against infection and clinical disease in a limited number of subjects selected for the higher incidence in their group than in the general target population. The studies are double-blind, randomized-controlled trials, and the selection of the efficacy endpoint is critical for their design. For example, the latter can consist in assessing the incidence of a disease in the vaccinated group compared to the incidence in the non-vaccinated group (tuberculosis, malaria, HIV) or measuring the presence of the infectious agent in the blood of the subjects in each group (e.g., CMV viremia).

Infectious human challenge studies involve the exposure of volunteers to infectious agents. Challenge trials aim to demonstrate efficacy of a vaccine candidate by comparing attack rates in vaccinated vs non-vaccinated volunteers. They might be considered for vaccine candidates against infectious agents that can be easily and rapidly diagnosed and treated efficiently (influenza, malaria, enteric diseases, etc.). Those studies allow for a greater understanding of the pathogen and the potency/efficacy of a new vaccine. Many ethical and safety considerations need to be addressed for such studies, and assessment is dependent on the pathogen, route of administration, and host species. WHO recently published specific regulatory considerations regarding human challenge trials during vaccine development (http://www.who.int/biologicals/expert_committee/WHO_TRS_1004_web_Annex_1.pdf?ua=1).

Prior to licensure of a new vaccine, regulatory agencies require proof that the vaccine production process is stable and that consistent lots can be produced. The difficulty is to produce consistently a biological product that, by essence, is a variable product. As part of this requirement, a so-called lot consistency or lot-to-lot consistency trial must be performed. The objective is to show that three consecutive produced lots (batches) are similar with respect to the induced immunogenicity. Subjects are randomly assigned vaccine doses from one of the three lots. The postvaccination blood samples of the subjects are assayed and antibody values are compared. Lot consistency is concluded if all three-paired-wise postvaccination geometric mean ratios are close to one. In some studies, a fourth group is added, either a placebo group or a reference vaccine. If there is a comparison with a reference vaccine, the study has to demonstrate that the investigational vaccine induces antibody titers that are at least as high as those induced by the reference vaccine. Safety assessment is usually added as a secondary objective, for example, to demonstrate that the investigational vaccine is tolerated as well as the reference vaccine, in terms of defined safety profile. On the clinical trial side, the rule is to follow GCPs like for any other clinical trial.

4 Conclusion

Vaccines are usually produced in small plants for phase 1 and 2 trials. When the decision is taken to continue development of a given vaccine, a specific plant has to be built to produce enough vaccine for phase 3 trials and further. On the production side, the manufacturer is required to comply with current Good Manufacturing Practice (cGMP) regulations, which concern personnel, buildings, equipment, production controls, records, and other aspects of the vaccine manufacturing process. Lot-to-lot consistency trials are only one step of the process for monitoring vaccine stability and quality. When clinical trials are nearing completion or have been completed and the sponsor believes that the product can be safe and effective for its intended use, the sponsor may apply for a license to manufacture and distribute the product commercially. In the meantime, production techniques should be developed and the manufacturing process standardized. Vaccine lots are subjects to pre-licensure, lot-release testing. After licensure, monitoring of the vaccine and production activities including periodic facility inspections must continue, as long as the manufacturer holds a license for the product.

References

1. Lebron JA, Wolf JJ, Kaplanski CV et al (2005) Ensuring the quality, potency and safety of vaccines during preclinical development. Expert Rev Vaccines 46:855–866
2. World Health Organization (2003) Guidelines on nonclinical evaluation of vaccines. World Health Organization, Geneva
3. The International Council for Harmonisation of Technical Requirements for Pharmaceuticals for Human Use (ICH) (1999) Specifications: test procedures and acceptance criteria for biotechnological/biological products, Q6B
4. Prescott MJ, Lidster K (2017) Improving quality of science through better animal welfare: the NC3Rs strategy. Lab Anim 46:152–156
5. Forster R (2012) Study designs for the nonclinical safety testing of new vaccine products. J Pharmacol Toxicol Methods 66:1–7

Chapter 13

The Advanced Development Pathway of the RTS,S/AS01 Vaccine

Lorenz von Seidlein

Abstract

Following successful phase 1 and 2 trials, RTS,S/AS01 was evaluated in a large phase 3 trial in 7 African countries in which 8922 young children and 6537 infants were enrolled and followed for a median of 48 and 38 months, respectively. The vaccine efficacy against uncomplicated malaria in children was 28% without booster and 36% with booster. The vaccine received the approval of the European Medical Agency in 2015, but two WHO expert committees requested more data before the programmatic use of RTS,S/AS01 in African children can be recommended. To provide such data, a very large, cluster randomized trial is currently in progress in three African countries. The integration of RTS,S/AS01 in national childhood vaccination programs will benefit the individual vaccinated child but is unlikely to make an impact on malaria transmission. Mass vaccination campaigns that include all age groups over short periods are more likely to harness the short but high protection afforded by RTS,S/AS01.

Key words RTS,S/AS01, Malaria, Vaccine, *P. falciparum*, Africa, Circumsporozoite protein CSP, WHO, GSK, WRAIR

1 Introduction

Vaccines play a critical role in the prevention of a range of infectious diseases including diphtheria, pertussis, tetanus, poliomyelitis, measles, rubella, and hepatitis B [1–6]. Universal vaccination has led to the elimination of polio and measles in many regions of the world and was essential in the eradication of smallpox [7]. Malaria control and elimination could be much accelerated if an ideal and affordable vaccine that is safe and confers lifelong, complete immunity were available. The only licensed antimalarial vaccine, RTS,S/AS01, has a number of strength which, if strategically harnessed, could facilitate the interruption of malaria transmission.

The original version of this chapter was revised. The correction to this chapter is available at https://doi.org/10.1007/978-1-4939-9550-9_21

Frédéric Ariey et al. (eds.), *Malaria Control and Elimination*, Methods in Molecular Biology, vol. 2013, https://doi.org/10.1007/978-1-4939-9550-9_13,

RTS,S is the product of a collaboration, initiated in 1987 between GlaxoSmithKline and the Walter Reed Army Institute of Research [8]. The vaccine antigen consists of two components, the carboxy-terminal half (amino acids 207 to 395) of circumsporozoite protein (CSP) of the NF54 *P. falciparum* strain and hepatitis B virus surface protein. The two proteins assemble into virus-like particles when simultaneously expressed in *Saccharomyces cerevisiae* yeast cells. It was recognized early on that the immunogenicity of this antigen on its own is insufficient to elicit a sufficiently strong, long-lasting, and appropriate immune response to succeed as a viable vaccine candidate. An adjuvant system had to be developed. AS01, the adjuvant system ultimately chosen, includes a liposomal formulation of the immune response enhancers MPL and QS21 [9].

2 Clinical Development

The early phase 1 and 2 trials of RTS,S/AS01 explored age de-escalation, dose optimization, immunogenicity, and safety. The early studies were followed by a series of phase 2/2b studies in the target population, African children [10–17]. The pivotal phase 3 study to assess safety and efficacy was a double-blind, individually randomized trial conducted between March 2009 and February 2014 in seven countries in sub-Saharan Africa [18]. Two groups of children 6–12 weeks and 5–17 months were randomly allocated to three study arms (1) RTS,S/AS01 at months 0, 1, and 2, followed by a booster dose at month 20 (R3R group); (2) RTS,S/AS01 primary vaccination series with a meningococcal serogroup C conjugate vaccine booster (R3C group); and (3) comparator vaccines: a rabies or a meningococcal vaccine depending on age of the participants (C3C group). The administration of the vaccines in the infants was timed to coincide with the childhood vaccinations included in the Expanded Program on Immunization (EPI). 8922 children and 6537 young infants were enrolled and followed for a median of 48 and 38 months, respectively. Malaria was detected by passive surveillance.

The vaccine was less protective when children were vaccinated between 6 and 12 weeks than between 5 and 17 months of age, and a booster vaccination at 20 months provided added protection. But even with a booster, the vaccine protection against uncomplicated malaria over 48 months was only 39% (Table 1).

Intensive investigation of adverse events following vaccination suggested that overall RTS,S/AS01 is safe. However, two safety signals were detected. Firstly, there were 22 meningitis cases, caused by meningococcus, pneumococcus, and *H. influenzae* reported during the follow-up period: 21 in the vaccine group compared to a single case in the control group. The meningitis cases occurred at variable times after vaccination. The range of pathogens and the variability in time to onset make a causal

Table 1
RTS,S/AS01 efficacy against uncomplicated and severe malaria in children 6–12 weeks and 5–17 months of age [19]

Study period	6–12 weeks		5–17 months	
Vaccine efficacy against	Clinical malaria	Severe malaria	Clinical malaria	Severe malaria
2.5–14 months (95% CI)	32.9% (26.3 to 38.9)	38.5% (7.8 to 59.0)	51.3% (47.5 to 54.9)	44.5% (23.8 to 59.6)
2.5–20 months (95% CI)	26.6% (20.3 to 32.4)	17.4% (−16.2 to 41.3)	45.7% (41.7 to 49.5)	37.7% (18.0 to 52.6)
2.5 months to se[a] 3 doses (95% CI)	18.2% (11.4 to 24.5)	16.0% (−14.5 to 38.4)	26.2% (20.8 to 31.2)	−2.2% (−31.3 to 20.4)
2.5 months to se[a] 4 doses (95% CI)	26.7% (20.5 to 32.4)	20.5% (−9.8 to 42.5)	39.0% (34.3 to 43.3)	31.5% (9.3 to 48.3)

[a]Study end—median 38 months for 6–12 weeks; 48 months for 5–17 months

relationship between RTS,S/AS01 vaccination and meningitis questionable. Because the meningitis incidence in the control group was lower than the background rates, it has been suggested that children who received meningococcal or rabies vaccines as control agents were more protected against meningitis than children randomized to receive RTS,S/AS01 [20, 21]. Secondly, following vaccination with RTS,S/AS01, all-cause mortality was higher in girls (mortality ratio, 1.91; 95% CI 1.30 to 2.79) compared to boys (MR 0.84; 95% CI, 0.61 to 1.17) [22, 23]. Whether these observations could be a chance finding needs to be explored in future studies. The currently ongoing phase 4 studies will closely monitor meningitis cases in relation to RTS,S/AS01 vaccinations and sex-ratio imbalances in morbidity and mortality.

Waning protection is a major challenge for inclusion of RTS,S/AS01 in EPI childhood vaccination programs. Following vaccination in the first 2 years of life, the vaccinated children may have less immunity against malaria than unvaccinated children and may be at an increased risk after the vaccine protection has worn off resulting in a rebound or age-shift of infections. To study the long-term benefits of the vaccine, Olotu and co-workers followed a group of 223 children who had received a three-dose regimen of RTS,S/AS01 without booster between 5 and 17 months of age and a control group of 224 children [24]. After 7 years, 164 of the vaccinated children and 148 of the children in the control group could be assessed. The protection against uncomplicated malaria was overall not significant 4% (95%CI -26% to 17%). Following protection during the first 4 years after vaccination, vaccinated children were at higher risk for malaria during year 5 and 6 compared to unvaccinated children. The investigators also observed lower levels of protection in children living in high-exposure areas than children living in low-exposure areas. In the low-exposure cohort, the overall vaccine efficacy was 26% (95%CI -9% to 50%) compared to 1.9% (95%CI -21 to 20) in the high-exposure cohort. There are no comparable long-term follow-up data of children who have received a booster dose of RTS,S. Based on the available information, it is reasonable to assume that a booster dose can delay but not prevent waning vaccine efficacy.

3 Phase 4 Effectiveness Trial

The vaccine dossier including the abovementioned phase 3 safety and efficacy data were submitted to the European Medicines Agency and received a positive scientific opinion in July 2015 [25, 26]. This assessment can be used by regulatory agencies in malaria-endemic countries to accelerate the local registration of RTS,S/AS01. Subsequently the dossier was reviewed by two expert committees (the Strategic Advisory Group of Experts, SAGE and the Malaria Policy Advisory Committee, MPAC) convened in a joint session by the World Health Organization [27]. In October 2015, the expert committees concluded that a very large effectiveness trial would have to be conducted, and its findings reviewed before the inclusion of RTS,S/AS01 in African childhood vaccination programs can be recommended. In contrast to the typical phase 3 efficacy trial that assesses the safety and protection of a vaccine when given under ideal conditions, an effectiveness trial estimates the impact of the vaccine when given under real public health conditions [28]. The individually randomized RTS,S/AS01 efficacy study showed the benefit an individual derives from the vaccine regimen. Such studies cannot predict how well the vaccine will perform when rolled out in a vaccination program. The impact may be reduced by poor adherence to the vaccine regimen or can be boosted through indirect protection (herd immunity or herd protection). To assess such indirect vaccine benefits, entire communities or clusters need to be randomized. Cluster randomized trials require much larger numbers of participants compared with individually randomized trials and also allow the detection of low-frequency adverse events not detected in smaller size, individually randomized trials.

In March 2017, an outline of a large cluster randomized trial, the Malaria Vaccine Implementation Programme, was presented to MPAC [29]. The trial will be conducted in Ghana, Kenya, and Malawi. In each country, 60 clusters with about 4000 children/cluster will be randomized. Children in the vaccine arm will be vaccinated at age 5, 6, 7, and 24 months. The major outcomes of this trial will be the operational feasibility of the vaccine regimen in target countries, the impact of the vaccine on all-cause mortality (overall and by gender), malaria-specific mortality, and severe malaria. The investigators have designed the trial to be able to detect all morbidity and mortality in trial participants, with specific attention to detect meningitis cases.

4 RTS,S/AS01 Deployment Scenarios

4.1 Inclusion of RTS,S/AS01 in Childhood Vaccination Programs in Sub-Saharan Africa

An ideal vaccine for a childhood vaccination program provides near-complete and lifelong protection. When such a vaccine is introduced in a national program and administered to all young children in a sustained fashion, even without catch-up vaccinations, the entire population will become protected in a few decades (Fig. 1). Depending on the protective efficacy of the vaccine, coverage of the population, and the basic reproductive number of the pathogen, transmission will be interrupted within a variable but limited time span.

In contrast, when a four-dose RTS,S/AS01 regimen that provides protection for less than 5 years is administered to all those 5–17 months of age in a sustained fashion, the number of protected individuals will remain constant over the years. Vaccinated

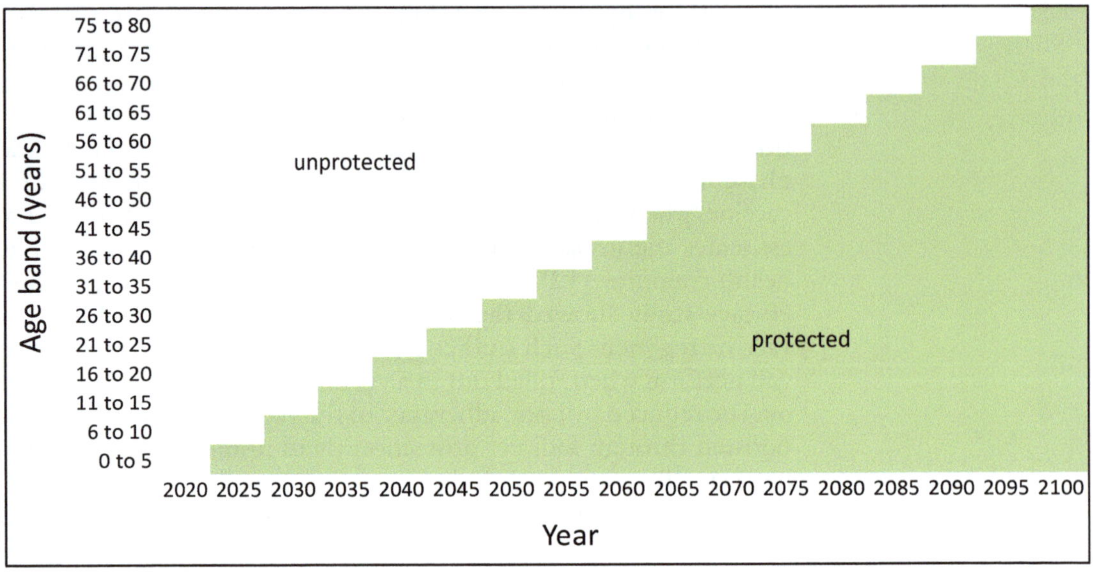

Fig. 1 Schematic representation of the progression of vaccine protection of a population participating in an ideal childhood vaccine program that confers lifelong immunity

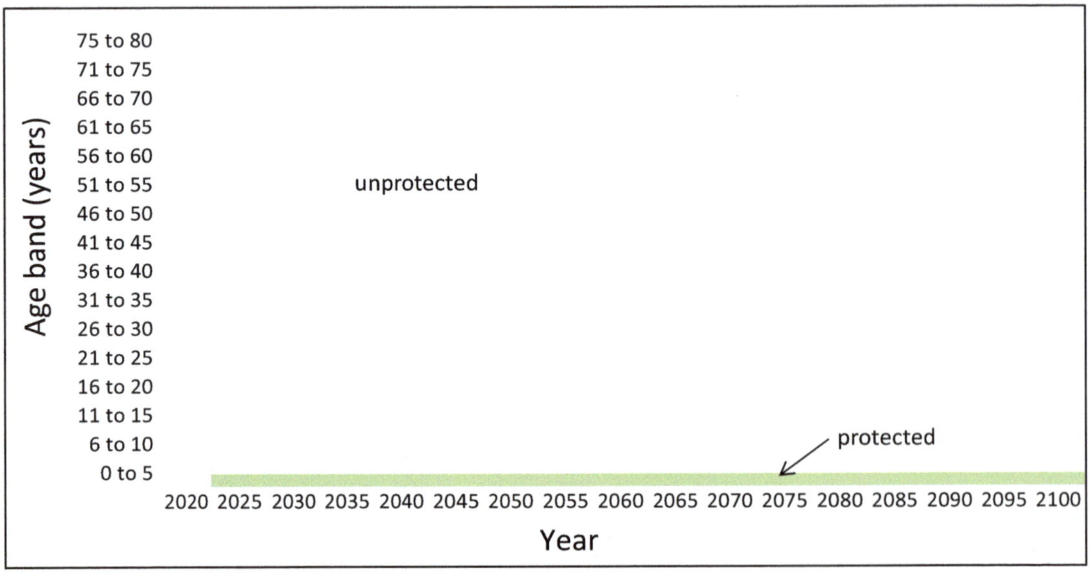

Fig. 2 Schematic representation of vaccine protection of a population participating in a less than ideal childhood vaccine program such as a RTS,S/AS01 childhood vaccination program

individuals will be protected for a short period then become susceptible again, so that at any given time, the large majority of the population is unprotected (Fig. 2).

The estimated number of averted malaria cases in the phase 3 trial RTS,S/AS01 suggests considerable individual health benefits for the vaccinated child. Considering the massive disease burden caused by malaria, the introduction of RTS,S/AS01 into childhood vaccination programs in sub-Saharan Africa is likely to make a major impact on the health of the vaccinated children.

However, there are several limitations with this deployment strategy. Firstly, the percentage of the African population under 5 years (60 months) of age is currently 8% [30]. Even if the majority of clinical malaria cases were to occur in younger children, which is no longer the case in many regions of Africa, inclusion of RTS,S/AS01 in African EPI programs would leave a large majority (92%) of the population (older children as well as adults) unprotected, resulting in sustained transmission. Since the inclusion of RTS,S/AS01 in African EPI programs would only protect a small fraction of the population at any given time and not interrupt transmission, use of RTS,S/AS01 in this fashion would not play to the strength of the vaccine. Secondly, with currently decreasing malaria transmission in many sub-Saharan African countries, the malaria disease burden has shifted from the youngest to older children. If RTS,S/AS01 were included in African EPI programs, there would be a risk that by the time the vaccinated children are most exposed, vaccine protection has waned. Inclusion of RTS,S/AS01 in African EPI programs would confine vaccine protection to a relatively narrow age band (children under five), which would make meaningful vaccine herd protection unlikely. Thirdly, potential benefits have to be weighed against the cost of the vaccine. Assuming a cost of USD $5/dose, a four-dose regimen will cost $20/child. Considering the characteristics of RTS,S/AS01, the implementation of a vaccine program should not replace other malaria control activities but has to be added to pre-existing activities such as early diagnosis and treatment, distribution of bednets, etc. National as well as international funds for malaria control and child health are limited. Hence the proposition to spend $20/child on the purchase of RTS,S/AS01 has to compete with other child health improvement strategies [31].

The work by Olotu and co-workers suggests the possibility that some of the health benefits resulting from a RTS,S/AS01 vaccination will be offset at a later stage by a rebound effect [24]. Releasing children into an unprotected environment at the end of their period of vaccine protection seems therefore unwise. Unprecedented progress is being made in the global reduction of malaria incidence. In the best of circumstances, malaria transmission will be reduced sufficiently in the coming years so that children with waning vaccine protection find themselves at a much lower risk for malaria than during earlier years [32]. A global reduction in malaria transmission could prevent a rebound or age shift. In less optimistic scenarios, it seems reasonable to consider annual RTS,S/AS01 booster doses in perpetuity following the initial four-dose regimen (5, 6, 7, 24 months). While intuitively attractive, such a perpetual vaccination program has not been tested. It is not known whether

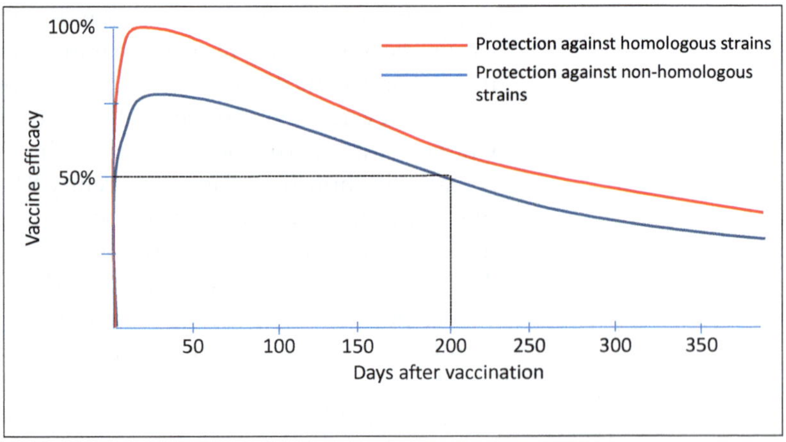

Fig. 3 The cumulative vaccine efficacy against primary or only malaria episode among children 5–17 months of age participating in the phase 3 RTS,S/AS01 trial [33]

repeated annual RTS,S/AS01 booster doses are either safe, efficacious, or feasible. If annual boosters are not implemented, other strategies including antimalarial prophylaxis have to be considered.

4.2 An Alternative Use of RTS,S/AS01

While highlighting the reasons why RTS,S/AS01 may not be ideal for an African EPI program, it is easy to overlook that this is the first vaccine which has consistently demonstrated protective efficacy and has made more progress toward registration than any other malaria vaccine candidate. Perhaps most importantly, RTS,S/AS01 provides high protection in the first 200 days after the completion of vaccination. Neafsey and co-workers explored the cumulative vaccine efficacy against first or only malaria episode depending whether the parasite strain was closely matched to the vaccine antigen (Fig. 3) [33]. Not surprising, they found that there was better protection against closely matched strains compared to more distant strains. More importantly for this discussion, they demonstrated that RTS,S/AS01 provides more than 50% protection against malaria episodes for 200 days.

An alternative use of RTS,S/AS01 would be in mass vaccination programs in areas with low malaria transmission toward the goal of elimination. To have an impact on transmission in a population, it would be critical to vaccinate all age groups of the entire population targeted for malaria elimination within a time window of less than 200 days (Fig. 4). RTS,S/AS01 has no effect on ongoing infections at the time of vaccination. In the presence of appropriate vectors, the transmission of subclinical infections seems therefore assured. To achieve an interruption of transmission, it would be mandatory to include the administration of a course of appropriate antimalarials with each vaccine dose. An ongoing trial explores whether there is an interaction between the administration

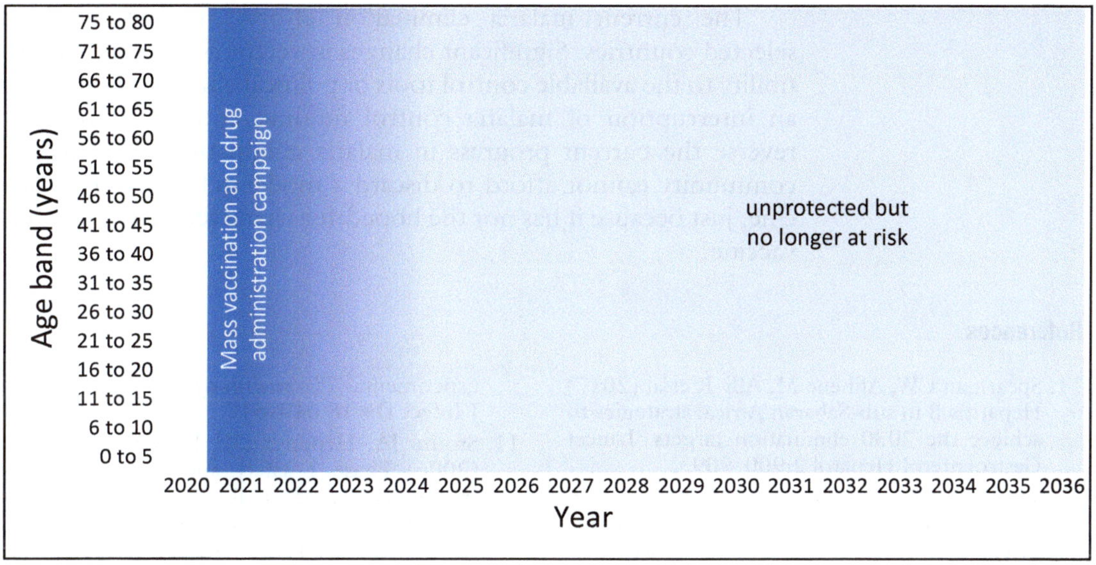

Fig. 4 A schematic representation of the impact of a combined mass vaccination and antimalarial drug administration campaign analogous to a large catch-up vaccination campaign

of dihydroartemisinin, piperaquine, and primaquine and the immunogenicity of RTS,S/AS01. Several countries in Africa, South America, and Southeast Asia have achieved very low falciparum malaria endemicity and are committed to malaria elimination. The spread of multidrug resistance in the Greater Mekong Subregion could stall and even upend these achievements [34]. In mathematical models, the combination of mass drug and vaccination campaigns can interrupt falciparum malaria transmission in a low endemicity region [35].

5 Conclusions

RTS,S/AS01 is globally the most advanced malaria vaccine. The vaccine has passed the pivotal phase 3 trial and received a positive scientific opinion from the European Medicines Agency in 2015. Confining the vaccine to a very narrow population target that foresees the use of RTS,S/AS01 exclusively in African EPI-based childhood vaccination programs would be misguided. The limited duration of protection leaves children unprotected when they are frequently most exposed. Furthermore, such programs are unlikely to have an impact on malaria transmission. A key strength of the vaccine is the early high protection afforded by the vaccine, which could be harnessed in vaccination campaigns that target all age groups within a short time window with the aim to interrupt malaria transmission.

The current malaria elimination efforts are promising in selected countries. Significant changes in vector or parasite susceptibility to the available control tools or political changes resulting in an interruption of malaria control funding could stall or even reverse the current progress in malaria elimination. The malaria community cannot afford to discard a moderately protective vaccine, just because it has not the hoped-for characteristics of an ideal vaccine.

References

1. Spearman CW, Afihene M, Ally R et al (2017) Hepatitis B in sub-Saharan Africa: strategies to achieve the 2030 elimination targets. Lancet Gastroenterol Hepatol 2:900–909
2. Wallace AS, Ryman TK, Dietz V (2014) Overview of global, regional, and national routine vaccination coverage trends and growth patterns from 1980 to 2009: implications for vaccine-preventable disease eradication and elimination initiatives. J Infect Dis 210(Suppl 1):S514–S522
3. Orenstein WA, Cairns L, Hinman A et al (2018) Measles and Rubella Global Strategic Plan 2012-2020 midterm review report: background and summary. Vaccine 36(Suppl 1): A35–A42
4. Orenstein WA, Hinman A, Nkowane B et al (2018) Measles and Rubella Global Strategic Plan 2012-2020 midterm review. Vaccine 36 (Suppl 1):A1–A34
5. Coughlin MM, Beck AS, Bankamp B et al (2017) Perspective on global measles epidemiology and control and the role of novel vaccination strategies. Viruses 9(1). https://doi.org/10.3390/v9010011
6. Thompson KM, Duintjer Tebbens RJ (2017) Lessons from the polio endgame: overcoming the failure to vaccinate and the role of subpopulations in maintaining transmission. J Infect Dis 216(suppl_1):S176–S182
7. Foege W (2011) House on fire: the fight to eradicate smallpox. University of California Press, Los Angeles, CA
8. Vekemans J, Leach A, Cohen J (2009) Development of the RTS,S/AS malaria candidate vaccine. Vaccine 27(Suppl 6):G67–G71
9. Didierlaurent AM, Laupeze B, Di Pasquale A et al (2017) Adjuvant system AS01: helping to overcome the challenges of modern vaccines. Expert Rev Vaccines 16:55–63
10. Kester KE, McKinney DA, Tornieporth N et al (2001) Efficacy of recombinant circumsporozoite protein vaccine regimens against experimental *Plasmodium falciparum* malaria. J Infect Dis 18:640–647
11. Stoute JA, Heppner DG Jr, Mason CJ et al (2006) Phase 1 safety and immunogenicity trial of malaria vaccine RTS,S/AS02A in adults in a hyperendemic region of western Kenya. Am J Trop Med Hyg 7:166–170
12. Abdulla S, Oberholzer R, Juma O et al (2008) Safety and immunogenicity of RTS,S/AS02D malaria vaccine in infants. N Engl J Med 359:2533–2544
13. Kester KE, Cummings JF, Ockenhouse CF et al (2008) Phase 2a trial of 0, 1, and 3 month and 0, 7, and 28 day immunization schedules of malaria vaccine RTS,S/AS02 in malaria-naive adults at the Walter Reed Army Institute of Research. Vaccine 26:2191–2202
14. Kester KE, Cummings JF, Ofori-Anyinam O et al (2009) Randomized, double-blind, phase 2a trial of falciparum malaria vaccines RTS,S/AS01B and RTS,S/AS02A in malaria-naive adults: safety, efficacy, and immunologic associates of protection. J Infect Dis 200:337–346
15. Kester KE, Gray Heppner D Jr, Moris P et al (2014) Sequential Phase 1 and Phase 2 randomized, controlled trials of the safety, immunogenicity and efficacy of combined pre-erythrocytic vaccine antigens RTS,S and TRAP formulated with AS02 Adjuvant System in healthy, malaria naive adults. Vaccine 32:6683–6691
16. Bejon P, Lusingu J, Olotu A et al (2008) Efficacy of RTS,S/AS01E vaccine against malaria in children 5 to 17 months of age. N Engl J Med 359:2521–2532
17. Bojang KA, Milligan PJ, Pinder M et al (2001) Efficacy of RTS,S/AS02 malaria vaccine against *Plasmodium falciparum* infection in semi-immune adult men in The Gambia: a randomised trial. Lancet 358:1927–1934
18. RTS,SCPT (2015) Efficacy and safety of RTS,S/AS01 malaria vaccine with or without a booster dose in infants and children in Africa:

final results of a phase 3, individually randomised, controlled trial. Lancet 386:31–45

19. Smith PG (2015) JTEG's summary of RTS,S/AS01 clinical trial data http://www.hoint/immunization/sage/meetings/2015/october/Smith_Malaria_Review_RTS_S_AS01_print.pdf
20. Gessner BD, Knobel DL, Conan A et al (2017) Could the RTS,S/AS01 meningitis safety signal really be a protective effect of rabies vaccine? Vaccine 35:716–721
21. Gessner BD, Wraith DC, Finn A (2016) CNS infection safety signal of RTS,S/AS01 and possible association with rabies vaccine. Lancet 387:1376
22. Aaby P, Rodrigues A, Kofoed PE et al (2015) RTS,S/AS01 malaria vaccine and child mortality. Lancet 386:1735–1736
23. Klein SL, Shann F, Moss WJ et al (2016) RTS,S malaria vaccine and increased mortality in girls. MBio 7:e00514–e00516
24. Olotu A, Fegan G, Wambua J et al (2016) Seven-year efficacy of RTS,S/AS01 malaria vaccine among young African children. N Engl J Med 374:2519–2529
25. World Health Organization (2018) Malaria vaccine: WHO position paper, January 2016 - Recommendations. Vaccine 36 (25):3576–3577. https://doi.org/10.1016/j.vaccine.2016.10.047
26. EMA (2015) European medicines agency: summary of opinion. http://www.ema europaeu/docs/en_GB/document_library/Medicine_for_use_outside_EU/2015/07/WC500190452.pdf
27. WHO (2016) Malaria vaccine: WHO position paper – January 2016. Wkly Epidemiol Rec 91 (4):33–52
28. Deen JL, Clemens JD (2006) Issues in the design and implementation of vaccine trials in less developed countries. Nat Rev Drug Discov 5:932–940
29. WHO (2017). http://www.who.int/malaria/mpac/mpac-mar2017-rtss-update-session2-presentation.pdf
30. PopulationPyramid.net (2017) Population pyramid Africa 2016. https://www.populationpyramid.net/visualizations
31. Winskill P, Walker PG, Griffin JT et al (2017) Modelling the cost-effectiveness of introducing the RTS,S malaria vaccine relative to scaling up other malaria interventions in sub-Saharan Africa. BMJ Glob Health 2:e000090
32. Bhatt S, Weiss DJ, Cameron E et al (2015) The effect of malaria control on *Plasmodium falciparum* in Africa between 2000 and 2015. Nature 526:207–211
33. Neafsey DE, Juraska M, Bedford T et al (2015) Genetic diversity and protective efficacy of the RTS,S/AS01 malaria vaccine. N Engl J Med 373:2025–2037
34. Imwong M, Suwannasin K, Kunasol C et al (2017) The spread of artemisinin-resistant *Plasmodium falciparum* in the Greater Mekong subregion: a molecular epidemiology observational study. Lancet Infect Dis 17:491–497
35. Tun STT, von Seidlein L, Pongvongsa T et al (2017) Towards malaria elimination in Savannakhet, Lao PDR: mathematical modelling driven strategy design. Malar J 16:483

Chapter 14

Live Vaccines Against Plasmodium Preerythrocytic Stages

Laura Mac-Daniel and Robert Ménard

Abstract

Vaccines that target the preerythrocytic phase of malaria hold great promise as elimination tools since they are the sole vaccines that can achieve sterile protection against a challenge. This chapter focuses on preerythrocytic stage vaccines based on live attenuated parasites. It first summarizes the main conclusions that have emerged from studies in rodents, which compared various parasite attenuation methods, and then presents the vaccination regimens that are currently being tested in humans.

Key words Malaria, Live vaccine, Subunit vaccine, Preerythrocytic stages, Radiation-attenuated sporozoites, Parasites attenuated by chemotherapy, Genetically attenuated parasites

1 Introduction

Vaccines are a highly desirable tool for reducing the burden of, and potentially eliminating, malaria. Of the three types of experimental malaria vaccines that target the preerythrocytic or erythrocytic stages in the vertebrate host, or parasite development in the mosquito, the former offer several advantages. The PE phase is the major bottleneck of the parasite life cycle, as only a few tens of sporozoites are deposited in the skin following a mosquito bite. This parasite form, which is extracellular, may be neutralized by specific antibodies before they invade hepatocytes. The ensuing liver stage of the parasite may then be targeted by cytotoxic T cells, since parasite epitopes can be processed and presented on the hepatocyte surface in association with MHC Class I molecules. Importantly, only PE vaccines have been shown capable of generating sterilizing immunity, defined as the complete clearance of challenge parasites in an immunized host. Therefore, an efficient PE vaccine prevents not only blood infection and the clinical symptoms but also parasite transmission.

Frédéric Ariey et al. (eds.), *Malaria Control and Elimination*, Methods in Molecular Biology, vol. 2013,
https://doi.org/10.1007/978-1-4939-9550-9_14,

2 Subunit Versus Live Vaccine Approaches

Malaria PE vaccine development has been dominated during the last three decades by subunit vaccines. Today, the most advanced subunit vaccine is RTS,S, which consists of the fusion of the hepatitis B surface antigen to epitopes of the *P. falciparum* CS protein. As detailed in a dedicated chapter, the RTS,S phase III field study displayed significant, though moderate, efficacy. Other subunit PE vaccine candidates have been tested, based on a handful of PE parasite antigens and using viral vectors in prime-boost approaches [1], which have also failed so far to generate convincing results. In contrast, vaccination with attenuated "whole organisms" is known to trigger broad immune responses against a large number of parasite antigens, which is hoped to help circumvent the problems posed by the diversity and polymorphism of parasite targets. In the last 15 years, attenuated parasites have eclipsed subunit preparations as an anti-malaria PE vaccine for humans, because of the increasingly recognized efficacy of the former and the suboptimal achievements of the latter.

3 Live PE Vaccine Approaches: Lessons from Rodents

Live PE vaccines are expected to develop sufficiently to generate protective immunity, without generating symptomatic blood infection. Three means of arresting parasite development in the liver, or immediately after, have been used: (a) irradiation of the sporozoite, causing the ensuing liver stage to arrest its development at the time of nuclear division; (b) co-delivery of normally infective sporozoite with an anti-malarial drug; or (c) genetic modification of the parasite, causing the immunizing parasite to arrest at a defined point. The three approaches have been studied in rodents, which are briefly summarized below.

3.1 Radiation-Attenuated Sporozoites (RAS)

The concept that irradiated sporozoites induce sterile protection was first demonstrated in rodents [2]. The intravenous injection of *P. berghei* X-radiation-attenuated sporozoites into mice protected 2 weeks later against an intravenous challenge with sporozoites, but not against blood-stage parasites. Subsequent RAS studies in rodents showed that (a) RAS were normally motile and cell invasive; (b) RAS-derived liver stages were blocked midway through their development; and (c) irradiated, blocked liver stages were the important immunogens that triggered protection. Immunological studies then showed that antibodies from RAS-immunized mice, especially those directed to the CS protein, could neutralize sporozoites and that cytotoxic T cells, primarily $CD8^+$ T cells, contributed to anti-liver stage immunity [3].

3.2 Parasites Attenuated by Chemotherapy

A number of drugs that impair parasite development in the liver and beyond have been used in protocols called chemoprophylaxis with sporozoites (CPS). The first drug used in CPS protocols was chloroquine (CQ) [4], which has no activity against sporozoites or liver stages but kills erythrocytic stages during their initial multiplication cycles. CQ-CPS-induced protection was found to be more robust than that induced by RAS and to depend purely on PE, not erythrocytic, immunity, indicating that the increased protection was due to the complete development of the immunizing parasites in the liver. Antibiotics that inhibit the replication of the apicoplast in the liver stage, namely, azithromycin and clindamycin, were also used in CPS approaches. These drugs cause the formation of hepatic merozoites that fail to replicate inside RBC. Azithromycin/clindamycin-CPS-induced protection was found to be stronger and more durable than that induced by CQ-CPS [5]. This is thought to be due to the suppressive effect of blood-stage multiplication, which occurs using CQ but not azithromycin or clindamycin, on PE immunity [6]. Therefore maximal liver-stage development and minimal blood-stage development appear to confer the strongest protection against liver stages [7].

3.3 Genetically Attenuated Parasites (GAP)

GAP of interest are genetically modified in erythrocytic stages and are developmentally arrested specifically after sporozoite invasion of hepatocytes. Since the report of the first protective GAP [8], many others were generated that can be divided into four groups, depending on the time of parasite arrest during its development in the liver [9]. The very early-blocked and early-blocked GAP lack a protein involved in the formation/maintenance (P36, P52, B9, SLARP/SAP1) or the function (UIS3, UIS4), respectively, of the parasitophorous vacuole membrane. As expected, these very early- or early-blocked GAP induce protection that is not stronger than that conferred by RAS. The late-blocked GAP, which regroup mutants devoid of the apicoplast-resident type II fatty acid synthesis (FAS II) pathway, and the very late-blocked GAP, such as the PALM-deficient mutant defective in liver merozoite formation, confer stronger protection than RAS. One late-blocked FASII mutant, the *P. yoelii* FABB/F^- GAP, was shown to induce broader $CD8^+$ T cell responses than RAS as well as some degree of cross-stage and cross-species (*P. berghei*) protection [10]. Therefore, late liver-stage development may enhance protective efficacy by allowing the presentation of a larger set of antigens to the immune system.

4 Live Approaches in Humans

The demonstration that RAS were also protective in humans was brought in the early 1970s [11]. However, RAS had to be delivered by mosquito bites, and the bites of more than thousand

P. falciparum RAS-infected mosquitoes, divided into 7–10 immunization sessions over a period of almost a year, were required for protection. The interest in live vaccination approaches in humans subsequently dropped as it was thought that, with the advent of molecular biology, the development of more practical subunit malaria vaccines was merely a question of time.

To date, only RAS and CPS methods have been tested in humans and exclusively in malaria naive adults. A single *P. falciparum* GAP entered a phase I clinical trial, the very early-blocked P56$^-$P32$^-$ double mutant [12]. However, it induced a breakthrough infection in one volunteer (subjected to ~200 bites of GAP-infected mosquitoes), which caused the trial to terminate. No other GAP was tested since.

4.1 CPS and Mosquito Bites

In the years 2000, the first success in protecting humans against malaria PE stages was achieved using a CQ-CPS trial conducted in the Netherlands (Table 1). Ten volunteers were immunized three times by the bites of 12–15 *P. falciparum*-infected mosquitoes, while under CQ cover; 8 weeks after the final immunization, all immunized volunteers were protected against a challenge by the bites of five mosquitoes [13]. Moreover, six of the ten volunteers protected at 8 weeks were rechallenged after 28 months, and four were still protected [14]. Protection was therefore remarkably solid and durable. The same group later showed that, like in rodents, CQ-CPS-induced immunity was directed exclusively at the liver-stage, as it protected against a sporozoite, but not blood-stage, challenge [15]. It also revealed that similar protection was obtained using CQ or mefloquine (MQ) and that the CQ/MQ-CPS approach was ~20 times more protective than RAS immunization [16].

4.2 RAS (PfSPZ^{irr}) and Parenteral Injection

The biotechnology company Sanaria was founded in 2003 to manufacture a vaccine based on cryopreserved, aseptic, purified, X-irradiated NF54 *P. falciparum* sporozoites, called here PfSPZ^{irr} [17], for parenteral inoculation into humans. The first vials of the PfSPZ^{irr} vaccine were produced in 2010 [18]. Similarly, cryopreserved, aseptic, purified, non-irradiated NF54 *P. falciparum* sporozoites, called here PfSPZ^{WT}, were also manufactured, for CPS regimens as well as quantitative challenges (controlled human malaria infection, CHMI).

Three clinical trials of the PfSPZ^{irr} vaccine have been conducted in adult, malaria-naive volunteers in the USA (Table 2). In the first trial [19], the PfSPZ^{irr} vaccine was administered intradermally (ID) or subcutaneously (SC). However, despite large immunizing doses, immunization was not protective against the bites of five *P. falciparum*-infected *Anopheles stephensi* mosquitoes 3 weeks after the last immunization. In the second trial [20], the PfSPZ^{irr} vaccine was injected IV. Five injections of 135,000 PfSPZ^{irr}

Table 1
CPS approach, immunization by mosquito bites

Immunization				Challenge 1			Challenge 2			
Drug	Parasite	Dose[a]	Interval[b]	Dose[c]	Time[d]	Protection	Dose[c]	Time[d]	Protection	Reference
CQ[e]	NF54	3 × 15	1 m	5 mos	8 w	10/10	5 m	28 m	4/6	[13, 14]
CQ[e]	NF54 + 3D7	3 × 15	1 m	5 mos	21 w	5/5				[15]
CQ[e]	NF54 + 3D7	3 × 15	1 m	iRBC[f]	21 w	0/9				[15]
CQ[g]	NF54	3 × 8	1 m	5 mos	20 w	3/5				[16]
MQ[h]	NF54	3 × 8	1 m	5 mos	20 w	7/10				[16]

[a]Three sessions of bites of 15 or 8 Pf-infected *Anopheles stephensi* mosquitoes for 15 min; starting 8 days after the start of CQ prophylaxis and 22 days after the start of MQ prophylaxis
[b]Interval between two immunizing doses (m, month)
[c]Challenge by bites of five *P. falciparum*-infected *Anopheles stephensi* mosquitoes or injection of infected red blood cells (iRBC)
[d]Time after the last immunization (w, week; m, month)
[e]CQ prophylaxis: loading dose of 300 mg on first and second day, then 300 mg once a week for 13 weeks
[f]Challenge by 1962 viable *P. falciparum*-infected RBC injected IV
[g]CQ prophylaxis: loading dose of 300 mg on first and fourth day, then 300 mg once a week for 12 weeks
[h]MQ prophylaxis: loading dose of 125 mg twice a week for 3 weeks, followed by 250 mg once a week for 12 weeks

Table 2
PfSPZ[irr]

Immunization			Challenge 1			Challenge 2			
Doses	Route	Interval[a]	Dose[b]	Time[c]	Protection	Dose[b]	Time[c]	Protection	Reference
4–6 × 7500–135,000	ID/SC	1 m	5 mosq	3 w	2/44				[19]
4 × 135,000	IV	1 m	5 mosq	3 w	6/9				[20]
5 × 135,000	IV	1 m[d]	5 mosq	3 w	6/6	5 mos	21 w	2/6	[20, 21]
3 × 270,000	IV	1 m	5 mosq	3 w	3/9	5 mos	25 w	2/3	[21]
4 × 270,000 (1)	IV	1 m	5 mosq	3 w	7/9	5 mos	24 w	3/4	[21]
4 × 270,000 (2)	IV	1 m	5 mosq	21 w	6/11	5 mos	59 w	5/5	[21]
4 × 2,200,000	IM	1 m	5 mosq	3 w	3/8	5 mos	25 w	0/3	[21]

[a]Interval between two immunizing doses (m, month)
[b]Bites of five *P. falciparum-infected Anopheles stephensi* mosquitoes
[c]Time after last immunization (w, week)
[d]Seven week-interval between fourth and fifth dose

protected all (6/6) volunteers against a challenge by the bites of five mosquitoes; however, of the six volunteers protected at 3 weeks, four were not protected upon rechallenge at 21 weeks [21]. In the third trial [21], the schedule of four IV injections of 270,000 PfSPZ^{irr} was found to be the most protective; in one group, it protected 6/11 volunteers at 21 weeks, and 5/5 of those protected at 21 weeks were still protected at 59 weeks. Decreasing immunization to three IV injections of 270,000 PfSPZ^{irr}, however, only protected 3/9 volunteers at 3 weeks. Despite much higher doses, IM inoculation of PfSPZ^{irr} was poorly protective.

These human trials also indicated a dose-dependent increase in the frequency of PfSPZ-specific antibodies as well as CD4$^+$ and CD8$^+$ memory T cells producing any combination of IFN-γ, IL-2, or TNFα. In addition they also suggested that CD8$^+$ T cells are primarily confined to the liver and that γδ T cells play an important role in protection [14, 20, 21].

4.3 CPS and Parenteral Injection of PfSPZ^{WT}

The PfSPZ^{WT} manufactured by Sanaria were also tested in a CQ-CPS protocol [22]. In this trial (Table 3), three doses of 512,000 PfSPZ^{WT} inoculated IV under CQ cover protected all volunteers against a challenge by 3200 PfSPZ^{WT} injected by direct venous inoculation (DVI) at 10 weeks. This confirmed the much stronger protection afforded by CQ-CPS than RAS, due to the complete development of PfSPZ^{WT} in the liver. Lower doses of PfSPZ^{WT}, however, failed to protect all volunteers.

4.4 Homologous Versus Heterologous Challenge

In all rodent and human trials conducted so far, all challenges were performed using the same strain as that used for immunization (homologous challenge). Two recent studies [23, 24] have addressed the question of whether immunization with PfSPZ^{irr} could protect against a challenge with a heterologous strain, i.e., whether it would potentially protect against the variety of strains

Table 3
CQ-CPS approach, immunization by PfSPZ^{WT}

Immunization				Challenge			
Drug	Dose	Route	Interval[a]	Dose[b]	Time[c]	Protection	Reference
CQ[d]	3 × 51,200	IV	1 m	3200 IV	10 w	9/9	[22]
CQ[d]	3 × 12,800	IV	1 m	3200 IV	10 w	6/9	[22]
CQ[d]	3 × 3200	IV	1 m	3200 IV	10 w	3/9	[22]

[a]Interval between two immunizing doses (m, month)
[b]Challenge by PfSPZ^{WT} injected IV
[c]Time after the last immunization (w, week)
[d]All volunteers received oral chemoprophylaxis with CQ starting with a loading of 620 mg two days before first PfSPZ inoculation followed by weekly maintenance doses (5 mg kg^{-1}) through five days after last PfSPZ inoculation

Table 4
PfSPZ[irr], homologous vs. heterologous challenge

			Challenge 1			Challenge 2			
Doses	Route	Interval[a]	Homo/ hetero[b]	Time[c]	Protection	Homo/ hetero[b]	Time[c]	Protection	Reference
5 × 270,000 (1)	IV	1 m[d]	Homo	3 w	12/13	Homo	24 w	7/10	[23]
5 × 270,000 (2)	IV	1 m[d]	Hetero	3 w	4/5[e]	Hetero	24 w	1/10[e]	[23]
3 × 900,000	IV	8 w	Homo	19 w	9/14	Hetero	33 w	5/6	[24]

[a]Interval between two immunizations
[b]Bites of five *Anopheles stephensi* mosquitoes infected by a homologous (3D7) or heterologous (7G8) strain of *P. falciparum*
[c]Time after last immunization (w, week)
[d]8 week-interval between fourth and fifth dose
[e]In this group subjected to heterologous challenge, several volunteers underwent challenge 2 in the absence of analysis of protective efficacy after challenge 1

found in nature (Table 4). To this end, challenges were performed with homologous parasites using the 3D7 clone derived from the NF54 strain, which are of African origin, or heterologous parasites using the 7G8 clone, which is of Brazilian origin. One study [23] indicated a significantly lower protection level when challenging with the heterologous strain. The second study [24], using much larger immunizing doses, showed strong protection upon challenge with the heterologous strain.

5 Conclusion

Although live attenuated parasites appear to have greater potential than subunit vaccines in stimulating strong and lasting PE immunity, their transformation into a usable human vaccine is not an easy task. One limiting factor is the requirement of a cold chain to deliver the cryopreserved parasites. Another is the need for IV administration of the vaccine, which is currently not approved for public health preventive interventions and, in any event, is impractical in infants. Hopefully, a very late-blocked GAP will be engineered that is much more protective than RAS and therefore allows for lower doses and possibly a skin administration route. Finding the right genes and ensuring the absence of breakthrough infection by the GAP is the major difficulty of this approach.

Two additional questions persist. One is the capacity of a live attenuated vaccine to confer strain-transcendent immunity, an issue that is still not clarified [23, 24]. Another question is whether responses in semi-immune individuals in endemic areas match those of naive adults in the West, i.e., whether pre-existing immunity affects the mounting of protective immunity. A recent study [25] addressed this question: 30 healthy, semi-immune young adults living in the malaria-endemic region of Bioko Island, Equatorial Guinea, immunized with three doses of 2.7×10^5 $PfSPZ^{irr}$ by IV inoculation, developed a significantly lower antibody responses than US adults who received the same immunization regimen. The next clinical trials that will be conducted in Africa will determine whether long-term exposure to natural infection indeed leads to the downregulation of immune responses against the parasite.

References

1. Ewer KJ, Sierra-Davidson K, Salman AM et al (2015) Progress with viral vectored malaria vaccines: a multi-stage approach involving 'unnatural immunity. Vaccine 33:7444–7451
2. Nussenzweig RS, Vanderberg J, Most H et al (1967) Protective immunity produced by the injection of X-irradiated sporozoites of *Plasmodium berghei*. Nature 216:161–163
3. Tse SW, Radtke AJ, Zavala F (2011) Induction and maintenance of protective CD8+ T cells against malaria liver stages: implications for vaccine development. Mem Inst Oswaldo Cruz 106(Suppl 1):172–178
4. Beaudoin RL, Strome CP, Mitchell F et al (1977) *Plasmodium berghei*: immunization of mice against the ANKA strain using the unaltered sporozoite as an antigen. Exp Parasitol 42:1–5
5. Friesen J, Silvie O, Putrianti ED et al (2010) Natural immunization against malaria: causal prophylaxis with antibiotics. Sci Transl Med 2:40ra49
6. Orjih AU, Nussenzweig RS (1979) *Plasmodium berghei*: suppression of antibody response to sporozoite stage by acute blood stage infection. Clin Exp Immunol 38:1–8
7. Nganou-Makamdop K, Sauerwein RW (2013) Liver or blood-stage arrest during malaria sporozoite immunization: the later the better? Trends Parasitol 29:304–310
8. Mueller AK, Labaeid M, Kappe SH et al (2005) Genetically modified *Plasmodium* parasites as a protective experimental malaria vaccine. Nature 433:164–167
9. Bijker EM, Borrmann S, Kappe SH et al (2015) Novel approaches to whole sporozoite vaccination against malaria. Vaccine 33:7462–7468
10. Butler NS, Schmidt NW, Vaughan AM et al (2011) Superior antimalarial immunity after vaccination with late liver stage-arresting genetically attenuated parasites. Cell Host Microbe 9:451–462
11. Clyde DF, Most H, McCarthy VC et al (1973) Immunization of man against sporozoite-induced falciparum malaria. Am J Med Sci 266:169–177
12. Spring M, Murphy J, Nielsen R et al (2013) First-in-human evaluation of genetically attenuated *Plasmodium falciparum* sporozoites administered by bite of *Anopheles* mosquitoes to adult volunteers. Vaccine 31:4975–4983
13. Roestenberg M, McCall M, Hopman J et al (2009) Protection against a malaria challenge by sporozoite inoculation. N Engl J Med 361:468–477
14. Roestenberg M, Teirlinck AC, McCall MB et al (2011) Long-term protection against malaria after experimental sporozoite inoculation: an open-label follow-up study. Lancet 377:1770–1776
15. Bijker EM, Bastiaens GJ, Teirlinck AC et al (2013) Protection against malaria after immunization by chloroquine prophylaxis and sporozoites is mediated by preerythrocytic immunity. Proc Natl Acad Sci U S A 110:7862–7867
16. Bijker EM, Schats R, Obiero JM et al (2014) Sporozoite immunization of human volunteers under mefloquine prophylaxis is safe, immunogenic and protective: a double-blind randomized controlled clinical trial. PLoS One 9: e112910
17. Luke TC, Hoffman SL (2003) Rationale and plans for developing a non-replicating, metabolically active, radiation-attenuated *Plasmodium falciparum* sporozoite vaccine. J Exp Biol 206:3803–3808
18. Hoffman SL, Billingsley PF, James E et al (2010) Development of a metabolically active, non-replicating sporozoite vaccine to prevent

Plasmodium falciparum malaria. Hum Vaccin 6:97–106

19. Epstein JE, Tewari K, Lyke KE et al (2011) Live attenuated malaria vaccine designed to protect through hepatic $CD8^+$ T cell immunity. Science 334:475–480
20. Seder RA, Chang LJ, Enama ME et al (2013) Protection against malaria by intravenous immunization with a nonreplicating sporozoite vaccine. Science 341:1359–1365
21. Ishizuka AS, Lyke KE, DeZure A et al (2016) Protection against malaria at 1 year and immune correlates following PfSPZ vaccination. Nat Med 22:614–623
22. Mordmüller B, Surat G, Lagler H et al (2017) Sterile protection against human malaria by chemoattenuated PfSPZ vaccine. Nature 542:445–449
23. Epstein JE, Paolino KM, Richie TL et al (2017) Protection against *Plasmodium falciparum* malaria by PfSPZ vaccine. JCI Insight 2: e89154
24. Lyke KE, Ishizuka AS, Berry AA et al (2017) Attenuated PfSPZ vaccine induces strain-transcending T cells and durable protection against heterologous controlled human malaria infection. Proc Natl Acad Sci U S A 114:2711–2716
25. Olutu A, Urbano V, Hamad A et al (2018) Advancing global health through development and clinical trials partnerships: a randomized, placebo-controlled, double-blind assessment of safety, tolerability, and immunogenicity of PfSPZ vaccine for malaria in healthy Equatoguinean men. Am J Trop Med Hyg 98:308–318

Chapter 15

Development of Blood Stage Malaria Vaccines

Aneesh Vijayan and Chetan E. Chitnis

Abstract

The blood stage of the malaria parasite life cycle is responsible for all the clinical symptoms of malaria. During the blood stage, *Plasmodium* merozoites invade and multiply within host red blood cells (RBCs). Here, we review the progress made, challenges faced, and new strategies available for the development of blood stage malaria vaccines. We discuss our current understanding of immune responses against blood stages and the status of clinical development of various blood stage malaria vaccine candidates. We then discuss possible paths forward to develop effective blood stage malaria vaccines. This includes a discussion of protective immune mechanisms that can be elicited to target blood stage parasites, novel delivery systems, immunoassays and animal models to optimize vaccine candidates in preclinical studies, and use of challenge models to get an early readout of vaccine efficacy.

Key words Malaria, Malaria vaccines, Immunity to malaria, Vaccine development, Blood stage vaccines

1 Introduction

Malaria remains a major public health problem in many parts of the tropical world. Intensive application of malaria control tools including insecticide-treated nets (ITNs), indoor residual spraying of insecticides (IRS), early detection with rapid diagnostic tests (RDTs), and treatment with artemisinin combined therapy (ACTs) has led to significant reduction in the number of malaria cases and malaria-related deaths over the past two decades. From an estimated 500 million cases of malaria each year in the 1990s that caused as many as 1 million deaths annually, malaria incidence and malaria-related deaths reduced to 210 million malaria cases in 2015 that resulted in 440,000 deaths [1]. However, in 2016, 215 million malaria cases and 445,000 malaria-related deaths were reported, suggesting that the effectiveness of current approaches for malaria control may have reached a plateau [2]. Moreover, the currently used control methods are highly resource intensive and require continuous application. Any reduction or interruption in the application of malaria control tools is followed with a rebound of malaria

Frédéric Ariey et al. (eds.), *Malaria Control and Elimination*, Methods in Molecular Biology, vol. 2013, https://doi.org/10.1007/978-1-4939-9550-9_15,

transmission. Also, while the currently used tools described above are effective at controlling *P. falciparum* infections, they are less effective at dealing with *Plasmodium vivax*, which represents more than 50% of malaria cases in many endemic regions of the tropics outside Africa [1, 2]. *P. vivax* is more difficult to control due to its unique biology, which includes the latent hypnozoite stage in the liver and the early appearance of gametocytes, which can be transmitted even before symptoms develop and the patient seeks antimalarial drug treatment [3]. For these reasons, the availability of effective vaccines that protect individuals as well as block transmission of *P. falciparum* and *P. vivax* would be valuable tools that could synergize with other control efforts to effectively control and eventually eliminate malaria.

Malaria parasites have a complex life cycle and infect two distinct cell types in humans. *Plasmodium* sporozoites traverse through host epithelial and endothelial cells following injection by the mosquito to finally invade hepatocytes in the liver, where they start to multiply and differentiate into merozoites that are released into the bloodstream. *Plasmodium* merozoites invade and multiply within host erythrocytes to establish a blood stage infection. All the clinical symptoms associated with malaria arise during the blood stage of the parasite life cycle. During the blood stage, some of the parasites differentiate into male and female gametocytes, which are responsible for parasite transmission. The gametocytes undergo the process of gametogenesis in the mosquito midgut to form male and female gametes, which fertilize to form zygotes. The zygotes transform into ookinetes that traverse the midgut epithelium to form oocysts. Thousands of sporozoites emerge from each oocyst and find their way to the salivary glands to complete the parasite life cycle. *Plasmodium* parasites thus have a complex life cycle with multiple stages and diverse morphological forms. Efforts to develop malaria vaccines have targeted the parasite either at the preerythrocytic stage to prevent infection, at the blood stage to target the form responsible for the clinical symptoms, or the sexual and mosquito stages to prevent transmission. Here, we will review the approaches used and progress made in the development of malaria vaccines that target the blood stage of malaria parasites.

2 Rationale for Blood Stage Vaccines for Malaria

The rationale for a blood stage malaria vaccine is based on the fact that individuals who are repeatedly exposed to *P. falciparum* in endemic areas develop immunity to clinical disease and blood stage infection [4]. Naturally acquired protective immune responses that develop following exposure to malaria parasites are primarily directed against *P. falciparum* blood stages. Seminal studies first conducted in the 1960s showed that passive transfer of immunoglobulins from malaria-exposed immune individuals to children infected with *P. falciparum* cleared blood stage parasites [5, 6]. Protection against blood stage parasites appears to primarily be dependent on acquisition of antibodies against parasite target antigens. Identification of the antigens that serve as targets of such protective immune responses has been the holy grail of blood stage malaria vaccine research.

One of the first approaches used to identify potential merozoite antigens that could be targeted by antibodies was to generate monoclonal antibodies against antigens on the surface of *P. falciparum* merozoites. The first merozoite proteins identified using this approach included the *P. falciparum* merozoite surface protein-1 (PfMSP1) and *P. falciparum* apical merozoite antigen-1 (PfAMA1) [7, 8]. While PfMSP1 is constitutively expressed on the merozoite surface, PfAMA1 is initially localized in internal apical organelles referred to as micronemes and is secreted to the merozoite surface during invasion. PfMSP1 is a 195 kDa protein that is proteolytically processed during invasion so that a C-terminal 42 kDa fragment is anchored to the merozoite surface and forms a complex with other proteolytic fragments of PfMSP1 as well as other merozoite surface proteins. Following a final proteolytic step, only a 19 kDa fragment of PfMSP1 (PfMSP1$_{19}$), which contains a conserved cysteine-rich region with homology to epidermal growth factor (EGF)-like domains, remains on the merozoite surface as it enters the RBC. Antibodies directed against PfMSP1$_{19}$ inhibit RBC invasion by merozoites [9]. PfAMA1 contains conserved cysteines that form three disulfide-linked subdomains. Antibodies directed against PfAMA1 also inhibit RBC invasion by *P. falciparum* merozoites [10]. Based on these observations, PfMSP1 and PfAMA1 were the first leading malaria vaccine candidates.

Other routes to identification of blood stage malaria vaccine candidates have taken a functional approach to identify parasite proteins that bind RBC receptors to mediate invasion. *P. falciparum* proteins identified using this approach include the erythrocyte-binding antigen family (EBA family) and the PfRH family [11]. The EBA family comprises of PfEBA175 that binds sialic acid residues on glycophorin A, its homologues PfEBA181 and PfEBA140 that bind other RBC receptors, as well as an orthologue from *P. vivax* referred to as the *P. vivax* Duffy binding protein (PvDBP), which binds the Duffy antigen to mediate invasion. The PfRH family, which includes PfRH1a/b, PfRH2a/b, PfRH4, and PfRH5, shares homology with the *P. vivax* reticulocyte-binding proteins. Antibodies to EBA and PfRH family proteins inhibit RBC invasion by *P. falciparum* and are therefore considered candidates worth exploring for malaria vaccine development. Of these proteins, PfRH5, which binds the receptor basigin on RBCs, is the only one that cannot be deleted by genetic manipulation suggesting that it plays a critical, essential role in invasion [12]. Moreover, PfRH5 is highly conserved, and antibodies raised against PfRH5 effectively block RBC invasion by diverse *P. falciparum* field isolates [13]. PfRH5 is thus the leading candidate for inclusion in blood stage malaria vaccines.

Another approach to identify *P. falciparum* and *P. vivax* blood stage vaccine candidates has used field-based longitudinal cohort studies to identify antigens that are the targets of protective antibody responses. Such studies have used longitudinal cohorts of children in malaria-endemic regions to identify associations between presence of antibodies against specific antigens and reduction in the risk of malaria incidence or infection with *P. falciparum* or *P. vivax*. These studies suggest that a broad repertoire of antibody responses against diverse merozoite antigens is associated with protection against malaria [14–19]. No single antigen stands out as the protective antigen in such studies. Some *P. falciparum* blood stage antigens that have shown strong association with protection include proteins such as PfRH2b, PfEBA175, PfEBA140, RON2, and RON4, all of which have been shown to play important functional roles in invasion. In other studies, naturally acquired antibodies to an essential protein complex, PfRH5-PfRIPR-PfCyRPA, on merozoites that aids RBC invasion were shown to be associated with protection [20–22]. Antibodies elicited against these highly conserved antigens are capable of inhibiting blood stage growth of diverse *P. falciparum* strains in vitro [22]. Identification of combinations of such key merozoite antigens [19, 23] that can synergize to control blood stage parasite growth effectively may be key to identifying antigens for a multicomponent vaccine for malaria. In case of *P. vivax*, a combinatorial analysis using data from a cohort study on immune responses to *P. vivax* identified that the following antigens, PvEBP, PvDBP, P41, PvCyrPA, PvRBP1a, and PVX_018550, were most commonly present in combinations of five antigens that had the most significant association with protection [16]. These studies in both *P. falciparum* and *P. vivax* suggest that development of an effective blood stage vaccine will require a combination of antigens that elicits antibody responses that act additively or synergistically to achieve significant levels of protection.

In addition to simply measuring antigen recognition titers by ELISA, the use of functional assays to analyze antibody responses can provide insights into potential mechanisms of protective immunity. For example, in vitro receptor-binding assays based on PvDBP-Duffy antigen [24] or PfEBA175-glycophorin A [25] interactions have demonstrated that presence of antibodies that inhibit these interactions is associated with protection against *P. vivax* and *P. falciparum*, respectively. In addition to antibodies that target receptor-ligand interactions to limit blood stage growth, antibodies that target parasites by other mechanisms have also been proposed. These include antibodies against merozoite surface proteins that elicit complement-mediated mechanisms that can lyse merozoites [26] as well as antibody-dependent cellular mechanisms such as opsonic phagocytosis of merozoites [17] or infected RBCs [27] and antibody-dependent cellular inhibition of blood stage parasite growth, which involves monocytes [28]. Some targets of such antibody responses include PfMSP1, PfMSP2, PfMSP3, glutamate rich protein (GLURP), and PfEMP1. Several vaccine candidates based on these antigens are in early phase clinical development.

The introduction of controlled human malaria infection (CHMI) has further extended our understanding of development of anti-parasite immunity. A trial in which volunteers were exposed to low doses of *P. falciparum* sporozoites delivered by infectious mosquito bites under cover of chloroquine resulted in the development of immune responses that provided complete protection against subsequent challenge with *P. falciparum* sporozoites [29]. Analysis of immune responses following CHMI showed that protection was mediated by effector memory T cells against infected erythrocytes that secrete multiple cytokines including INF-γ, TNF-α, and IL2 [29]. Furthermore, it was observed that antibodies against blood stage antigens such as PfMSP1 and PfAMA1 did not correlate with protection in this model. In an alternative approach, repeated administration of "ultralow" doses of *P. falciparum*-infected RBCs followed by drug treatment before parasites reached patency also elicited complete protection against subsequent blood stage challenge. Immunity elicited in this model also did not involve antibodies and was completely dependent on CD4+ and CD8+ T cells and secretion of IFN-γ [30]. These approaches suggest the possibility of developing attenuated blood stage parasites as vaccines to elicit protection against malaria. Moreover, they demonstrate the possibility of protective T-cell responses against blood stage malaria parasites. Figure 1 shows a summary of naturally acquired and vaccine-induced immune responses that may play a role in protection against blood stage malaria parasites.

3 Blood Stage Malaria Vaccine Candidates Under Clinical Development

A number of clinical trials have evaluated blood stage malaria vaccine candidates in recent years. The major *P. falciparum* merozoite antigens that have been evaluated for their vaccine potential in clinical trials include PfMSP1, PfMSP3, PfAMA1, GLURP, SERA5, EBA175, and PfRH5. In case of *P. vivax*, the only blood stage antigen tested in clinical trials is PvDBP. Here, we will review results of some of the clinical trials with these blood stage antigens.

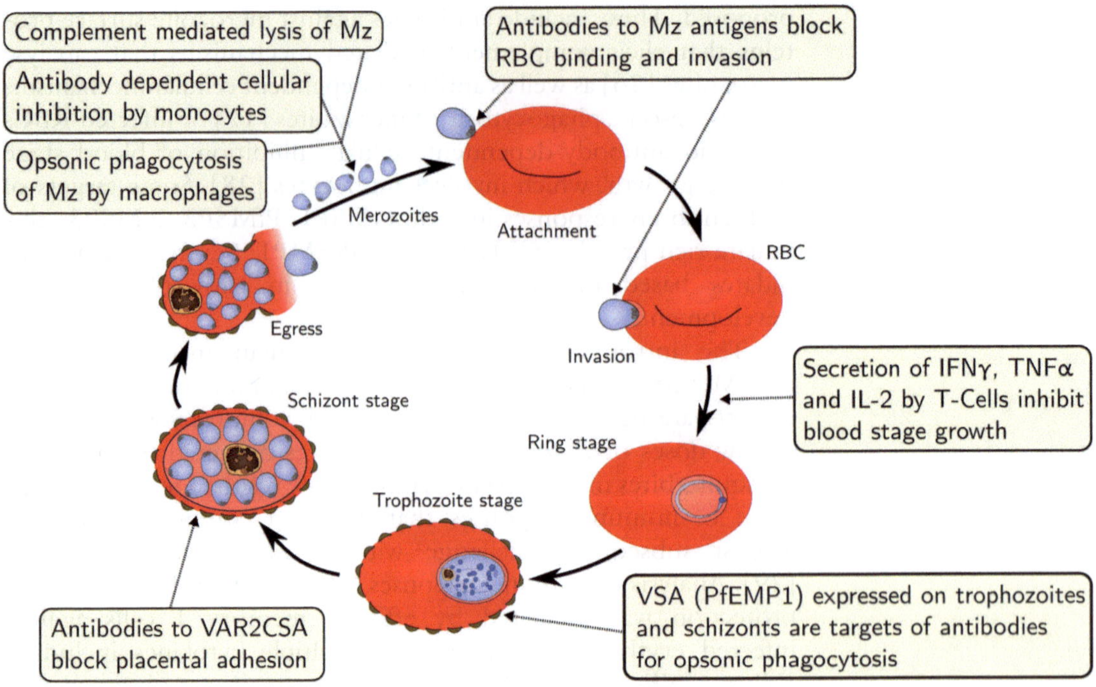

Fig. 1 Host immune responses associated with protection against *P. falciparum* blood stage parasites. Different mechanisms that may contribute toward protective immunity against blood stage *P. falciparum* parasites. Mz, merozoites; VSA, variant surface antigens; PfEMP1, *P. falciparum* erythrocyte membrane protein-1; RBC, red blood cells; VAR2CSA, VSA expressed on surface of *P. falciparum*-infected erythrocytes that adhere to placenta during malaria in pregnancy

3.1 PfMSP1

PfMSP1, the 195 kDa antigen that is found on the surface of merozoites, is proteolytically processed into 83, 30, 38, and 42 kDa fragments that form a complex on the merozoite surface [7]. The C-terminal 42 kDa PfMSP1 fragment ($PfMSP1_{42}$) is processed in a final proteolytic cleavage step to yield a 19 kDa fragment ($PfMSP1_{19}$) that is attached to the merozoite surface with a glycophosphatidyl inositol (GPI) anchor as it enters the RBC [31, 32]. Vaccine development efforts have focused on the C-terminal $PfMSP1_{42}$ or $PfMSP1_{19}$ fragments. Preclinical studies in *Aotus* monkey model demonstrated that immunization with $PfMSP1_{42}$ formulated with Freund's adjuvant, Montanide ISA720 or AS02A, can elicit partial protection against *P. falciparum* blood stage challenge with the homologous parasite strain [33]. Level of protection in the *Aotus* monkey model depended on the adjuvant used and correlated with the ELISA titers and invasion inhibitory activity of antibodies elicited by the vaccine formulation [33]. Phase 1 and 2 trials in humans indicated that recombinant $PfMSP1_{42}$ formulated with adjuvants such as AS02 was immunogenic and elicited antibodies that recognized native PfMSP1 [34–36]. However, immunization of individuals residing in *P. falciparum* endemic regions of Africa with $PfMSP1_{42}$ formulated with AS02 did not protect against natural challenge in the field [35]. The lack of protection observed in these studies was due to the inability of the vaccine to elicit high-titer growth inhibitory antibodies against *P. falciparum* blood stage parasites. Moreover, analysis of antigenic polymorphisms in $PfMSP1_{42}$ in the circulating strains demonstrated that the *P. falciparum* 3D7 allele on which the $PfMSP1_{42}$ vaccine was based was actually rare in the field sites where the vaccine candidate was tested [36]. Novel approaches such as designing recombinant antigens that cover major allelic forms will be needed to overcome the problem of polymorphisms in such vaccine candidate antigens. Recently, a nonhuman primate study with a chimeric recombinant protein of $PfMSP\text{-}1_{19}$ and PfMSP-8 produced high-titer anti-PfMSP-1 neutralizing antibodies [37, 38]. Studies that use novel delivery platforms such as nanoparticles and viral vectors demonstrate enhanced immunogenicity with $PfMSP\text{-}1_{42}$ antigen [39, 40]. Such approaches that use new vaccine delivery platforms to elicit high-titer functional antibodies that achieve high rates of growth inhibition may be necessary to improve the efficacy of vaccine candidates based on PfMSP-1.

3.2 PfAMA1

The *P. falciparum* apical membrane antigen 1 (PfAMA1) is an essential microneme protein that mediates RBC invasion by merozoites [41, 42]. This 83 kDa protein is processed to a 66 kDa protein, which involves proteolytic cleavage of its N-terminal region, before it translocates to the merozoite surface [41, 42]. Further proteolytic processing of the molecule produces 48 and 44 kDa fragments that are released during invasion. Antibodies that disrupt the proteolytic processing of the 66 kDa form of PfAMA1 can block RBC invasion [43]. Antibodies raised against the protein by immunization in preclinical animal models or as a result of natural infection are associated with protection [44–46]. However, PfAMA1 is highly polymorphic and like other blood stage antigens requires high antibody titers for efficient inhibition of blood stage growth. This is reflected by the disappointing results from PfAMA1 based vaccines in CHMI and phase 2 field trials in which recombinant PfAMA1 formulated with adjuvants failed to elicit protection against *P. falciparum* artificial or natural challenge [47–49]. A recent initiative, AMA1-DiCo, to address the problem of PfAMA1 polymorphism is under development to produce recombinant chimeric PfAMA1 constructs that will together cover most of the naturally occurring alleles. The results from the phase 1 trial of the recombinant AMA1-DiCo vaccine adjuvanted with Alhydrogel or GLA-SE elicits antigen-specific antibodies that recognize native PfAMA1 from different *P. falciparum* isolates by immunofluorescence assays

[50]. However, the neutralizing capacity of antibodies against diverse alleles remains to be tested.

PfAMA1 interacts with the rhoptry neck protein 2 (PfRON2), which is secreted from the rhoptries into the host RBC membrane during the process of invasion [51]. It has been demonstrated that a vaccine comprised of PfAMA1 and PfRON2 produced significant levels of protection in a nonhuman primate model that was mediated by antibodies against the PfAMA1/PfRON2 complex [52, 53]. These studies support the evaluation of PfAMA1/PfRON2 complex in clinical trials.

3.3 PfRH5

The *P. falciparum* reticulocyte binding-like homologue protein 5 (PfRH5) is a merozoite protein that is essential for RBC invasion [54]. Unlike other members of the PfRH family, the PfRH5 protein is relatively small (~60 kDa) and highly conserved among diverse strains. It has now been established that PfRH5 exhibits a novel kite-like architecture and binds to basigin on RBCs through its tip [55, 56]. Antibodies that bind PfRH5 at the tip block the PfRH5-basigin interaction and block invasion. Limited antigenic diversity and the association of naturally acquired PfRH5 antibodies with protection make it an ideal vaccine candidate [20–22, 56]. Recently, it was reported that PfRH5 forms a complex with two other *P. falciparum* blood stage proteins, PfCyRPA and PfRIPR [57, 58]. In addition, a third merozoite protein, P113, was identified that anchors the PfRH5-PfCYRPA-PfRIPR complex on the parasite [59]. Consequently, antibodies raised against these proteins neutralized the parasite in an in vitro growth inhibition assay [60, 61]. A recent study elucidates the association of PfRH5 antibodies with protection against heterologous challenge in an *Aotus* monkey model [13]. These studies were recently extended into humans using prime boost strategies employing ChAd63 and MVA viral vectors that expressed full-length PfRH5. Even though vaccinees seroconverted, the antibody levels attained were low and were mostly IgG1 with moderate levels of IgG3 [62]. However, it is promising that the antibodies were neutralizing and strain transcending in a GIA. Furthermore, the antibodies were able to disrupt the PfRH5 complex formation with P113, basigin, and PfCyRPA [63]. In the same vein, it was demonstrated that IgG3 antibodies and not IgG1 against PfRH5 were significantly associated with protection in a longitudinal study in Papua New Guinea [22]. The ongoing controlled human challenge study with recombinant PfRH5 in AS01 adjuvant should provide proof of concept for a vaccine based on PfRH5 and further help us understand the role of PfRH5 antibodies in protection against *P. falciparum* blood stages (ClinicalTrials.gov: NCT02927145).

3.4 PfSERA5

PfSERA5, a member of a multigene family of putative proteases, plays an important role in parasite exit from infected RBCs. PfSERA5 is essential for *Plasmodium* survival [64, 65]. In field studies, antibodies that target the N-terminal region of PfSERA5 are associated with inhibition in an in vitro GIA [64, 66, 67]. In a phase 1 clinical trial, the vaccine candidate, BK-SE36, based on recombinant PfSERA5 protein formulated with alum elicited high-titer antibodies in a malaria naïve Japanese population [68]. However, in a cohort of malaria-exposed Ugandan individuals, the antibody titers were lower than in the Japanese cohort [68, 69]. The antibody titers were higher in children who had low malaria exposure in the Ugandan cohort, indicating that pre-existing immunity may have a negative effect on the vaccine [68, 69]. Although the Ugandan study was not designed to evaluate efficacy of the vaccine, follow-up of the volunteers for 1 year provided preliminary data that suggests that immunization with BK- SE36 was protective [69]. The results of another ongoing clinical trial with BK-SE36/CpG vaccine in healthy malaria-exposed children aged 1–5 in Burkina Faso, which is designed to study efficacy of the vaccine, are anticipated by 2019.

3.5 GLURP and MSP3 (GMZ2)

GMZ2 malaria vaccine is a recombinant fusion protein of conserved domains of *Plasmodium falciparum* blood stage antigens, $GLURP_{27\text{-}500}$ and $MSP3_{212\text{-}380}$. Immuno-epidemiological studies associate GLURP and MSP3 antibodies with reduced risk for malaria [28, 70–73]. A study in nonhuman primates indicated a significant correlation between antibody titers and partial protection [74]. The cytophilic functional antibodies elicited by the vaccine inhibit parasite growth through antibody-dependent cellular inhibition (ADCI) [75, 76]. Results from recently concluded phase 2b clinical trial of GMZ2 vaccine using alum adjuvant elicited a modest efficacy of 14% in children aged 12–60 months [77]. Significant association of anti-GMZ2 antibodies with reduction in clinical malaria cases was observed in vaccinees [77] that warrants further development of this antigen with novel delivery platforms to improve immunogenicity and efficacy.

3.6 PvDBP

The *P. vivax* Duffy binding protein (DBP), which binds the Duffy antigen receptor for chemokines (DARC), plays an essential role in invasion by *P. vivax* merozoites [78]. Similar to other members of the erythrocyte-binding protein family, the conserved N-terminal cysteine-rich region within PvDBP, region II (PvDBPII), mediates receptor binding [78]. Although significant polymorphisms are reported in PvDBPII, the binding residues are conserved across diverse *P. vivax* isolates [79–81]. Studies on acquisition of antibodies against PvDBP in children residing in *P. vivax* endemic regions have shown that although antibodies to PvDBPII are commonly observed, most children develop antibodies with poor binding inhibitory activity that is strain-specific [24]. Only a minority of children (<10%) develop high-titer, strain-transcending binding inhibitory antibodies against PvDBPII. Acquisition of such high-titer binding inhibitory anti-PvDBPII antibodies is associated with protection against *P. vivax* [24] providing support for the development of a vaccine based on PvDBPII. Moreover, preclinical immunogenicity studies have demonstrated that it is possible to elicit high-titer strain-transcending binding inhibitory antibodies against PvDBPII by immunization both with viral vector-based delivery strategies [82] and recombinant PvDBPII protein formulated with adjuvants such as GLA-SE [83]. Phase 1 clinical trials to evaluate the safety and immunogenicity of PvDBPII have demonstrated that PvDBPII delivered either using viral vectors [84] or recombinant protein formulated with GLA-SE [85] elicits high-titer binding inhibitory antibodies that are strain-transcending and block DARC binding by diverse polymorphic PvDBPII domains. Efforts have also been made to engineer a recombinant PvDBPII antigen that directs the antibody response to the conserved residues in the polymorphic region [86, 87]. The resulting antigen elicits broadly neutralizing antibodies albeit at lower levels in comparison to the native antigen. The next step is to test the efficacy of PvDBPII-based *P. vivax* vaccine candidates in *P. vivax* blood stage challenge model or field trials for protection of individuals residing in endemic regions against natural *P. vivax* challenge.

3.7 VAR2CSA

Pregnancy-associated malaria (PAM) is a serious manifestation of *P. falciparum* malaria that results in maternal anemia and complications during pregnancy including increased risk of abortion, premature delivery, and underweight babies at birth. The pathogenesis of PAM is associated with the sequestration of *P. falciparum*-infected RBCs in the placenta. Adhesion of *P. falciparum*-infected RBCs to the placenta is mediated by binding with chondroitin sulfate A (CSA) on proteoglycans in the placenta through interaction with the variant surface antigen VAR2CSA expressed on the surface of infected RBCs [88]. Identification of naturally acquired antibodies against the N-terminal region of VAR2CSA and their association with better outcomes in PAM strongly support the development of a vaccine based on VAR2CSA to protect against malaria in pregnancy [89–91]. In recent studies the association of strain-specific VAR2CSA antibodies to PAM indicates that a vaccine based on VAR2CSA should address the presence of polymorphisms in order to elicit strain-transcending neutralizing antibodies [92, 93]. The results of two different ongoing phase 1 a/b clinical trials, PRIMALVAC and PlacMalVac, that targets DBL1X-DBL2X domain from *P. falciparum* 3D7 strain and 1D1- DBL2x-ID2a domain from *P. falciparum* FCR3 strain, respectively, are highly anticipated by the malaria vaccine community [94].

4 Improving Efficacy of Blood Stage Malaria Vaccines

Despite significant efforts toward clinical development of malaria vaccines over the past couple of decades, an effective blood stage malaria vaccine remains elusive. Here, we will discuss some directions that could be pursued that could lead to development of blood stage malaria vaccines that elicit protection with high efficacy.

4.1 Antigen Combinations and Delivery Platforms to Enhance Immunogenicity and Efficacy of Blood Stage Vaccines

It is clear that a vaccine based on a single blood stage antigen is unlikely to yield high efficacy. It will be necessary to combine blood stage antigens to achieve synergy and high rates of growth inhibition or parasite clearance. Combining antigens will also reduce the likelihood of development of variants that may escape immune responses elicited by a vaccine based on a single antigen. Combining antigens may also allow us to elicit diverse immune mechanisms. For example, one antigen may elicit receptor-blocking antibodies that inhibit invasion, whereas another antigen may elicit antibodies that mediate opsonic phagocytosis or complement-mediated lysis of merozoites. Such diverse mechanisms may yield an additive or synergistic effect to inhibit parasite growth with high efficiency.

Growth inhibition assays using sera or antibodies from clinical trials show that it is difficult to elicit high-titer, long-lasting antibodies that inhibit growth with high efficiency. Recombinant proteins formulated with adjuvants have failed to elicit and sustain the levels of antibodies required for high rates of blood stage growth inhibition. There is a need to improve the immunogenicity of available vaccine antigens with novel vaccine delivery platforms. A number of efforts to improve immunogenicity have used virus-like particles (VLPs) that display parasite-derived peptide antigens on their surface. This can be achieved either by creating genetic fusions that express peptide antigens fused to viral surface proteins that assemble to form chimeric VLPs. Conformational changes in the antigen or misfolding of the viral surface protein can adversely affect the antigenicity of the vaccine candidate or the ability of the virus protein to form VLPs. An alternative approach is to cross-link the antigen to the surface of VLPs by chemical conjugation so that the VLPs are decorated with the vaccine antigen on their surface. The cross-linking process and antigen to VLP ratio need to be optimized to ensure that the protective epitopes on the antigen are retained and remain accessible to antibodies on the surface of the chimeric VLPs. Recent progress using SpyTag-SpyCatcher technology has made it possible to take such a modular approach to combine antigens with VLPs using click chemistry with limited risk of destroying antigen conformation [95, 96]. Moreover, this approach is amenable to developing combination vaccines relatively easily by simply mixing multiple antigen-VLP conjugates.

Preclinical studies using such antigen-VLP conjugates demonstrate the ability to elicit potent antibody responses [95]. Development of nanoparticles coated with recombinant blood stage antigens or protein-protein conjugates has also been explored [40, 97–99]. Although a number of such particle-based vaccine development approaches elicit high levels of antibodies that are long-lasting in preclinical animal models, whether these results transfer to humans remains to be tested. For example, while a malaria transmission blocking vaccine based on Pfs25 conjugated with ExoProtein-A (EPA) elicited high-titer functional antibodies in phase 1 trials, the antibody titers dropped to baseline levels within a year [99, 100]. Identifying an optimal delivery system and formulation that elicits long-lasting potent antibody responses in humans will be a key breakthrough to enable development of blood stage malaria vaccines with high efficacy.

4.2 Use of Functional Immunoassays and Novel Preclinical Models to Evaluate Blood Stage Vaccine Candidates

Pre-screening of vaccine candidates using relevant immunoassays at an early stage is essential to promote progress of the most promising vaccine candidates. Currently, we do not have an established assay or model that can clearly predict the success of blood stage vaccine candidates in clinical trials. A brief overview of assays and models that can guide the development of blood stage vaccines is provided below.

Most blood stage vaccine candidates aim to elicit high-titer antibodies against the native antigen. The ELISA continues to be the most widely used method to screen antibody responses in field studies to identify potential vaccine candidates as well as to evaluate immune responses in preclinical studies and clinical trials. However, the ELISA does not always predict efficacy of the vaccine candidate accurately because it reports average reactivity of polyclonal sera and does not focus only on functional antibodies that are associated with protection. The use of assays that quantify presence of antibodies to specific functional conformational epitopes on an antigen or that measure inhibition in functional receptor-binding assays or growth inhibition assays (GIA) may more accurately predict association of antibodies against specific antigens with protection [24, 55, 56, 101–103]. For example, the PvDBPII-DARC receptor- binding assay was used to demonstrate that naturally acquired antibodies capable of blocking the binding of PvDBPII to DARC are associated with protection against *P. vivax* infection [24, 81]. The assay was also used to demonstrate that vaccine candidates based on PvDBPII using either viral vector-based prime boost approaches or recombinant PvDBPII formulated with GLA-SE elicit potent strain-transcending binding inhibitory antibodies in preclinical studies as well as phase 1 trials [82–85]. Use of this assay to analyze sera from a phase 2a challenge trial may allow us to define a neutralization titer using the PvDBPII-DARC binding assay, which could guide further clinical development. The GIA measures the relative enzymatic activity of parasite lactate dehydrogenase [104] and can give a direct readout of the capacity of antibodies to inhibit replication of blood stage parasites. A limitation of the GIA is that it does not report on inhibition of parasite growth by antibodies through other mechanisms such as opsonic phagocytosis, complement-mediated lysis, or antibody-dependent cellular inhibition involving monocytes. These mechanisms have been shown to play a role in naturally acquired immunity to *P. falciparum* blood stage parasites [26, 105–108]. It would be valuable to develop assays that could be used in medium- to high-throughput format to screen for antigens that could serve as targets of such protective immune responses. Combining antigens that elicit antibody responses by diverse immune mechanisms may yield synergy to achieve high levels of protective efficacy.

In addition to development of novel assays to evaluate immune responses to malaria parasite antigens, the availability of animal models that mimic immune responses in humans would greatly help advance malaria vaccine development. The development of humanized mouse models to obtain proof of concept in preclinical studies would greatly help overcome the barrier of expensive trials in nonhuman primates or challenge trials in humans that currently limit our ability to screen multiple vaccine candidates to identify formulations that yield high efficacy. Early efforts to develop a mouse model of blood stage malaria were hindered by practical difficulties such as requirement of daily injection with human erythrocytes and rapid clearance of infected human RBCs by the mouse immune system [109, 110]. Development of a mouse model that supports erythropoiesis of human erythrocytes and mimics natural infection also paves the way to grow *P. vivax*, which preferentially infects reticulocytes. Recent advances have made it possible to develop humanized murine models that have both human organs as well as a human immune system [108–112]. The model, which supports a chimeric human liver and a humanized immune system and mimics human erythropoiesis, has been shown to sustain the entire parasite life cycle starting with infection of hepatocytes with sporozoites, release of merozoites and infection of RBCs, replication in RBCs, and transmission of gametocytes. Such models can be used to test if immune responses made by the humanized immune system in the mouse can protect against *P. falciparum* infection.

4.3 Use of Controlled Human Malaria Infection (CHMI) Model for Evaluation of Blood Stage Malaria Vaccines

The potential of CHMI for pre-screening malaria vaccine candidates was demonstrated in the 1980s at the Walter Reed Army Institute of Research [113]. However, most CHMI studies were based on infectious mosquito bites and focused on preerythrocytic stages of malaria parasite life cycle. A couple of drawbacks of the conventional CHMI is the mandatory requirement to treat the subjects before they develop high blood parasitemia and the difficulty in controlling the number of infectious merozoites released following the liver stage. This limits the potential of CHMI for testing blood stage vaccines. A well-established model for experimental blood stage infection was developed at the Queensland Institute of Medical Research (QIMR), Brisbane, which is currently used to screen blood stage vaccines and anti-malaria drugs [114, 115]. As with other assays used to screen blood stage vaccines, blood stage CHMI has its own drawbacks. When compared to natural infection, the starting inoculum used to initiate the infection is very low, which could potentially influence the outcome. Nevertheless, this is a cost-effective alternative to expensive and time-consuming field trials to test the efficacy of blood stage vaccine candidates. For instance, a study with PfAMA1 based vaccine candidate, FMP2.1/AS01, failed to protect in a blood stage CHMI even though it elicits growth inhibitory antibodies providing an early phase readout of the efficacy of this blood stage vaccine candidate [116]. This highlights the need to improve the immunogenicity of FMP2.1 before launching into field trials to test efficacy against natural challenge.

5 Conclusion

The application of our improved understanding of the biology of RBC invasion together with the development of functional immunoassays should enable us to identify the most promising novel blood stage malaria vaccine candidates. Evaluation of such novel vaccine candidates in humanized preclinical mouse models followed by clinical testing in phase 1 safety and immunogenicity studies and phase 2a challenge trials should provide an efficient path to evaluate efficacy of blood stage vaccine candidates before initiating field trials to test vaccines for protection against natural challenge in malaria-endemic areas. Following this path should enable development of blood stage malaria vaccines that elicit protection with high efficacy in the coming years.

Acknowledgments

Work on malaria vaccine development in the laboratory of CEC has been supported over the years by Department of Biotechnology (DBT), Government of India, Biotechnology Industry Research Advisory Council (BIRAC), PATH Malaria Vaccine Initiative, European Vaccine Initiative, and Institut Pasteur. AV was supported by a Marie-Curie Fellowship.

References

1. WHO (2016) World malaria report 2016. WHO, Geneva
2. WHO (2017) World malaria report 2017. WHO, Geneva
3. Mueller I, Galinski MR, Baird JK et al (2009) Key gaps in the knowledge of *Plasmodium vivax*, a neglected human malaria parasite. Lancet Infect Dis 9:555–566
4. Riley EM, Stewart VA (2013) Immune mechanisms in malaria: new insights in vaccine development. Nat Med 19:168–178
5. Cohen S, McGregor IA, Carrington S (1961) Gamma-globulin and acquired immunity to human malaria. Nature 192:733–737
6. McGregor IA (1964) The passive transfer of human malarial immunity. Am J Trop Med Hyg 13:237–239
7. Holder AA, Freeman RR (1984) The three major antigens on the surface of *Plasmodium falciparum* merozoites are derived from a single high molecular weight precursor. J Exp Med 160:624–629
8. Deans JA, Alderson T, Thomas AW et al (1982) Rat monoclonal antibodies which inhibit the in vitro multiplication of *Plasmodium knowlesi*. Clin Exp Immunol 49:297–309
9. John CC, O'Donnell RA, Sumba PO et al (2004) Evidence that invasion-inhibitory antibodies specific for the 19-kDa fragment of merozoite surface protein-1 (MSP-1 19) can play a protective role against blood-stage *Plasmodium falciparum* infection in individuals in a malaria endemic area of Africa. J Immunol 173:666–672
10. Kennedy MC, Wang J, Zhang Y et al (2002) In vitro studies with recombinant *Plasmodium falciparum* apical membrane antigen 1 (AMA1): production and activity of an AMA1 vaccine and generation of a multiallelic response. Infect Immun 70:6948–6960
11. Lopaticki S, Maier AG, Thompson J et al (2011) Reticulocyte and erythrocyte binding-like proteins function cooperatively in invasion of human erythrocytes by malaria parasites. Infect Immun 79:1107–1117
12. Baum J, Chen L, Healer J et al (2009) Reticulocyte-binding protein homologue 5 – an essential adhesin involved in invasion of human erythrocytes by *Plasmodium falciparum*. Int J Parasitol 39:371–380
13. Douglas AD, Baldeviano GC, Lucas CM et al (2015) A PfRH5-based vaccine is efficacious against heterologous strain blood-stage *Plasmodium falciparum* infection in aotus monkeys. Cell Host Microbe 17:130–139
14. Nebie I, Diarra A, Ouedraogo A et al (2008) Humoral responses to *Plasmodium falciparum* blood-stage antigens and association with incidence of clinical malaria in children living in an area of seasonal malaria transmission in Burkina Faso, West Africa. Infect Immun 76:759–766
15. Richards JS, Arumugam TU, Reiling L et al (2013) Identification and prioritization of merozoite antigens as targets of protective human immunity to *Plasmodium falciparum* malaria for vaccine and biomarker development. J Immunol 191:795–809
16. França CT, White MT, He W-Q et al (2017) Identification of highly-protective combinations of *Plasmodium vivax* recombinant proteins for vaccine development. Elife 6:e28673
17. Osier FH, Feng G, Boyle MJ et al (2014) Opsonic phagocytosis of *Plasmodium falciparum* merozoites: mechanism in human immunity and a correlate of protection against malaria. BMC Med 12:108
18. Daou M, Kouriba B, Ouédraogo N et al (2015) Protection of Malian children from clinical malaria is associated with recognition of multiple antigens. Malar J 14:56
19. Bustamante LY, Powell GT, Lin Y-C et al (2017) Synergistic malaria vaccine combinations identified by systematic antigen screening. Proc Natl Acad Sci U S A 114:12045–12050
20. Patel SD, Ahouidi AD, Bei AK et al (2013) *Plasmodium falciparum* merozoite surface antigen, PfRH5, elicits detectable levels of invasion-inhibiting antibodies in humans. J Infect Dis 208:1679–1687
21. Tran TM, Ongoiba A, Coursen J et al (2014) Naturally acquired antibodies specific for *Plasmodium falciparum* reticulocyte-binding protein homologue 5 inhibit parasite growth and predict protection from malaria. J Infect Dis 209:789–798
22. Weaver R, Reiling L, Feng G et al (2016) The association between naturally acquired IgG subclass specific antibodies to the PfRH5 invasion complex and protection from *Plasmodium falciparum* malaria. Sci Rep 6:33094
23. Pandey AK, Reddy KS, Sahar T et al (2013) Identification of a potent combination of key *Plasmodium falciparum* merozoite antigens that elicit strain-transcending parasite-neutralizing antibodies. Infect Immun 81:441–451

24. King CL, Michon P, Shakri AR et al (2008) Naturally acquired Duffy-binding protein-specific binding inhibitory antibodies confer protection from blood-stage *Plasmodium vivax* infection. Proc Natl Acad Sci U S A 105:8363–8368
25. Irani V, Ramsland PA, Guy AJ et al (2015) Acquisition of functional antibodies that block the binding of erythrocyte-binding antigen 175 and protection against *Plasmodium falciparum* malaria in children. Clin Infect Dis 61:1244–1252
26. Boyle MJ, Reiling L, Feng G et al (2015) Human antibodies fix complement to inhibit *Plasmodium falciparum* invasion of erythrocytes and are associated with protection against malaria. Immunity 42:580–590
27. Chan JA, Fowkes FJI, Beeson JG (2014) Surface antigens of *Plasmodium falciparum*-infected erythrocytes as immune targets and malaria vaccine candidates. Cell Mol Life Sci 71:3633–3657
28. Druilhe P, Spertini F, Soesoe D et al (2005) A malaria vaccine that elicits in humans antibodies able to kill *Plasmodium falciparum*. PLoS Med 2:e344
29. Roestenberg M, McCall M, Hopman J et al (2009) Protection against a malaria challenge by sporozoite inoculation. N Engl J Med 361:468–477
30. Pombo DJ, Lawrence G, Hirunpetcharat C et al (2002) Immunity to malaria after administration of ultra-low doses of red cells infected with *Plasmodium falciparum*. Lancet 360:610–617
31. Blackman MJ, Whittle H, Holder AA (1991) Processing of the *Plasmodium falciparum* major merozoite surface protein-1: identification of a 33-kilodalton secondary processing product which is shed prior to erythrocyte invasion. Mol Biochem Parasitol 49:35–44
32. Harris PK, Yeoh S, Dluzewski AR et al (2005) Molecular identification of a malaria merozoite surface sheddase. PLoS Pathog 1:e29
33. Singh S, Miura K, Zhou H et al (2006) Immunity to recombinant *Plasmodium falciparum* merozoite surface protein 1 (MSP1): protection in *Aotus nancymai* monkeys strongly correlates with anti-MSP1 antibody titer and in vitro parasite-inhibitory activity. Infect Immun 74:4573–4580
34. Malkin E, Long CA, Stowers AW et al (2007) Phase 1 study of two merozoite surface protein 1 (MSP1(42)) vaccines for *Plasmodium falciparum* malaria. PLoS Clin Trial 2:e12
35. Ogutu BR, Apollo OJ, McKinney D et al (2009) Blood stage malaria vaccine eliciting high antigen-specific antibody concentrations confers no protection to young children in western Kenya. PLoS One 4:e4708
36. Thera MA, Doumbo OK, Coulibaly D et al (2006) Safety and allele-specific immunogenicity of a malaria vaccine in Malian adults: results of a phase I randomized trial. PLoS Clin Trial 1:e34
37. Alaro JR, Partridge A, Miura K et al (2013) A chimeric *Plasmodium falciparum* merozoite surface protein vaccine induces high titers of parasite growth inhibitory antibodies. Infect Immun 81:3843–3854
38. Burns JM, Miura K, Sullivan J et al (2016) Immunogenicity of a chimeric *Plasmodium falciparum* merozoite surface protein vaccine in *Aotus* monkeys. Malar J 15:159
39. Douglas AD, de Cassan SC, Dicks MD et al (2010) Tailoring subunit vaccine immunogenicity: maximizing antibody and T cell responses by using combinations of adenovirus, poxvirus and protein-adjuvant vaccines against *Plasmodium falciparum* MSP1. Vaccine 28:7167–7178
40. Parween S, Gupta PK, Chauhan VS (2011) Induction of humoral immune response against PfMSP-119 and PvMSP-119 using gold nanoparticles along with alum. Vaccine 29:2451–2460
41. Triglia T, Healer J, Caruana SR et al (2000) Apical membrane antigen 1 plays a central role in erythrocyte invasion by *Plasmodium* species. Mol Microbiol 38:706–718
42. Bannister LH, Hopkins JM, Dluzewski AR et al (2003) *Plasmodium falciparum* apical membrane antigen 1 (PfAMA-1) is translocated within micronemes along subpellicular microtubules during merozoite development. J Cell Sci 116:3825–3834
43. Dutta S, Haynes JD, Moch JK et al (2003) Invasion-inhibitory antibodies inhibit proteolytic processing of apical membrane antigen 1 of *Plasmodium falciparum* merozoites. Proc Natl Acad Sci U S A 100:12295–12300
44. Kariuki S, Nahlen BL, Kolczack M et al (2001) Longitudinal study of natural immune responses to the *Plasmodium falciparum* apical membrane antigen (AMA-1) in a holoendemic region of malaria in western Kenya: Asembo Bay Cohort Project VIII. Am J Trop Med Hyg 65:100–107
45. Miura K, Zhou H, Muratova OV et al (2007) In immunization with *Plasmodium falciparum* apical membrane antigen 1, the specificity of antibodies depends on the species immunized. Infect Immun 75:5827–5836

46. Remarque EJ, Roestenberg M, Younis S et al (2012) Humoral immune responses to a single allele PfAMA1 vaccine in healthy malaria-naive adults. PLoS One 7:e38898
47. Ouattara A, Mu J, Takala-Harrison S et al (2010) Lack of allele-specific efficacy of a bivalent AMA1 malaria vaccine. Malar J 9:175
48. Thera MA, Doumbo OK, Coulibaly D et al (2011) A field trial to assess a blood-stage malaria vaccine. N Engl J Med 365:1004–1013
49. Sheehy SH, Duncan CJ, Elias SC et al (2012) ChAd63-MVA-vectored blood-stage malaria vaccines targeting MSP1 and AMA1: assessment of efficacy against mosquito bite challenge in humans. Mol Ther 20:2355–2368
50. Sirima SB, Durier C, Kara L et al (2017) Safety and immunogenicity of a recombinant *Plasmodium falciparum* AMA1-DiCo malaria vaccine adjuvanted with GLA-SE or Alhydrogel® in European and African adults: a phase 1a/1b, randomized, double-blind multi-center trial. Vaccine 35:6218–6227
51. Srinivasan P, Beatty WL, Diouf A et al (2011) Binding of *Plasmodium* merozoite proteins RON2 and AMA1 triggers commitment to invasion. Proc Natl Acad Sci U S A 108:13275–13280
52. Srinivasan P, Ekanem E, Diouf A et al (2014) Immunization with a functional protein complex required for erythrocyte invasion protects against lethal malaria. Proc Natl Acad Sci U S A 111:10311–10316
53. Srinivasan P, Baldeviano GC, Miura K et al (2017) A malaria vaccine protects *Aotus* monkeys against virulent *Plasmodium falciparum* infection. NPJ Vacc 2:14
54. Crosnier C, Bustamante LY, Bartholdson SJ et al (2011) Basigin is a receptor essential for erythrocyte invasion by *Plasmodium falciparum*. Nature 480:534–537
55. Wright KE, Hjerrild KA, Bartlett J et al (2014) Structure of malaria invasion protein PfRH5 with erythrocyte basigin and blocking antibodies. Nature 515:427–430
56. Chen L, Xu Y, Healer J et al (2014) Crystal structure of PfRh5, an essential *P. falciparum* ligand for invasion of human erythrocytes. Elife 3:e04187
57. Chiu CY, Healer J, Thompson JK et al (2014) Association of antibodies to *Plasmodium falciparum* reticulocyte binding protein homolog 5 with protection from clinical malaria. Front Microbiol 5:314
58. Reddy KS, Amlabu E, Pandey AK et al (2015) Multiprotein complex between the GPI-anchored CyRPA with PfRH5 and PfRipr is crucial for *Plasmodium falciparum* erythrocyte invasion. Proc Natl Acad Sci U S A 112:1179–1184
59. Volz JC, Yap A, Sisquella X et al (2016) Essential role of the PfRh5/PfRipr/CyRPA complex during *Plasmodium falciparum* invasion of erythrocytes. Cell Host Microbe 20:60–71
60. Galaway F, Drought LG, Fala M et al (2017) P113 is a merozoite surface protein that binds the N terminus of *Plasmodium falciparum* RH5. Nat Commun 8:14333
61. Favuzza P, Blaser S, Dreyer AM et al (2016) Generation of *Plasmodium falciparum* parasite-inhibitory antibodies by immunization with recombinantly-expressed CyRPA. Malar J 15:161
62. Ntege EH, Arisue N, Ito D et al (2016) Identification of *Plasmodium falciparum* reticulocyte binding protein homologue 5-interacting protein, PfRipr, as a highly conserved blood-stage malaria vaccine candidate. Vaccine 34:5612–5622
63. Payne RO, Silk SE, Elias SC et al (2017) Human vaccination against RH5 induces neutralizing antimalarial antibodies that inhibit RH5 invasion complex interactions. JCI Insight 2:e96381
64. Aoki S, Li J, Itagaki S et al (2002) Serine repeat antigen (SERA5) is predominantly expressed among the SERA multigene family of *Plasmodium falciparum*, and the acquired antibody titers correlate with serum inhibition of the parasite growth. J Biol Chem 277:47533–47540
65. McCoubrie JE, Miller SK, Sargeant T et al (2007) Evidence for a common role for the serine-type *Plasmodium falciparum* serine repeat antigen proteases: implications for vaccine and drug design. Infect Immun 75:5565–5574
66. Apio Okech B, Nalunkuma A, Okello D et al (2001) Natural human immunoglobulin G subclass responses to *Plasmodium falciparum* Serine Repeat Antigen in Uganda. Am J Trop Med Hyg 65:912–917
67. Yagi M, Bang G, Tougan T et al (2014) Protective epitopes of the *Plasmodium falciparum* SERA5 malaria vaccine reside in intrinsically unstructured N-terminal repetitive sequences. PLoS One 9:e98460
68. Horii T, Shirai H, Jie L et al (2010) Evidences of protection against blood-stage infection of *Plasmodium falciparum* by the novel protein vaccine SE36. Parasitol Int 59:380–386
69. Palacpac NMQ, Ntege E, Yeka A et al (2013) Phase 1b randomized trial and follow-up study in Uganda of the blood-stage malaria

vaccine candidate BK-SE36. PLoS One 8: e64073
70. Oeuvray C, Theisen M, Rogier C et al (2000) Cytophilic immunoglobulin responses to *Plasmodium falciparum* glutamate-rich protein are correlated with protection against clinical malaria in Dielmo, Senegal. Infect Immun 68:2617–2620
71. Kana IH, Adu B, Tiendrebeogo RW et al (2017) Naturally acquired antibodies target the glutamate-rich protein on intact merozoites and predict protection against febrile malaria. J Infect Dis 215:623–630
72. Soe S, Theisen M, Roussilhon C et al (2004) Association between protection against clinical malaria and antibodies to merozoite surface antigens in an area of hyperendemicity in Myanmar: complementarity between responses to merozoite surface protein 3 and the 220-kilodalton glutamate-rich protein. Infect Immun 72:247–252
73. Amoah LE, Nuvor SV, Obboh EK et al (2017) Natural antibody responses to *Plasmodium falciparum* MSP3 and GLURP (R0) antigens are associated with low parasite densities in malaria patients living in the Central Region of Ghana. Parasit Vectors 10:395
74. Carvalho LJ, Alves FA, Bianco C et al (2005) Immunization of *Saimiri sciureus* monkeys with a recombinant hybrid protein derived from the *Plasmodium falciparum* antigen glutamate-rich protein and merozoite surface protein 3 can induce partial protection with Freund and Montanide ISA720 adjuvants. Clin Diagn Lab Immunol 12:242–248
75. Theisen M, Soe S, Oeuvray C et al (1998) The glutamate-rich protein (GLURP) of *Plasmodium falciparum* is a target for antibody-dependent monocyte-mediated inhibition of parasite growth in vitro. Infect Immun 66:11–17
76. Oeuvray C, Bouharoun-Tayoun H, Gras-Masse H et al (1994) Merozoite surface protein-3: a malaria protein inducing antibodies that promote *Plasmodium falciparum* killing by cooperation with blood monocytes. Blood 84:1594–1602
77. Sirima SB, Mordmüller B, Milligan P et al (2016) A phase 2b randomized, controlled trial of the efficacy of the GMZ2 malaria vaccine in African children. Vaccine 34:4536–4542
78. Chitnis CE, Miller LH (1994) Identification of the erythrocyte binding domains of *Plasmodium vivax* and *Plasmodium knowlesi* proteins involved in erythrocyte invasion. J Exp Med 180:497–506
79. Singh SK, Hora R, Belrhali H et al (2006) Structural basis for Duffy recognition by the malaria parasite Duffy-binding-like domain. Nature 439:741–744
80. VanBuskirk KM, Sevova E, Adams JH (2004) Conserved residues in the *Plasmodium vivax* Duffy binding protein ligand domain are critical for erythrocyte receptor recognition. Proc Natl Acad Sci U S A 101(44):15754–15759
81. Hans D, Pattnaik P, Bhattacharyya A et al (2005) Mapping binding residues in the *Plasmodium vivax* domain that binds Duffy antigen during red cell invasion. Mol Microbiol 55:1423–1434
82. de Cassan SC, Shakri AR, Llewellyn D et al (2015) Preclinical assessment of viral vectored and protein vaccines targeting the duffy-binding protein region II of *Plasmodium vivax*. Front Immunol 6:348
83. Wiley SR, Raman VS, Desbien A et al (2011) Targeting TLRs expands the antibody repertoire in response to a malaria vaccine. Sci Transl Med 3:93ra69
84. Payne RO, Silk SE, Elias SC et al (2017) Human vaccination against *Plasmodium vivax* Duffy-binding protein induces strain-transcending antibodies. JCI Insight 2: e93683
85. Singh K, Mukherjee P, Shakri AR et al (2018). A malaria vaccine candidate based on Duffy binding protein elicits high titer strain transcending functional antibodies in a Phase I clinical trial. NPJ Vaccines. 3:48. doi: 10.1038/s41541-018-0083-3.
86. Ntumngia FB, Pires CV, Barnes SJ et al (2017) An engineered vaccine of the *Plasmodium vivax* Duffy binding protein enhances induction of broadly neutralizing antibodies. Sci Rep 7:13779
87. Chen E, Salinas ND, Huang Y et al (2016) Broadly neutralizing epitopes in the *Plasmodium vivax* vaccine candidate Duffy Binding Protein. Proc Natl Acad Sci U S A 113:6277–6282
88. Fried M, Duffy PE (2015) Designing a VAR2CSA-based vaccine to prevent placental malaria. Vaccine 33:7483–7488
89. Staalsoe T, Shulman CE, Bulmer JN et al (2004) Variant surface antigen-specific IgG and protection against clinical consequences of pregnancy-associated *Plasmodium falciparum* malaria. Lancet 363:283–289
90. Ndam NT, Denoeud-Ndam L, Doritchamou J et al (2015) Protective antibodies against placental malaria and poor outcomes during pregnancy, Benin. Emerg Infect Dis 21:813–823

91. Dechavanne S, Srivastava A, Gangnard S et al (2015) Parity-dependent recognition of DBL1X-3X suggests an important role of the VAR2CSA high-affinity CSA-binding region in the development of the humoral response against placental malaria. Infect Immun 83:2466–2474

92. Patel JC, Hathaway NJ, Parobek CM et al (2017) Increased risk of low birth weight in women with placental malaria associated with *P. falciparum* VAR2CSA clade. Sci Rep 7:7768

93. Doritchamou JY, Herrera R, Aebig JA et al (2016) VAR2CSA domain-specific analysis of naturally acquired functional antibodies to *Plasmodium falciparum* placental malaria. J Infect Dis 214:577–586

94. Chêne A, Houard S, Nielsen MA et al (2016) Clinical development of placental malaria vaccines and immunoassays harmonization: a workshop report. Malar J 15:476

95. Janitzek CM, Matondo S, Thrane S et al (2016) Bacterial superglue generates a full-length circumsporozoite protein virus-like particle vaccine capable of inducing high and durable antibody responses. Malar J 15:545

96. Thrane S, Janitzek CM, Matondo S et al (2016) Bacterial superglue enables easy development of efficient virus-like particle based vaccines. J Nanobiotechnol 14:30

97. Pusic K, Aguilar Z, McLoughlin J et al (2013) Iron oxide nanoparticles as a clinically acceptable delivery platform for a recombinant blood-stage human malaria vaccine. FASEB J 27:1153–1166

98. Karch CP, Doll TA, Paulillo SM et al (2017) The use of a *P. falciparum* specific coiled-coil domain to construct a self-assembling protein nanoparticle vaccine to prevent malaria. J Nanobiotechnol 15:62

99. Radtke AJ, Anderson CF, Riteau N et al (2017) Adjuvant and carrier protein-dependent T-cell priming promotes a robust antibody response against the *Plasmodium falciparum* Pfs25 vaccine candidate. Sci Rep 7:40312

100. Talaat KR, Ellis RD, Hurd J et al (2016) Safety and immunogenicity of Pfs25-EPA/Alhydrogel®, a transmission blocking vaccine against *Plasmodium falciparum*: an open label study in malaria naïve adults. PLoS One 11:e0163144

101. Crossey E, Frietze K, Narum DL et al (2015) Identification of an immunogenic mimic of a conserved epitope on the *Plasmodium falciparum* blood stage antigen AMA1 using virus-like particle (VLP) peptide display. PLoS One 10:e0132560

102. Chia WN, Goh YS, Rénia L (2014) Novel approaches to identify protective malaria vaccine candidates. Front Microbiol 5:586

103. Douglas AD, Williams AR, Knuepfer E et al (2014) Neutralization of *Plasmodium falciparum* merozoites by antibodies against PfRH5. J Immunol 192:245–258

104. Makler MT, Ries JM, Williams JA et al (1993) Parasite lactate dehydrogenase as an assay for *Plasmodium falciparum* drug sensitivity. Am J Trop Med Hyg 48:739–741

105. Chan JA, Howell KB, Reiling L et al (2012) Targets of antibodies against *Plasmodium falciparum*-infected erythrocytes in malaria immunity. J Clin Invest 122:3227–3238

106. Ghumra A, Khunrae P, Ataide R et al (2011) Immunisation with recombinant PfEMP1 domains elicits functional rosette-inhibiting and phagocytosis-inducing antibodies to *Plasmodium falciparum*. PLoS One 6:e16414

107. Zhou J, Feng G, Beeson J et al (2015) CD14hiCD16+ monocytes phagocytose antibody-opsonised *Plasmodium falciparum* infected erythrocytes more efficiently than other monocyte subsets, and require CD16 and complement to do so. BMC Med 13:154

108. Jafarshad A, Dziegiel MH, Lundquist R et al (2007) A novel antibody-dependent cellular cytotoxicity mechanism involved in defense against malaria requires costimulation of monocytes FcgammaRII and FcgammaRIII. J Immunol 178:3099–3106

109. Arnold L, Tyagi RK, Mejia P et al (2010) Analysis of innate defences against *Plasmodium falciparum* in immunodeficient mice. Malar J 9:197

110. Tsuji M, Ishihara C, Arai S et al (1995) Establishment of a SCID mouse model having circulating human red blood cells and a possible growth of *Plasmodium falciparum* in the mouse. Vaccine 13:1389–1392

111. Amaladoss A, Chen Q, Liu M et al (2015) De novo generated human red blood cells in humanized mice support *Plasmodium falciparum* infection. PLoS One 10:e0129825

112. Wijayalath W, Majji S, Villasante EF et al (2014) Humanized HLA-DR4.RagKO.IL2RγcKO.NOD (DRAG) mice sustain the complex vertebrate life cycle of *Plasmodium falciparum* malaria. Malar J 13:386

113. Carter R, Ballou WR, Schneider I et al (1986) Malaria transmitted to humans by mosquitoes infected from cultured *Plasmodium falciparum*. Am J Trop Med Hyg 35:66–68

114. Cheng Q, Lawrence G, Reed C et al (1997) Measurement of *Plasmodium falciparum* growth rates in vivo: a test of malaria vaccines. Am J Trop Med Hyg 57:495–500

115. Engwerda CR, Minigo G, Amante FH et al (2012) Experimentally induced blood stage malaria infection as a tool for clinical research. Trends Parasitol 28:515–521

116. Payne RO, Milne KH, Elias SC et al (2016) Demonstration of the blood-stage *Plasmodium falciparum* controlled human malaria infection model to assess efficacy of the *P. falciparum* Apical Membrane Antigen 1 vaccine, FMP2.1/AS01. J Infect Dis 213:1743–1751

Part V

Vector Control

Chapter 16

Insecticide-Treated Mosquito Nets

Pierre Carnevale and Frédérick Gay

Abstract

The coherent and coordinated strategy put in place since the beginning of the century to fight malaria has led to a significant reduction in the global burden of the disease. Of the various elements composing this strategy, it appears that vector control and, in the first place, the massive distribution of LLIN (long-lasting impregnated nets) have contributed significantly to this success. The idea, a priori trivial, of impregnating nets with insecticide to make them more effective, emerged in the late 1980s in Benin. Since then, thanks to the ongoing support of WHO and collaboration with industry, there has been a paradigm shift that puts LLIN at the forefront of malaria control. This chapter summarizes, in chronological order, the different steps that led to the use of LLIN, starting with simple mosquito nets. It provides a brief overview of the studies that have shown their effectiveness both from the entomological and the morbidity and mortality point of view. Finally, it presents the limitations and challenges that will need to be overcome if LLIN are to remain an effective tool in the fight against malaria.

Key words Mosquito nets, Impregnating nets, Insecticide, Malaria control strategy

1 Introduction

Since the year 2000, an enormous amount of work and resources has been devoted to malaria control to meet one of the United Nations Millennium Development Goal (halting malaria progress by year 2015) as well as the WHO target of reducing malaria incidence by 75% relative to the levels of the year 2000. The 20-fold increase in international finances allowed (1) the distribution of millions of LLIN, (2) insecticide residual spraying (IRS), (3) a significant improvement in case management (CM) with widespread availability of reliable rapid detection tests (RDT), and (4) efficient and low-cost artemisinin-combination therapies (ACT)—while waiting for an operational vaccine [1].

The effect of different interventions in the various epidemiological and socioeconomical situations of sub-Saharan African countries remains poorly understood owing to the absence of reliable surveillance data. Therefore, there is a clear need to investigate these aspects in the context of interventions implemented

Frédéric Ariey et al. (eds.), *Malaria Control and Elimination*, Methods in Molecular Biology, vol. 2013, https://doi.org/10.1007/978-1-4939-9550-9_16,

against vectors and parasite. A spatiotemporal Bayesian geo-statistical model was recently developed [2] to evaluate the recent evolution of *Plasmodium falciparum* parasite rate (PfPR) and malaria disease incidence. Authors built a large database of malaria field surveys with detailed reconstructions of changing intervention coverage to directly evaluate trends from 2000 to 2015 and quantify the effect of malaria control efforts. They found that (1) PfPR in children (2–10 years) in endemic Africa halved, with around three-quarters of this decline occurring after 2005; (2) the incidence of clinical disease fell by 40%; (3) interventions averted 663 (542–753 credible interval) million clinical cases since 2000; and (4) insecticide-treated nets, the most widespread intervention, were by far the largest contributor (68% of cases averted), while ACT and IRS contributed to 19% and 13%, respectively. From such estimations it is possible to consider that some 450 million (369–512) malaria cases were averted thanks to the scaling-up of insecticide-treated mosquito nets in the last decade.

Despite this impressive progress, Dr Tedros Adhanom Ghebreyesus, Director General of the WHO, underlines in the WHO 2017 report [3] that in 2016 just over half (54%) of the people at risk of malaria in sub-Saharan Africa were sleeping under an insecticide-treated mosquito net—the primary prevention method. This level of coverage represents a considerable increase since 2010 but is far from universal. In the absence of an efficient vaccine, vector control remains the main method of prevention at the community level, and it is worth revisiting how this "old" mosquito net became the "key" element of malaria control.

2 The First Steps of the Mosquito Net

Mosquito nets (MN) have a long history. As recounted by Masefield, utilization of mechanical protection to secure relief from the attacks of mosquitoes is an ancient practice in Europe. Herodotus (484–425 BC) observed that in parts of Egypt above the marshes, the inhabitants were, at night, accustomed to retire in lofty towers as gnats are unable to fly to any height because of the winds. The ancient Romans were also familiar with the net (*canopeum*). In India, Marco Polo observed that the wealthier residents of the Coromandel Coast used bedsteads provided with curtains, which could be closed by pulling a string to prevent annoyance by fleas and other small vermins [4].

With a growing understanding of the epidemiology of malaria, personal protection against bites of mosquitoes improved, due mainly to the availability of wire gauze and of woven cotton MN [5, 6]. In The Gambia, MN were used for a long time for protection against biting insects [7]. At the end of 1980s, a randomized intervention trial showed that children (1–9 years old) sleeping under MN had approximately 30% less malaria episodes than children without MN, even if the reduction was not statistically significant [8]. In the 1990s, a comparison of the efficacy of insecticide-treated and untreated bed nets for the prevention of malaria in children aged 1–4 years showed that children who slept regularly under an untreated bed net had lower parasite and spleen rate and higher mean packed cell volume (PCV) than children who did not use a net [9].

To test whether untreated bed nets protected against malaria, cross-sectional prevalence surveys were implemented in 48 villages of The Gambia involving children (6 months to 5 years), comparing children with untreated nets in good condition ($n = 481$) and children with no net ($n = 252$). The presence of a net reduced *P. falciparum* prevalence by 51%, parasitemia >5000 parasites/mL by 52%, the association fever and parasitemia by 46%, fever and high-density parasitemia by 35%, enlarged spleens by 19%, and moderate to severe anemia by 40% [10]. These authors concluded that an untreated net, provided in relatively good condition, could protect against malaria. However, as already mentioned, in typical situations, nets are frequently not in good condition, and holed nets no longer confer any protection to sleepers.

3 Pyrethroid-Treated Nets

MNs are largely used in tropical regions but their limitations are well known. Therefore, adding a chemical dimension to the physical barrier was tested to improve their efficacy. During World War II, in the Pacific Ocean theater, US Armies treated the nets with DDT. The Chinese army did the same during the 1960s. However, this chemical does not induce the knockdown (KD) effect required to quickly stop mosquitoes when seeking their blood meal. In contrast, pyrethroids, made available in the 1960s and 1970s, are suitable compounds for such effect (*see* **Note 1**).

4 First ITN

Since 1968, the Medical Entomology Department of the Muraz Centre of Bobo-Dioulasso (Burkina Faso) has been a WHO Pesticide Evaluation Scheme (WHOPES) Collaborative Centre, where different house insecticides spraying were tested in experimental huts of the Soumousso field station (*see* Photos 1 and 2). In June 1983, for the first time, cotton-made MN were dipped in aqueous solution of permethrin (CE 20%) to get a concentration of 80 mg a.i./m^2, as proposed by Hervy and Sales, thus making the first pyrethroid-treated nets (ITN) to be tested in the experimental huts of Soumousso [11]. Two models were used, "single"

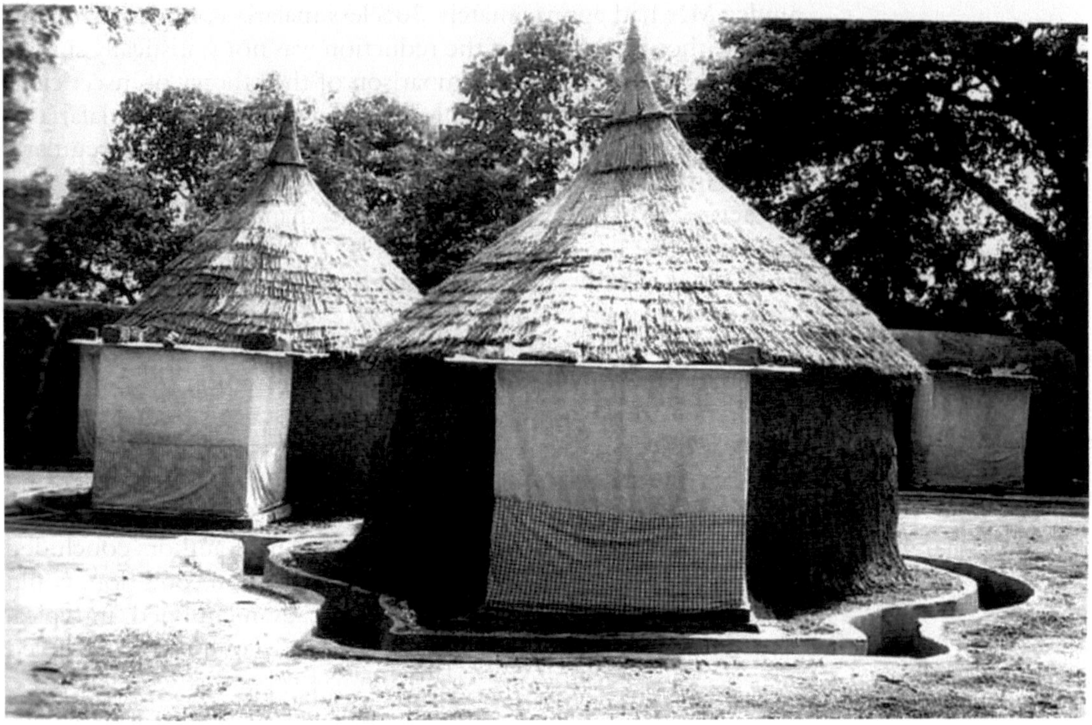

Photo 1 Soumousso Field Station, experimental hut, Mossi model where the first permethrin-treated nets were tested (picture F. Darriet)

one (10 m^2) and "collective" (13.5 m^2), and hung in two types of experimental huts, round "Mossi" and cubic "Bobo." Half of these nets were holed (5% of the whole surface of the net), and half remained intact. Untreated nets were used as control. Four entomological parameters were evaluated in comparing huts with permethrin-treated nets versus untreated nets: deterrence, i.e., the number of mosquitoes caught inside huts; blood-feeding behavior, i.e., the number of fully blood-fed females; and exophilic-induced behavior, i.e., the number of specimens caught in verandah-trap and mortality induced, either immediate or delayed. The free-flying *Anopheles* population was mainly composed of *An. funestus* and *An. gambiae*. Other species of *Anopheles* (*nili*, *flavicosta*, *rufipes*) were caught as well as some *Mansonia*. When comparing samples collected in huts with permethrin-treated nets (PTN) and with untreated nets (control), four important entomological conclusions were reached: (1) high deterrence effect, with 69% fewer *An. gambiae* and 73% fewer *An. funestus* collected; (2) high exophilic effect, with 96% *An. gambiae* and 97% *An. funestus* collected in verandah traps compared to 33% and 27% in control hut, respectively; (3) 15–20% blood-feeding reduction, since 81% *An. gambiae* and 84% *An. funestus* were found blood-fed in huts with holed treated nets compared to

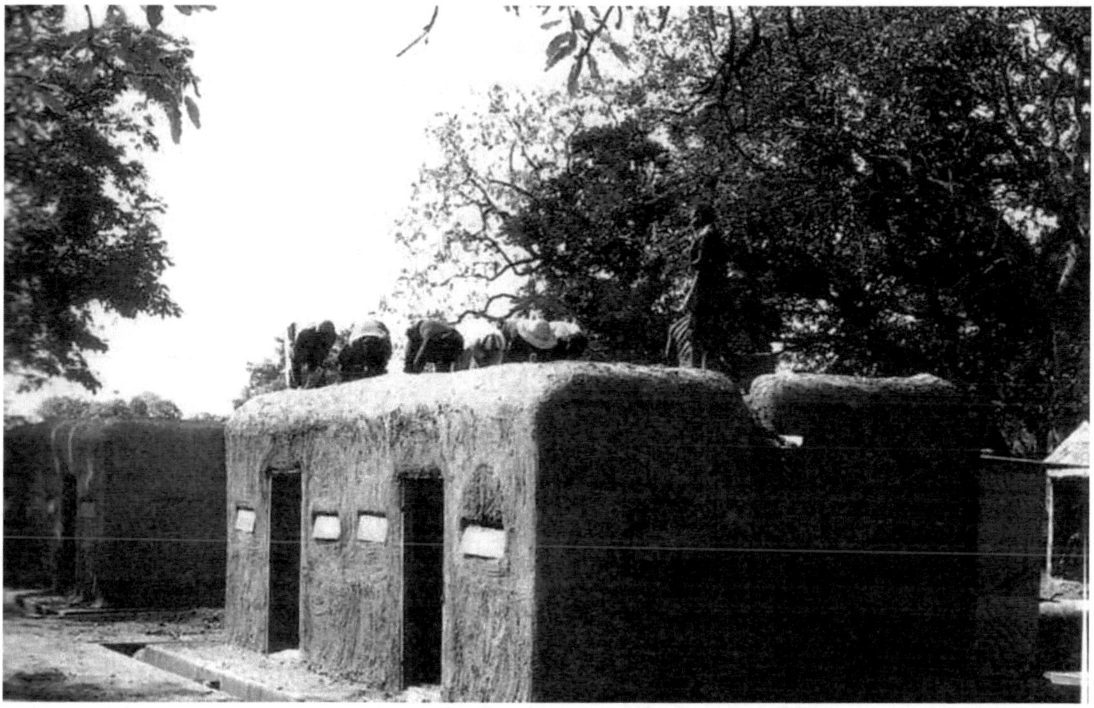

Photo 2 Soumousso Field Station, experimental hut, Bobo model where the first permethrin-treated nets were tested (picture F. Darriet)

99% and 98% in huts with untreated and holed nets; and (4) mortality reached 15–20% for *An. gambiae* and *An. funestus* with holed or intact treated nets.

Bobo-Dioulasso soon became a "cradle" of training on handling mosquito nets. At the end of the 1980s and during the 1990s, numerous trials of permethrin- or deltamethrin-treated nets were performed in sub-Saharan Africa [8, 12–27], Southeast Asia [28–32], the Pacific region [33, 34], South America [35–37], and others. Overall, results converged to indicate a major impact of ITN, i.e., ~90% reduction in transmission and ~50% reduction in morbidity.

The next question was that of the actual efficacy of ITN on malaria mortality. A first report in The Gambia found a 63% reduction in the mortality of children (1–4 years) caused by ITN [38]. Subsequently, a large-scale multicountry ITN program was launched, with TDR support, in Ghana [39], Kenya [40], and The Gambia [41], which showed a reduction of overall infant mortality of 17%, 33%, and 25%, respectively. A fourth trial was performed in Burkina Faso, with impregnated curtains, which provided a similar level of protection with a reduction of 15% [42].

Therefore, a growing body of evidence confirmed the efficacy of ITN interventions in reducing mortality and malaria-specific disease among children and suggested that ITN should be promoted for vector control in National Malaria Control Programs [43]. Nonetheless, several issues remained. It was unclear whether ITN could have an actual impact in "real-life" conditions. An unexpected problem was the low percentage of ITN retreatment, which is required every 6–8 months, and was often not done. Consequently, under WHO pressure, work was devoted to develop "do-it-yourself" kits for impregnating nets. However, impregnation is not easily scalable, which underscored the need for new material.

5 LLIN: Long-Lasting Insecticide-Treated Nets

To address the issue of low compliance in retreating classical ITN, WHO promoted the development of long-lasting industrialized treated nets that could remain effective for several years rather than the 6–8 months of ITN. The concept of long-lasting nets, i.e., the need and feasibility of such nets, was discussed in Montpellier, in 1999, by researchers and heads of chemicals factories.

These industrialized treated nets had to fulfill the requirements of the WHOPES (WHO Pesticide Evaluation Scheme) [44]: 3 years of efficacy under field conditions, resistance to 20 standardized washes, mortality >80%, and KD >95%. Data were examined by working group experts in various meetings to elaborate the WHO recommendations. In January 2011, nine LLIN had received the WHO label, by either full or interim recommendation. Since then, other LLIN types have been analyzed by the WHOPES. Indeed, it must be noted that various types of nets and methods of insecticide treatment exist: coating or incorporating the insecticide into the thread, using polyester, polyethylene, etc. However, all insecticides used were of the pyrethroid class (permethrin, deltamethrin, alpha-cypermethrin, lambda-cyhalothrin).

Thus, since the first publication of permethrin-treated nets in 1984, much work has been devoted to ITN and then LLIN. It is obviously beyond the scope of this chapter to make a comprehensive analysis of this work (*see* web page for a list of WHO recommended long-lasting insecticidal nets at https://www.who.int/neglected_diseases/vector_ecology/vector-control/Long-lasting_insecticidal_nets_June_2017).

The availability of industrialized long-lasting insecticide-treated nets had a crucial impact in the implementation of large-scale vector control programs in a two-step policy: before 2007, the recommendation was to target "at risk" groups (i.e., children <5 years and pregnant women) with LLIN distribution. Subsequently, the WHO issued a statement to promote universal coverage [45].

6 LLIN and Insecticide Resistance (IR)

For two decades now, ITN-LLIN has constituted the main tools for vector control in malaria control programs. However, pyrethroid resistance in main malaria vectors has been reported in many African countries [46–50], which complicate the situation [51, 52]. Indeed, the current spread of pyrethroid resistance (Fig. 1), especially in sub-Saharan Africa where over 90% of the malaria cases occur, is of great concern since pyrethroid, for the time being, is the only insecticide used for net impregnation.

One has to remember that the failure of the great Malaria Eradication Program (MEP) (1955–1969) was mainly due to the resistance of main vectors, such as *An. gambiae*, to DDT. Resistance to DDT was known since 1953, i.e., before the start of the MEP itself, and it was hoped that vector elimination would go faster than the spread of resistance. This hope was misplaced and the program collapsed. Current LLIN are entirely dependent on a single class of insecticide, the pyrethroids, and pyrethroid resistance has been reported in 29 countries in 2010–2015, raising the question as to whether LLIN are still effective [53].

In Benin, a 2-month trial in experimental huts compared the efficacy of lambda-cyhalothrin-treated nets (λTN) (lambda-cyhalothrin Icon, 2.5% CS, 18 mg a.i./m^2) and indoor residual spraying (IRS) (lambda-cyhalothrin, 10% WP) in Ladji (*An. coluzzii*,

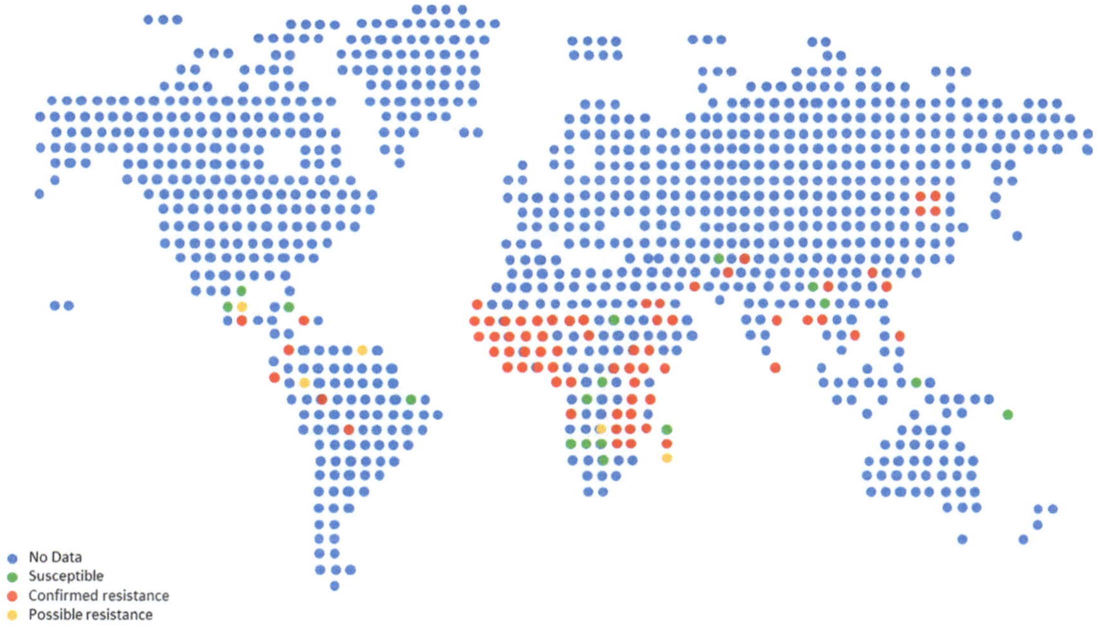

Fig. 1 Reported insecticide susceptibility status for malaria vectors (2010–2014), from WHO, 2016

high-frequency kdr, pyrethroid resistance) and Mallanville (*An. coluzzii*, low kdr, pyrethroid susceptible) [54].

It clearly appeared that the efficacy of λTN was almost complete against pyrethroid susceptible *An. coluzzii* of Mallanville but was strikingly reduced in Ladji where *An. coluzzii* free-flying population is highly resistant to pyrethroid and displays a high kdr frequency. However, the corresponding impact on morbidity was not clear. A meta-analysis of 60 studies was done comparing efficacy of untreated net (UTN), conventionally treated nets (CTN), and LLIN in areas were mosquito resistance varied [50]. Strode and collaborators concluded: "What is clear from the results is that ITN continue to have a substantive effect compared to UTN in many studies," and "ITN continue to have an effect in all categories of resistance."

Another study performed in 2015 sampled mosquitoes in 21 villages in Southern Benin, where mosquitoes have high levels of insecticide resistance, concluded that LLIN continue to offer individual protection against malaria in an area of high resistance. It was therefore considered that malaria vector control still mattered despite insecticide resistance and that it was worth maintaining LLIN as they still protect children against malaria in an insecticide resistance area [55].

To confirm these results, a large-scale pluridisciplinary study was then implemented (June 2012 to November 2016) to evaluate the efficacy of LLIN (PermaNet® 2.0 and Olyset®) on prevalence of infection and incidence of the disease. The study took place in five countries (Benin, Cameroon, Kenya, Sudan, and India) displaying various levels and mechanisms of pyrethroid resistance among the main vectors: *An. gambiae s.s.*, *An. coluzzii*, *An. arabiensis* and *An. funestus* in African countries, and *An. culicifacies* in India [1]. After the follow-up of 40,000 children of 279 clusters in these five countries, it was concluded that (1) long-lasting insecticidal net users had lower infection prevalence (adjusted odds ratio [OR] = 0.63, 95% CI [0.51–0.78]) as well as disease incidence (adjusted rate ratio [RR] = 0.62, [0.41–0.94]) compared to nonusers, across a range of resistance levels; and (2) there was no evidence of an association between insecticide resistance and infection prevalence (adjusted OR = 0.86, [0.70–1.06]) or incidence (adjusted RR = 0.89, [0.72–1.10]).

Consequently, it is now accepted that irrespective of insecticide resistance, populations in malaria endemic areas should continue to use LLIN to reduce their risk of infection and that universal access to LLIN, together with information campaigns to achieve greater use of nets, should continue in malaria endemic areas even in the presence of insecticide resistance.

7 Conclusion

When, in June 1983, at the Muraz Centre in Bobo-Dioulasso, cotton nets were dipped in a plastic basin containing water and a little permethrin and hung in the trap huts of the experimental station of Soumousso and shown to reduce human/*Anopheles* contacts; who would have thought that these ITN, soon after changed into LLIN, would end up being the only actual and operational tool for control of malaria vectors? Who would have thought that a few decades later, hundreds of millions of such LLIN would have been distributed in all countries where malaria is still present and be part of all National Malaria Control Programs? Who would have thought that they would constitute the pinnacle of the fight against vectors, complementing improved case management with rapid detection tests (RDT) and artemisinin-combination therapies (ACT)? Who would have thought that the scaling-up of LLIN, as it has been done these last years, would have prevented hundreds of millions of malaria cases in children and tens of thousands of malaria deaths? Recent figures estimate that half a billion LLIN were distributed in Africa from 2012 to 2014. Considering the number of malaria cases avoided because of individual vector control, one could state: 1 net given = 1 malaria episode averted. In any case, these gains need to be sustained, although the current spread and increase in pyrethroid resistance among main malaria vectors are threatening malaria control programs.

At present, three main issues deserve special attention: biological, i.e., insecticide resistance; ethological, i.e., the behavior often referred to as "misusage of nets"; and economical, considering that nets, even when long-lasting, have a life of about 3 years and must be changed, which implies vast financial resources. Therefore, any vector control program must be conceived and implemented as Integrated Vector Control, often translated as Integrated Vector Management. Teams involved in these actions must be pluridisciplinary and include biological, social, and environmental experts, engineers, etc. Importantly, LLIN are only a part of such multipurpose program. They are not a "magic bullet" but a useful and efficient tool that must be correctly used. Finally, in view of their large-scale use, it will be important to test whether nets confer protection to other vector-borne diseases such as leishmaniasis, Chagas disease, etc. and if they contribute to the quality of sleep and therefore quality of life.

8 Note

1. Pyrethroids are neurotoxins that prevent the closure of the voltage-gated sodium channels in the axonal membranes. They inhibit the repolarization process, leaving the axonal

membrane permanently depolarized, thereby paralyzing the organism. In the 1950s, Rothamsted Research, an agricultural research institution, identified the most active components of pyrethrum, extracted from East African Chrysanthemum flowers that had long been known to have insecticidal property. The first generation of pyrethroids was developed in the 1960s and included bioallethrin, tetramethrin, resmethrin, and bioresmethrin, which are still largely used as domestic insecticides to kill flies and other domestic insects. By the 1970s, the Rothamsted team had discovered a second generation of more persistent compounds, notably permethrin (1973), cypermethrin (used for domestic purposes against household ants and cockroaches), and deltamethrin (which is one of the most popular and widely used insecticides in the world). Later, fenvalerate, lambda-cyhalothrin (used to treat MN), and beta-cyfluthrin were developed. Due to its safety, permethrin was the first pyrethroid used for treating MN.

References

1. Kleinschmidt I, Bradley J, Knox T et al (2018) Implications of insecticide resistance for malaria vector control with long-lasting insecticidal nets: a WHO-coordinated, prospective, international, observational cohort study. Lancet Infect Dis 18:640–649
2. Bhatt S, Weiss D, Cameron E et al (2015) The effect of malaria control on *Plasmodium falciparum* in Africa between 2000 and 2015. Nature 526:207–211
3. WHO (2017) Annual report 2017. WHO, Geneva
4. Partington W (1923) The war against malaria. Ross Research Institute, London
5. Ronald R (1897) On some peculiar pigmented cells found in two mosquitoes fed on malarial blood. Br Med J 18:1786–1788
6. Bruce-Chwatt LJ (1985) Essential malariology. William Heinemann Medican Books Ltd, London
7. MacCormack C (1984) Human ecology and behaviour in malaria control in tropical Africa. Bull World Health Org 62:81–87
8. Snow R, Rowan K, Lindsay S et al (1988) A trial of bed nets (mosquito nets) as a malaria control strategy in a rural area of The Gambia, West Africa. Trans R Soc Trop Med Hyg 82:212–215
9. D'Alessandro U, Olaleye B, McGuire W et al (1995) A comparison of the efficacy of insecticide-treated and untreated nets in preventing malaria in Gambian children. Trans R Soc Trop Med Hyg 89:568–598
10. Clarke S, Bogh C, Brown R et al (2001) Do untreated bednets protect against malaria? Trans R Soc Trop Med Hyg 95:457–462
11. Carnevale P, Bitsindou P, Diomandé L et al (1992) Insecticide impregnation can restore the efficiency of torn bed nets and reduce man-vector contact in malaria endemic areas. Trans R Soc Trop Med Hyg 86:362–364
12. Carnevale P, Robert V, Snow RW et al (1991) L' impact des moustiquaires imprégnées sur la prévalence et la morbidité liée au paludisme en Afrique sub-saharienne. Ann Soc Belg Med Trop 71:127–150
13. Beach R, Ruebush T, Sexton J et al (1993) Effectiveness of permethrin impregnated bednets and curtains for malaria control in a holoendemic area of western Kenya. Am J Trop Med Hyg 49:290–300
14. Karch S, Garin B, Asidi N et al (1993) Moustiquaires imprégnées contre le paludisme au Zaïre. Ann Soc Belg Med Trop 73:37–53
15. Snow RW, Rowan KM, Greenwood BM (1987) A trial of permethrin-treated bed nets in the prevention of malaria in Gambian children. Trans R Soc Trop Med Hyg 81:563–567
16. Lindsay S, Snow R, Bloomfield G et al (1989) Impact of permethrin-treated bed nets on malaria transmission by the *Anopheles gambiae* complex in the Gambia. Med Vet Entomol 3:263–271
17. Sexton J, Ruebush T, Brandling-Bennett A et al (1990) Permethrin-impregnated curtains

and bednets prevent malaria in western Kanya. Am J Trop Med Hyg 43:11–18

18. Lindsay S, Adiamah J, Miller J et al (1991) Pyrethroid treated bednets effects on mosquitoes of the *Anopheles gambiae* complex in The Gambia. Med Vet Entomol 5:477–483
19. Lyimo E, Msuya F, Rwegoshora R et al (1991) Trial of pyrethroid impregnated bednets in an area of Tanzania holoendemic for malaria. Part 3. Effects on the prevalence of malaria parasitaemia and fever. Acta Trop 49:157–163
20. Magesa SM, Wilkes TJ, Mnzava AEP et al (1991) Trial of pyrethroid impregnated bednets in an area of Tanzania holoendemic for malaria. Part 2: effects on the malaria vector population. Acta Trop 49:97–108
21. Njau R, Mosha F, Nguma J (1993) Field trials of pyrethroid impregnated bednets in northern Tanzania. I. Effects on malaria transmission. Insect Sci Appl 5:575–584
22. Pleass R, Armstrong J, Curtis C et al (1993) Comparison of permethrin treatments for bednets in The Gambia. Bull Entomol Res 83:133–140
23. Winch P, Makemba A (1993) Bagamoyo bed net project. Muhimbili Medical Centre. Dar es salaam, Tanzania
24. Jaenson J, Gomes M, Barreto dos Santos R et al (1994) Control of endophagic *Anopheles* mosquitoes and human malaria in Guinea Bissau, West Africa by use of permethrin-treated bed nets. Trans R Soc Trop Med Hyg 88:620–624
25. Stich A, Maxwell C, Haji A et al (1994) Insecticide-impregnated bed nets reduce malaria transmission in rural Zanzibar. Trans R Soc Trop Med Hyg 88:150–154
26. Vulule J, Beach R, Ayieli F et al (1994) Reduced susceptibility of *Anopheles gambiae* to permethrin associated with the use of permethrin-impregnated bednets and curtains in Kenya. Med Vet Entomol 8:71–75
27. Premji Z, Lubega P, Hamisi Y et al (1995) Changes in malaria-associated morbidity in children using insecticide treated mosquito nets in the Bagamoyo District of coastal Tanzania. Trop Med Parasitol 46:147–153
28. Li Z, Zhang C, Wu Y et al (1989) Trial of deltamethrin impregnated-bed nets for the control of malaria transmitted *Anopheles sinensis* and *Anopheles anthropophagus.* Am J Trop Med Hyg 40:356–359
29. Kere N, Parkinson A, Samrawickrema W (1993) The effect of permethrin impregnated bednets on the incidence of *Plasmodium falciparum* in children of north Guadalcanal, Solomon Islands. Southeast Asian J Trop Med Public Health 24:130–137
30. Luo D, Lu D, Yao R et al (1994) Alphamethrin-impregnated bed nets for malaria and mosquito control in China. Trans R Soc Trop Med Hyg 88:625–628
31. Cheng H, Yang W, Kang K et al (1995) Large-scale spraying of bednets to control mosquito vectors and malaria in Sichuan, China. Bull World Health Org 73:321–328
32. Jana-Kara B, Jihullah W, Shahi B et al (1995) Deltamethrin impregnated bednets against *Anopheles minimus* transmitted malaria in Assam. Ind J Trop Med Hyg 98:73–83
33. Charlwood J (1986) A differential response to mosquito nets by *Anopheles* and *Culex* mosquitoes from Papua New Guinea. Trans R Soc Trop Med Hyg 80:958–960
34. Hii JL, Kanai L, Foligela A et al (1993) Impact of permethrin impregnated mosquito nets compared with DDT house-spraying against malaria transmission by *An. farauti* and *An. punctulatus* in the Solomon Islands. Med Vet Entomol 7:333–338
35. Richards F, Klein R, Zea Flores R et al (1993) Permethrin-impregnated bed nets for malaria control in northern Guatemala: epidemiological impact and community acceptance. Am J Trop Med Hyg 49:410–418
36. Charlwood JD, Alecrim WD, Fe N et al (1995) A field trial with lambda-cyhalothrin (Icon) for the intradomiciliary control of malaria transmitted by Anopheles darlingi Root in Rondonia, Brazil. Acta Trop 60:3–13
37. Kroeger A, Mancheno M, Alarcon J et al (1995) Insecticide-impregnated bed nets for malaria control: varying experiences from Ecuador, Colombia, and Peru concerning acceptability and effectiveness. Am J Trop Med Hyg 53:313–323
38. Alonso P, Lindsay S, Armstrong J et al (1991) The effect of insecticide treated bed nets on mortality of Gambian children. Lancet 337:1499–1502
39. Binka FN, Kubaje A, Adjuik M et al (1996) Impact of permethrin impregnated bednets on child mortality in Kassena-Nankana district, Ghana: a randomized controlled trial. Trop Med Int Health 1:147–154
40. Nevill C, Some E, Mungala V et al (1996) Insecticide-treated bed nets reduce mortality and severe morbidity from among children on the Kenyan Coast. Trop Med Int Health 1:139–146
41. D'Alessandro U, Olaleye B, McGuire W et al (1995) Mortality and morbidity from malaria in Gambian children after introduction of an impregnated bednet programme. Lancet 345:479–483

42. Diallo D, Habluetzel A, Cuzin-Ouattara N et al (1999) Widespread distribution of insecticide-impregnated curtains reduces child mortality, prevalence and intensity of malaria infection, and malaria transmission in rural Burkina Faso. Parassitologia 41:377–381
43. Lengeler C (1998). Insecticide-treated bed nets and curtains for malaria control. The Cochrane Library Edition, 3, Oxford Update Software
44. WHO (2007) Insecticide-treated nets: a WHO position statement. World Health Organization, Geneva
45. WHO (2017) Achieving and maintaining universal coverage with long-lasting insecticidal nets for malaria control. WHO reference number: WHO/HTM/GMP/2017.20. WHO, Geneva
46. Etang J, Chandre F, Guillet P et al (2005) Reduced bio-efficacy of permethrin EC impregnated bed nets against an Anopheles gambiae strain with oxidase-based pyrethroid tolerance. Malar J 3:46
47. Ranson H, N'guessan R, Lines J et al (2011) Pyrethroid resistance in African anopheline mosquitoes: what are the implications for malaria control? Trends Parasitol 27:91–98
48. Edi C, Koudou B, Jones C et al (2012) Multiple-insecticide resistance in *Anopheles gambiae* mosquitoes, southern Côte d'Ivoire. Emerg Infect Dis 18:1508–1500
49. Churcher T, Lissenden N, Griffin J et al (2016) The impact of pyrethroid resistance on the efficacy and effectiveness of bednets for malaria control in Africa. Elife 5:e16090
50. Strode C, Donegan S, Garner P et al (2014) The impact of pyrethroid resistance on the efficacy of insecticide-treated bed nets against African anopheline mosquitoes: systematic review and meta-analysis. PLoS Med 11: e1001619
51. Ranson H, Lissende N (2016) Insecticide resistance in African anopheles mosquitoes: a worsening situation that needs urgent action to maintain malaria control. Trends Parasitol 32:187–196
52. Kisinza WN, Nkya TE, Kabula B et al (2017) Multiple insecticide resistance in *Anopheles gambiae* from Tanzania: a major concern for malaria vector control. Malar J 16:439
53. Haji K, Khatib B, Smith S et al (2013) Challenge for malaria elimination in Zanzibar: pyrethroid resistance in malaria vectors and poor performance of long-lasting insecticide nets. Parasit Vectors 6:82
54. N'Guessan R, Corbel V, Akogbeto M et al (2007) Reduced efficacy of insecticide-treated nets and indoor residual spraying for malaria control in pyrethroid resistance area, Benin. Emerg Infect Dis 13:199–206
55. Bradley J, Ogouyèmi-Hounto A, Cornélie S et al (2017) Insecticide-treated nets provide protection against malaria to children in an area of insecticide resistance in southern Benin. Malar J 16:225

Chapter 17

Sampling Adult Populations of *Anopheles* Mosquitoes

Julie-Anne A. Tangena, Alexandra Hiscox, and Paul T. Brey

Abstract

For the control and elimination of malaria, information on the local vector dynamics is essential. This information provides guidance on appropriate and timely deployment of vector control tools and their subsequent success. The data on the dynamics of local mosquito populations can be collected using many different *Anopheles* sampling methods. Dependent on the objectives, resources, time, and local environment, different traps and methods can be chosen. This chapter describes the sampling of adult populations, focusing on the important preparatory stages and some of the widely used sampling methods. The trapping methods discussed in this chapter are the human landing catch, human-baited net trap, animal landing catch, animal-baited net trap, CDC miniature light trap, Biogents Suna trap, peripheral net collection, pyrethrum collection, exit/entry trap, and resting shelter. For optimal deployment in the field, a step-by-step description of the sampling methods is given.

Key words *Anopheles*, Mosquito traps, Human landing catch, Human-baited net trap, Animal landing catch, Animal-baited net trap, CDC miniature light trap, Biogents Suna trap, Peripheral net collection, Pyrethrum collection, Exit-entry trap, Resting shelter

1 Introduction

The essence of malaria control and elimination is to treat existing cases and limit further transmission. To guide malaria control programs, disease transmission risk and transmission intensity measures (such as the entomological inoculation rate) are estimated by identifying the vectors and studying their bionomics [1–4]. This data is also used to measure the success of vector control programs, to monitor insecticide resistance development, and to identify changes in vector populations due to changes in climate and land use [5–10]. Gathering entomological data is challenging, as even in seemingly homogenous areas, species composition, sex ratios, biting periodicity, and gonotrophic age of populations can vary considerably over time and in space [11–18]. Proper implementation of mosquito sampling methods is essential to collect reliable vector data and for the subsequent control and elimination of malaria. The aim of this chapter is to provide starting medical entomologists and

Frédéric Ariey et al. (eds.), *Malaria Control and Elimination*, Methods in Molecular Biology, vol. 2013,
https://doi.org/10.1007/978-1-4939-9550-9_17,

non-experts with clear guidelines on the use of several important mosquito sampling methods.

Dependent on the objective, many different sampling methods, attractants, and locations can be used to collect mosquito data. It is important to keep in mind that there is no mosquito sampling method without bias, with every technique collecting data from a different proportion of the population. To address the objectives properly, it is important to recognize which proportion of the vector population needs to be sampled (endophilic, exophilic, host seeking, blood fed, etc.) and to link this requirement to the sampling methods that best achieve this (Table 1). Literature and regional experts should be consulted to collect information on the local malaria vectors and sampling methods previously used. If feasible, a preliminary study is useful to identify the most suitable collection method, fine-tune its setup, and finalize the study design.

One of the earliest methods with which malaria vectors were collected was the hand collection, the collection of resting mosquitoes from shaded/humid sites in and around the houses using an aspirator [19, 20]. The hand collections were designed to sample the indoor-resting population. Newer methods have largely replaced the use of hand collections, as they can collect a similar proportion of the mosquito population with greater efficiency [19, 20]. All mosquitoes rely on olfactory cues during host-seeking activity [21], with human baits, animal baits, light, carbon dioxide (CO_2), and nylon socks with human, animal, or synthetic odors mainly used to attract mosquitoes to traps. There are also opportunities in the forms of auditory and heat cues. The success of these lures is highly dependent on the local mosquito population, the trapping method used, the distance from the source, the emission rates, and the attractant placement within a trap.

Human-baited collections are an important means of collecting malaria vectors. They not only provide information on which species are anthropophilic (prefer human blood meals); they are also essential for the identification of biting times and locations. The strength of using a human bait is also its weakness, as it can expose the human participants to the bites of disease-transmitting mosquitoes. These ethical concerns can be minimized for diseases like malaria and Japanese encephalitis by using chemoprophylaxis and vaccines [22, 23]. However, no treatments or highly effective vaccines exist for many arboviral diseases. Worryingly, increasing levels of drug resistance in Southeast Asian *Plasmodium* strains are also making the use of malaria chemoprophylaxis more controversial [24, 25] (*see* **Note 1**). Despite the development of innovative trapping methods, human landing catches are still considered the gold standard for collecting mosquitoes. The human-baited net trap is an important alternative to the human landing catch, as it limits the exposure of human volunteers to mosquito-borne diseases and is less labor-intensive. The human-baited net trap has

Table 1
Description of mosquito sampling methods

		Human-baited		Animal-baited		Attractant-baited		Non-attractant			
		Landing catches	Net trap	Landing catches	Net trap	CDC light trap	Suna trap	Peripheral net collections	Pyrethrum collection	Entry/ exit trap	Resting shelter
Collection location	Indoor	ΔΔ	Δ			ΔΔ	ΔΔ		ΔΔ	ΔΔ	Δ
	Outdoor	ΔΔ	ΔΔ	ΔΔ	ΔΔ	Δ	ΔΔ	ΔΔ			Δ
Additional use of CO_2						Yes	Yes				
Mosquito specimen physical condition		***	***	***	***	*	*	***	**	**	***
Data required on:	Morphological identification	***	***	***	***	*	*	***	**	**	***
	Physiological status	*	*	*	*	*	*	**	**	**	**
	Blood index					**	**	**	**	**	**
	Dissections	***	***	***	***	*	*	***	**	**	***
	Estimating man-biting rate	***	**			**	**		*	*	
Research objective:	Malaria vector species composition	++	++			+	+		+	+	
	Location of biting (indoor/outdoor)	+++	++			+	+		++	++	
	Time of biting	+++	++	+	+	+	+				
	Resting behavior							+	+	+	+
	Monitor success of vector control	++	++	++	++	++	++	+	++	++	+
	Insecticide susceptibility status	+	+	+	+			+		+	+
	Early warning systems			+	+	++	++	+		+	+
	Mass-trapping and push-pull systems					+	++				

Δ Challenging, ΔΔ Suitable, *Acceptable, **OK, ***good, +Acceptable, additional trapping methods needed, ++OK, additional trapping methods advised, +++ good, other trapping methods not necessary been used all over the world in slightly different setups with varying success [20, 26–29]. The net trap, compared to the landing catches, has several important limitations: host attraction does not imply host feeding, mosquitoes have to overcome challenges to enter the trap, mosquitoes can enter the trap looking for shelter, mosquitoes can accidentally enter the trap, and mosquitoes can escape the net trap after failing to blood feed [29–32]. Animals can substitute human baits in both human landing catches and human-baited net traps, if the main malaria vectors are known to be both anthropophilic and zoophilic (prefer both human and animal blood meals). Animal-baited net traps have been especially useful for long-term surveillance studies, vector control effectiveness studies, and insecticide susceptibility tests [29, 30].

Fan-powered traps with attractants have been used extensively to collect anopheline mosquitoes in the field. These traps are generally preferred to human- and animal-baited traps, as they provide standardized collections with little labor investment. Fan-powered traps are easy to set up, are not reliant on the collecting efficacy of individuals, and are not affected by the varying attractiveness of the baits. Different fan-powered traps and attractants may be used depending on the local mosquito ecology, the target mosquito species, and their physiological status. Studies to date have indicated that human biting rates can only be estimated using fan-powered traps, if comparison studies are made with human landing catches. The identification of the best trap setup is time-consuming and requires extensive studies. Fan-powered traps also require a high financial investment and a reliable source of electrical power [33]. Examples of widely used attractant-baited traps are the CDC miniature light trap and Biogents Suna trap. The CDC miniature light trap is one of the most widely used traps for the collection of anopheline mosquitoes. All around the world, CDC light traps have replaced the human- and animal-baited sampling methods, with a wide variety of mosquito species collected at low labor cost [34–36]. However, care should be taken when analyzing the light trap data, as these traps may fail to sample important malaria vectors in representative numbers [15, 37]. The Biogents Suna trap is a relatively new trap [38–40]. In combination with a synthetic attractant blend that mimics human skin odors (referred to as the MB 5 lure) and a CO_2 supplement, the Suna trap has been successfully utilized to reduce mosquito entry rates, to collect *Anopheles gambiae* mosquitoes outdoors, and for mass trapping control efforts in Kenya [38, 39].

Non-attractant sampling methods collect mosquitoes in their flight path or in their resting area. Methods suitable for sampling without the use of attractant stimuli include peripheral net collections, pyrethrum spray collections, exit/entry traps, and resting shelters. Peripheral net collections, also referred to as barrier screen collections, are an outdoor collection method with which mosquitoes are intercepted during their flight by setting a net barrier in their flight path. This allows the collection of both blood-fed mosquitoes and host-seeking mosquitoes from opposite sides of the netting [41, 42]. The pyrethrum spray collections collect mosquitoes by spraying a room with pyrethrum insecticide, after which all knocked down mosquitoes are collected from the floor and other surfaces. Mosquito collections with pyrethrum spraying are highest in rooms with few exit points and a high number of endophagic and/or endophilic mosquitoes. They are a reliable way to identify indoor-resting mosquitoes and to recognize the seasonal changes in resting densities [29, 43, 44]. However, they do not collect all endophilic mosquitoes in an area; some mosquitoes might escape, rest underneath other shelters, or might not be found [30]. Exit/entry traps are cages attached to a window or door, which collect mosquitoes either entering or exiting rooms. The physiological state of the mosquitoes collected in the exit/entry traps provides information on the feeding and resting preference of the vector mosquitoes in an area [43, 45]. Resting shelters are artificial resting locations developed to attract mosquitoes that rest either before host seeking or when blood fed and developing eggs [30, 46]. Resting shelters can come in different shapes and sizes and can be used with or without the addition of attractants [30, 44, 47–50]. The shelters can be created by digging into the ground (pit trap) or by placing containers in which the malaria vectors are likely to rest such as fiber pots, clay pots, woven baskets, or boxes. Number of mosquitoes collected in the shelters may be low, as they are unable to compete with the great number of natural resting sites [45, 51].

In this chapter we describe the most commonly used adult *Anopheles* mosquito collection methods. Subheading 2 highlights the important aspects that need to be considered prior to deployment of the trapping methods in the field. Subheading 3 gives a step-by-step description of sampling adult populations of *Anopheles* mosquitoes.

2 Materials

2.1 Study Design

2.1.1 Sample Size Calculations

Collections performed at only a few sites or for a small number of nights are unlikely to be representative of the local mosquito population, while using a large number of collection sites or collection nights might not be feasible due to limited time, personnel, and other resources. To ensure the available resources are used optimally to reach the objectives of a study, the minimum required sample size should be calculated at the commencement of any entomological study. The sample size is calculated using the study objective. Going back to the basics of statistics, the objective of a study is focused on hypothesis testing. The null hypothesis (H_0) is

Table 2
Hypothesis testing

	H_0 is true	H_0 is false
Decision: reject	Type I error, probability = α	Correct decision, probability = $1-\beta$ (power)
Decision: fail to reject	Correct decision, probability = $1-\alpha$	Type II error, probability = β

that the observations recorded result from chance. An example is "there is no difference between trap A and trap B." The alternative hypothesis (H_1 hypothesis) is "there is a difference between trap A and trap B."

Using statistical analysis we can identify whether H_0 should be rejected in favor of the alternative hypothesis or not. There are two important errors that can occur when rejecting or not rejecting the H_0; the first error is that H_0 is rejected, while in reality it should not have been (i.e., the results lead to a conclusion that there is a difference between trap A and trap B when in reality there is not). This is called a false-positive or Type I error (Table 2). The probability of a Type I error occurring is noted with α. Generally α is set at 5% (0.05), indicating that a 5% probability of a false positive is acceptable for a given study (*see* **Note 2**). The second type of error is that the H_0 is not rejected, while in reality it should have been (i.e., the results lead to a conclusion that there is no difference between trap A and trap B where in reality there is). This is called a false-negative or Type II error (Table 2). The Type II error rate is noted with β and is related to the power of a test, the probability of correctly rejecting a false null hypothesis ($1-\beta$). Generally, the power of a study is set at 80% (0.8) probability of correctly rejecting a false null hypothesis.

When comparing two sets of data (e.g., catch size of a given mosquito species in trap A and trap B), the following sample size calculation formula is used (1) [52]. The results from the sample size calculation represent the total number of comparisons that need to be performed (which could be divided by two if two sets of traps are used simultaneously). To identify the expected variation in mosquito catch sizes, data from a preliminary study or other studies in the area are essential. If such data is not available, existing data taken from the literature should be used to make the sample size calculations:

$$\text{Sample size} = \frac{\left(\sigma_A^2 + \sigma_B^2\right)\left(z_{1-\alpha/2} + z_{1-\beta}\right)^2}{\Delta^2}. \tag{1}$$

σ_A^2 =Variance of trap data A.

σ_B^2 = Variance of trap data B.

$\alpha = 0.05$.

$1-\beta = 0.8$.

$Z_{1-\alpha/2} = 1.96$ (a standardized number).

$Z_{1-\beta} = 0.84$ (a standardized number).

$\Delta = |\mu_B - \mu_A|$.

μ_A= Mean of trap data A.

μ_B= Mean of trap data B.

The sample size calculation formula assumes (1) equal sample sizes in both data sets, (2) normally distributed data, and (3) a two-sided significance test will be performed to analyze the data.

2.1.2 Latin Square Design

An important and recommended study design for mosquito sampling methods is the Latin square design. This balanced design is especially useful for the comparison of mosquito sampling methods or when human participants are involved. It enables the number of collection days to be limited as the location of the trap and the collection days can be controlled for. A Latin square design consists of a square with Latin letters, with each letter corresponding to a certain treatment or trap. In one column and one row, every letter is only present once (Table 3). The Latin square design can be increased in size dependent on the number of sampling methods or participants involved. If ten traps are compared, the design will be a 10 × 10 square. An example of a Latin square design for the comparison of five trapping methods is shown in Table 4. Depending on the minimum number of comparisons necessary, which is calculated using the sample size calculations, the Latin square design can be repeated. For a sample size of 13, the 5 × 5 Latin square needs to be repeated three times to generate sufficient statistical power to address the question while keeping a balanced design. The same order can be used in the three Latin square replicates, or the three squares can be designed separately, to increase the number of different combinations. If a human volunteer is used as a trapping method, it is recommended to link the variation in attractiveness of the participant and its collection efficacy to one geographical position. It is also possible to account for differences between participants by rotating their positions throughout the collection period. However, variation between

Table 3
An example of a 4 × 4 Latin square design

A	B	C	D
B	C	D	A
C	D	A	B
D	A	B	C

Table 4
An example of a Latin square design for the comparison of five trapping methods

	Location 1	Location 2	Location 3	Location 4	Location 5
Day 1	A	B	C	D	E
Day 2	B	C	D	E	A
Day 3	C	D	E	A	B
Day 4	D	E	A	B	C
Day 5	E	A	B	C	D

The Latin letters describe five different trapping methods

the collection days will need to be identified using traps that do not differ in attraction (i.e., light traps).

2.1.3 Selection of Study Area

A suitable study area is selected using data on the malaria disease dynamics and the local environment. If several villages are compared, they should be of comparable demographics and habitat surroundings. The study design and selected study area should be discussed with the appropriate governmental authorities (*see* **Note 3**). After receiving appropriate administrative approval, the study should be discussed with the village leaders, opinion leaders, and other key stakeholders in the community (*see* **Note 4**). Observational data should be collected from the local community on the mosquito dynamics (mosquito nuisance, mosquito breeding sites, etc.) and mosquito-borne disease dynamics. This information is valuable for the identification of the mosquito collection sites where catch sizes may be highest. Building a good relationship with the local population is essential for the successful implementation of mosquito sampling methods. Time and care should be taken to involve the local community as much as possible in the design and implementation of a study. This involvement also provides an opportunity for training of the local population in mosquito-borne disease dynamics and mosquito control.

2.2 Ethical Approval

At the start of the study, it needs to be determined whether ethical approval is necessary as regulations can differ considerably between countries and between different funding organizations. Approval might be necessary even when human participants are not directly involved. Apart from country regulations, ethical approval from the organizations associated with the project including sponsors and research institutions might be required. Investigate this beforehand, including the dates when the committees meet and when the deadlines for protocol submissions are. The submission and approval often takes time. It may require the completion of forms and approvals specific for a particular region. Ensure this application process is started directly after the research protocol is finalized and at least 6 months before the start of the study. Allow sufficient budget to cover the fees for the ethical review of a study. The use of animals requires different approvals than for human participants, and these applications may also take time and should be made as soon as possible.

2.3 Safety of Fieldworkers

To ensure the safety of all fieldworkers, the following aspects should be considered:

- Fieldworkers should be provided with the appropriate vaccinations before the start of the study. This should be at no cost to the fieldworkers.
- During activities in the field, all fieldworkers should have good medical insurance provided by the institution running the study.
- A first aid box should be available in the field. The content of the box should be assembled in close collaboration with local medical doctors. The first aid box should at least include all commonly used medicines, a thermometer, stethoscope, blood pressure meter, sterilizing products, cotton wool, and Band-Aids. Furthermore, if collections are done in an area with venomous snakes, antivenoms and appropriate fluids should be included. Depending on the local epidemiology, rapid diagnostic tests for malaria (*Plasmodium falciparum* and *P. vivax*) and dengue should also be included.
- The fieldworkers should not use any repellent or insecticide-treated clothing during the collection period. They are protected from mosquito bites by wearing thick, long-sleeved clothing and closed shoes.
- The field supervisors, but preferably all fieldworkers, should have successfully completed a basic first aid training. If the collections are done in an area with venomous snakes, the training should include how to administer antivenom.
- Fieldworkers should receive a short training on the different endemic diseases in the area, including their symptoms and treatment.
- A clear emergency protocol should be in place for fieldworkers in case of an emergency. The protocol should include the contact information for the nearest health center, hospital, and police station.
- Depending on the selected collection sites, a satellite phone might be necessary.

2.4 Selection of Human Participants and Animal Baits

2.4.1 Supervisor and Participant Selection

1. A clear plan is made regarding the protection of participants against local vector-borne diseases using vaccines and/or chemoprophylaxis (*see* **Note 1**).
2. A meeting is organized in the study area with the village leaders to explain the project and receive their approval. During this time one or two supervisors are selected from the local population (*see* **Note 5**).
3. A general village meeting is organized to present the project and sensitize the community.
4. A fieldworker fluent in the local language clearly explains the project aims and methodology and that human participants are sought from the local population. The requirements for participation are highlighted. Participants in human landing catches should be non-smoking healthy males >18 years (*see* **Note 6**). They should not drink alcohol nor eat spiced and garlic-containing food 24 h before and during the collection period (*see* **Note 7**). Both the risks and benefits of participation are explained.
5. Community members are given the opportunity to ask questions and to receive full answers to these questions.
6. At a set date and time, supervisors and human landing catch participants are invited for a health check. If necessary, multiple visits to the study area are planned to recruit a sufficient number of participants.
7. One by one a fieldworker fluent in the local language informs the participants and supervisors about the project, highlighting the risks and benefits. Opportunity is given to ask questions concerning the study. The participants are informed that they can leave the project at any time without penalty, even after signing the consent form (*see* **Note 8**).
8. Supervisors' and participants' health is checked. Participants with fever are excluded. Eyesight is tested by asking participants to read a number plate that is about 10 m away or to thread a large needle. To reduce the potential harm related to secondary exposure to dengue, participants with a history of dengue fever are excluded from the study in regions where dengue transmission occurs.
9. Participants and supervisors that pass the health check are provided with an information sheet in their local language. The information sheet contains all information about the project: the risks, the benefits, and the contact information of the fieldworkers (Fig. 1). Illiterate participants are explained what the document entails and encouraged to call if they have any questions during the study period.

Information sheet for study participants (translated into the local language)

<< PROJECT NAME; Title of project >>

Information sheet for the collection of mosquitoes using *<<mosquito trapping method>>*

Responsible scientists: *<<Name, function and organisation, contact details>>*

Introduction:

You are invited to take part in a research study. Before you decide if you want to take part, it is important that you understand why the research is being done. Allow me to explain what the study is about and what it will involve. Please take your time to listen to the information carefully. Ask us if there is anything that is not clear.

Purpose:

<<Describe situation of vector-borne diseases in study area>> People get sick when bitten by a certain type of mosquito. The mosquito spits the disease into you, making you sick. *<<Describe the objective of the study>>*. This information is important for us to find ways of stopping the diseases where you live.

What will happen if you agree to participate?

- You may be exposed to mosquito bites, which could make you sick.
- *<<Describe the collection method that is used by participants>>*. You will collect mosquitoes using an aspirator and transfer them into holding cups.
- We will need you to help us collect mosquitoes in the months of *<<xx to xx>>* for a total of *<<xx>>* times.
- You will be asked to collect mosquitoes during the day and/or night for *<<xx>>* consecutive hours. Starting time will be *<<xx : xx>>* h or *<<xx : xx>>* h.
- You will have a <<xx>> minute break each hour.
- You will be asked to collect mosquitoes in *<<describe the different study sites>>*.
- You must not drink alcohol or smoke before or during the collection period.
- *<<Mention if insecticides or repellents are used in the study>>*.

Benefits: The results of the study will help us understand how *<<malaria and dengue>>* can be controlled in the area where you live and work.

You will receive:

- Payment for this work of *<<xx 'local currency'>>* for day collections and *<<xx 'local currency'>>* for night collections.
- *<<Medical insurance for the duration of the project>>*. If you feel unwell during the field work or within three weeks after mosquito collections, you will receive prompt medical treatment free of charge. If you are feverish or feel unwell, please contact

Fig. 1 Information sheet for human-baited collections

the local health office/hospital/clinic directly and call ***<<Head of project; Tel: xx-xxxx>>.***

- *<<Vaccination for protection against Japanese encephalitis>>*
- *<<Medicine to protect you from malaria throughout the study duration>>*

Risks: Mosquitoes you are collecting in the different habitats may carry diseases. You may be exposed to *<<malaria, dengue, chikungunya, Zika, West Nile etc.>>*, for which no treatment exists.

Participation: You have the right not to join the study and to leave the study at any time without penalty or loss of benefits to which you are otherwise entitled.

Confidentiality: Your individual information will be kept private. No personal information will be stored in a computer file. The paperwork showing your name will be kept in a locked cupboard and not digitalised.

Payment: There is payment for participation in this study of *<<xx 'local currency'>>* for day collections and *<<xx 'local currency'>>* for night collections.

Research sponsor: This research is sponsored by the *<<funders of the study>>*

Ethical Approval: This study has been approved by *<<ethics committee name>>*, whose task it is to make sure that research participants are protected. If you wish to find out more about the local ethics committee, please contact *<<name, address and telephone number>>*

Please feel free to ask questions, if you have any. You can always reach us by calling << *Head of project; Tel: xx-xxxx*>>

Fig. 1 (continued)

10. Supervisors and participants are asked to sign a consent form in their local language (Fig. 2). If they are illiterate, a witness consent is signed by a fellow community member who has witnessed the fieldworker explain the nature of the study and has witnessed the participant agreeing to participate (*see* **Note 9**).
11. In areas where malaria is endemic, all participants receive free access to malaria chemoprophylaxis using the locally recommended drug (*see* **Note 10**). All are provided with the appropriate vector-borne disease vaccinations for the area (*see* **Note 11**).
12. Phone numbers, names, and addresses of the supervisors and participants are collected (*see* **Note 12**). They receive a schedule of the collection days and times.
13. Before the start of the study, supervisors and participants are educated on the basics of vector-borne diseases. They are taught how to collect mosquitoes with an aspirator.

Consent form for human-baited collections (translated into the local language)

<< PROJECT NAME; Title of project >>
Identification number participant: ....
Name Village ....
Name of participant.. consents to participate in the above research study.

Participant Statement

I, the participant named above, have witnessed a << Project name >> staff member explaining the nature of the study as described on the information sheet. The purpose of the research study has been explained and opportunity has been given to ask questions concerning this study. Any such questions have been answered in full. Should any further questions arise concerning this study, I know to contact **<< Head of project; Tel: xx-xxxx >>.** I consent voluntarily to participate as a participant in this research and I understand that I may withdraw from this study at any time without penalty.

Name of Participant ....

signature/thumb print.................................Date............... (day / month / year)

Person obtaining consent ....

signature/thumb print.................................Date............... (day / month / year)

Witness consent, if applicable

Witness Statement: I have witnessed the << Project name >> staff member explaining the nature of the study as described on the information sheet to the person named above. The purpose of the research study has been explained and opportunity has been given to ask questions concerning this study. Any such questions have been answered in full. Should any further questions arise concerning this study the participant knows to contact **<< Head of project; Tel: xx-xxxx >>.** The participant understands that he/she may withdraw from this study at any time without penalty.

I confirm that the individual has given consent freely.

Name of witness ....

signature/thumb print.................................Date............... (day / month / year)

Person obtaining consent ....

signature/thumb print.................................Date............... (day / month / year)

Fig. 2 Consent form for human-baited collections

14. If the participants agree, their names could be shared with the local health offices in advance so that they are aware of who is taking part in the study which involves human landing catches and/or human-baited net trapping.
15. If the collection sites are far away from the village, transportation is arranged for the participants.

2.4.2 Animal Bait Selection

1. A meeting is organized in the study area with the village leaders to explain the project and receive their approval.
2. The village leaders are asked to identify community members who may be willing to provide the animals. If necessary, payment to the owner of the animals per time period is discussed.
3. One or more animal owners are identified who can easily transport their animals to the mosquito collection site. It is confirmed that animals have not been given medicine that can influence the host-seeking behavior of mosquitoes, such as ivermectin and acaricides. Owners of the animals are asked for approval to use their animals.
4. The owners of the animals receive a schedule of the collection days, and (if available) their phone numbers are noted.

2.5 Field Laboratory

If the mosquito collections are done far away from the research institute (more than 3 h one way), a field laboratory should be established close to the collection site for rapid handling of specimens. The field laboratory should minimally consist of a clean room with a table, fridge, and – 20 °C freezer. Samples which are to be molecularly analyzed for virus identification need to be stored at −80 °C after collection in the field or stored in RNA stabilization solution. Choose a field laboratory that stays cool during the day (easier working environment) and which is not facing a main road (to limit dust). Below, a short description of possible activities that could be performed in the field laboratory is given.

2.5.1 Morphological Identification of Mosquito Samples

The holding cups or collection bags containing mosquitoes are transported back to the laboratory and placed inside the –20 °C freezer for ~1 h to kill the mosquitoes. One collection cup/bag is emptied on to a large piece of white paper. The mosquitoes are carefully placed inside a petri dish using forceps. The petri dish with mosquitoes is placed underneath the stereo microscope. All mosquitoes are identified morphologically using mosquito identification keys. Mosquitoes collected from electric traps generally go through the fan blades before reaching the collection cup. The morphological identification of the collected samples is then challenging. This is further complicated by the samples easily drying out in the collection cups.

The mosquitoes are transferred to labelled Eppendorf tubes where they are kept dry by placing a few beads of silica gel covered with cotton wool in the Eppendorf tube. Generally, mosquitoes of the same species and sex and with the same abdominal condition collected at one site on one date are placed in one Eppendorf tube (referred to as a mosquito pool). However, depending on the study objectives, the samples can be stored individually. A maximum of ten samples are placed in one 1.5 mL Eppendorf tube, after which a second tube should be used. The collection site data from the holding cup/collection bag are copied into the data form (Fig. 3). Next, the information of each individual mosquito is recorded in a notebook: the date of morphological identification, the mosquito species name, the abdominal condition, and the Eppendorf tube number in which the sample is stored. The data form is an example for mosquito samples that have been dissected. Each row represents one mosquito in one storage tube. If dissections are not done, one row can represent a mosquito pool in one storage tube. An additional column should be added to quantify the number of mosquitoes. The Eppendorf tube is retained in a storage box inside the freezer for future transportation back to the central laboratory. The next holding cup/collection bag is emptied and the process repeated. At the end, the dissecting kit is cleaned with a piece of cotton wool and 80% alcohol.

2.5.2 Blood Meal

To understand the host preference of vector species, the blood meal of the blood-fed mosquitoes can be analyzed. After morphological identification, the abdomen of the mosquito is squashed with a clean needle on a piece of Whatman no. 3 filter paper [43]. The bloodstain is numbered by writing on the paper with a pencil, and the blood meal squash number is included in the data file (Fig. 3). Until analysis, the filter papers can be stored at room temperature in a dark dry place with silica gel and no access for insects.

2.5.3 Dissections

Freshly collected mosquitoes can be dissected if they are in good condition (not desiccated). Dissections can be used to determine gonotrophic status [53] or to test for malaria infection by identification of oocysts or sporozoïtes. If the mosquitoes are not yet knocked down, they are cooled in the fridge for 5 min. The samples are transferred to a petri dish on ice and morphologically identified. One by one the mosquitoes are carefully dissected on a glass slide with a drop of distilled water or phosphate-buffered saline (PBS) solution [43]. A cover slip is placed on top of the dissected area, and the area is examined with a compound microscope. The data is included in the data file (Fig. 3). The remaining pieces of the mosquito are carefully transferred to a clean empty Eppendorf tube. The Eppendorf number is noted in the data file (Fig. 3).

Example of a data form for mosquito sampling results

Unique ID #	Trap set	Trap collected	Location N′	Location E′	Habitat	Room sampling form	Room ID #	Time of collection	Participant or Fieldworker #	Identification dd/mm/yy	Genus	Species	Abdominal conditions	Blood meal - squash #	Dissections				Storage tube #
	dd/mm/yy		(GPS)												Spermatheca	Oocysts #	sporozoïtes	Parity	
1	22/11/17	23/11/17	19°40′34.30″N	102°6′24.10″E	Forest			18.00	P1	24/11/17	*Anopheles*	*gambiae* s.s	gravid		positive	5	positive	parous	1
2	22/11/17	23/11/17	19°40′34.30″N	102°6′24.10″E	Forest			18.00	P1	24/11/17	*Anopheles*	*gambiae* s.s	Blood fed	1	positive	0	positive	parous	2
3	22/11/17	23/11/17	19°40′56.80″N	102°7′1.80″E	Village	1	1	18.00	F1	24/11/17	*Anopheles*	*gambiae* s.s	unfed		negative	0	negative	nulliparous	3
4																			
5																			
6																			

Fig. 3 Example of a data form for mosquito sampling results

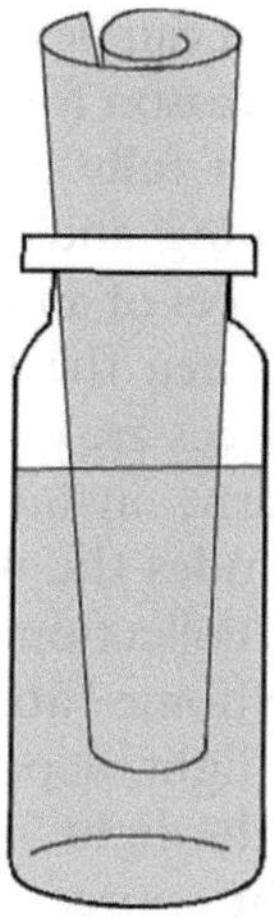

Fig. 4 A piece of filter paper in a small bottle with 10% sugar water for mosquito feeding

2.5.4 Insecticide Susceptibility Tests

For insecticide susceptibility tests, live adult mosquitoes or adults emerged from larval collections are carefully released into a holding cage (30 × 30 × 30 cm). The holding cage is placed on a table at 27 °C ± 2 °C with 75% ± 5% relative humidity or other conditions depending on the preference of the mosquito species. If humidity in the room is too low, damp towels are placed on top of the cages. The table is made inaccessible for ants by placing the legs in large cups of water/vegetable oil or by coating them with petroleum jelly. The table should be checked daily to ensure the ants have no access. A small container with 10% sugar water is placed inside the holding cage, with a piece of filter paper rolled up inside (Fig. 4). This provides the mosquitoes with access to sugar water to feed on. The mosquitoes are left in the cage for at least 24 h before exposure tests are performed.

Only actively flying mosquitoes are used for susceptibility testing. In order to select mosquitoes for the tests, lightly tap the cage and softly breathe into the cage. A hand is held about 2 cm from the cage, and only mosquitoes that exhibit host-seeking behavior are selected for the susceptibility tests. Host-seeking behavior is regarded as landing and/or probing close to the hand. One by one the mosquitoes are aspirated to morphologically identify them to species before releasing them in the bioassays. For detailed description of the bioassay procedures, please check the World Health Organization guidelines on test procedures for insecticide resistance monitoring in malaria vector mosquitoes [54].

2.6 Attractants

2.6.1 Light

Light can be an attractant for host-seeking mosquitoes [55] though the reason for attraction of mosquitoes to UV or incandescent light is not fully understood. Light is used as an attractant during the evening and night. The trap is placed in an area with no other sources of ambient light (e.g., an unlit room) to avoid competition between the trap and other light sources. If other external light sources are present in the collection area, they should be described clearly, including changes throughout the study period. This includes the moon phase, which can have a significant impact on the collection success, and the use of electrical light by residents of the home [56]. Mosquito species differ greatly in their response to the light, dependent on their distance from the source, the intensity of the light source, and the wavelength of the light source. The light source is generally attractive for mosquitoes from afar but repellent once the mosquitoes are closer. It is thus recommended that a preliminary field or literature study is done to select the best collection method for sampling the local vector population.

2.6.2 Carbon Dioxide

Carbon dioxide (CO_2) is one of the most commonly used attractants for mosquitoes. CO_2 is a universal attractant which activates mosquitoes' host-seeking behavior [57]. Because CO_2 is a long-range attractant, it may allow for a greater freedom in trapping placement. The efficacy of CO_2 is dependent on the mosquito species, the type of trap used, gas emission rate, and location of attractant placement relative to the trap. High CO_2 emission rates attract mosquitoes from afar but repel them once they are closer to the source. Low emission only attracts mosquitoes that are already in close proximity to the trap. It is important to conduct preliminary studies or refer to existing literature to identify the right emission rate of CO_2. Carbon dioxide can be produced for mosquito collections using one of the three methods described below.

1. *The sublimation of CO_2 from dry ice*: 0.5 kg of dry ice is placed in an insulated 1 L box with an open pour spout, which is connected to the trap entrance using a flexible tube (0.5 cm diameter). Aluminum foil and/or newspapers can be used to cover the dry ice. There is little control over the emission rates, and the sublimation of CO_2 is highly dependent on the ambient temperatures. The cold gas also decreases the temperature of the air around the trap. It is therefore important to measure variations in temperature during the collection period. If dry ice is easily obtainable in the study area, the sublimation of CO_2 is a suitable method.
2. *Sugar/molasses fermentation*: at least 1 h before trapping commences, 250 g of sugar or 250 mL of sugarcane-derived molasses should be mixed with 17.5 g dry instant yeast and 2 L of water in a clean 5 L plastic jerry can or glass bottle with lid [58]. The container is vigorously shaken for 30 s to mix all the

ingredients properly. A large container is used for the fermentation process to ensure there is enough space for foam production that is a by-product of the fermentation. A hole slightly larger than 0.5 cm diameter is made in the lid for introduction of a silicone tube (0.5 cm diameter). The gaps between the lid and tube are sealed using Para film and Vaseline to ensure that all gas release is through the silicone tube. After about 30 min, an average of 80.63 mL CO_2/min is released from the jerry can, with highest fermentation rates occurring during the first 11 h [58, 59]. The silicone tube from the jerry can is attached to the trapping device, near the trap entrance. Similar to dry ice, the production of CO_2 from sugar/molasses is highly dependent on the ambient temperatures. It is thus important to measure variations in temperature during the collection period. Sugar fermentation is a suitable method to implement in the field due to the use of easily accessible materials. However, the emission rate of CO_2 cannot be controlled, and the transportation of the jerry can be challenging.

3. *Compressed gas*: a cylinder with CO_2 is placed next to the trap with the release tube located near the trap entrance with a flow rate of 80 mL CO_2/min. The bulkiness and cost of the cylinders make this method more challenging in the field. However, the emission rate can be constant and controlled, which is not possible for the other two methods. This method can be used if CO_2 cylinders are easily obtainable in the field.

A possible alternative to the use of CO_2 for some mosquito species may be 2-butanone, an organic solvent [60]. This alternative can be useful in formulation with other human-derived volatiles impregnated on nylon strips [61].

2.6.3 Human and Animal Odor

Nylon socks with human or animal odor can be used as an attractant in traps [62, 63]. This is one of the easiest methods to activate the local host-seeking mosquitoes. If human odor is required, a local volunteer is asked to wear a 15 denier nylon sock for 24 h. While wearing the nylon sock, the volunteer is not allowed to use scented products or shower. They are also asked to abstain from smoking, drinking alcohol, and eating strongly spiced foods or foods containing large amounts of garlic. For animal odor collections, the nylon sock is bound on the upper leg of an animal for 24 h. It is confirmed with the animal owner that the animal has not been given medicine that could influence the host-seeking behavior of mosquitoes (ivermectin and acaricides). After 24 h the nylon sock with odor is stored in a clean glass bottle at –20° using latex gloves. About 30 min before use, the glass bottles are taken out of the freezer and acclimatized. The nylon socks are taken out of the glass bottle using latex gloves and attached to the trap. The wearing of gloves is important to avoid contamination with the odor of the person handling the odor samples. The nylon sock can be used for at least 8 days of collection [64]. The attractiveness of the nylon sock is likely longer. However, no experiments have been done to confirm this.

2.6.4 Synthetic Odor Blends

Chemicals, including octanol, L-lactic acid, ammonium, and 2-butanone, are attractive for some mosquito species during their host-seeking phase [55, 60, 65–67]. These semiochemicals can be blended to create an even more attractive blend which closely mimics the odor of a human host as it is perceived by malaria vector mosquitoes. The addition of CO_2 to the use of the blends can further increase mosquito attraction and numbers trapped [60]. The development of a synthetic odor blend mimicking human skin odors is challenging. It takes time and many trials, both in the laboratory and in the field. An example of a successful synthetic blend is the MB 5 blend. This blend is more attractive than a human odor for some mosquito species in Africa, especially as a long-range attractant [68, 69]. The identification of this blend has opened doors to mass-trapping systems for malaria vectors [40]. In the Suna trap, it resulted in reduced mosquito house entry rates [38]. More studies are necessary to improve the blend and to identify other attractive blends. This includes studies in Asia and South America, where local mosquito species will have adapted to be attracted to the odors of their local host.

The MB 5 blend production method is adapted from the SOP "Production of odour bait-MB5-2015," courtesy of Wageningen University and Research, Laboratory of Entomology, the Netherlands, and the International Centre of Insect Physiology and Ecology, Kenya.

1. The blend is produced in a clean workspace, preferably in a fume hood. Gloves are worn at all times.
2. The odor bait MB 5 is comprised of 1 mL of five different components, impregnated as a mixture on one strip of nylon. The components of the blend and their dilutions are described in Table 5. The compounds are pre-diluted in a solvent to the right concentrations, to create stock solutions.
3. Nylon strips (26.5 cm × 5 cm) are cut from 15 denier ladies' stockings/tights made from 90% polyamide and 10% spandex (or 100% polyamide).
4. The nylon strips are cleaned by putting them in a bottle with 70% ethanol. The bottle is shaken vigorously. The nylon strips are taken out and hung from a rack inside the fume hood to dry (Fig. 5).
5. For one bait, 1 mL of each of the five stock solutions is added to a 10 mL plastic vial (Table 5). Dependent on the number of baits that are produced, several vials can be prepared simultaneously.

Table 5
Description of the five MB 5 blend components

Compound	Concentration	Solvent	Nylon sock impregnation
Ammonia	2.5% (v/v)	Water	1 mL
L-(+)-lactic acid	85% (W/W)	Water	1 mL
Tetradecanoic acid	0.00025 g/L	Ethanol	1 mL
3-Methyl-1-butanol	0.000001% (v/v)	Water	1 mL
Butan-1-amine	0.001% (v/v)	Paraffin oil	1 mL

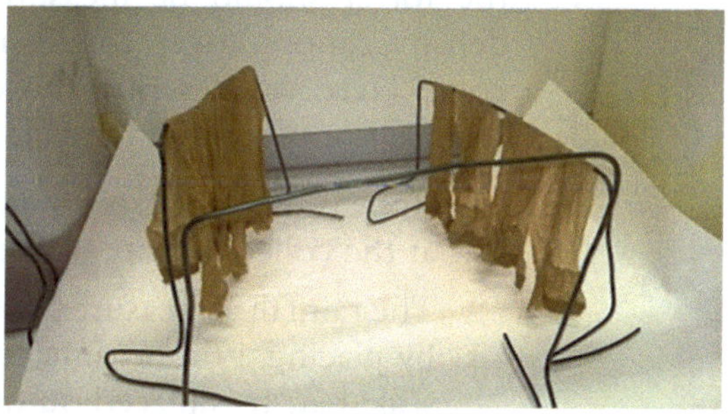

Fig. 5 Nylon strips drying on a rack after incubation with MB 5 blend

6. The vials are vortexed to mix the solutions.
7. One nylon strip is added to each vial. With clean forceps the nylon strip is moved inside the vial until the solution is absorbed.
8. The glass vial is closed and incubated at 20 °C ± 2 °C for approximately 3 h.
9. After the incubation period, the strips are taken out of the vial and air-dried on a rack for ~3 h (Fig. 5). A filter paper is placed underneath the racks to absorb droplets of odor bait. The rack should be air-permeable, to allow air to circulate around the strips (*see* **Note 13**).
10. After drying, the strips are wrapped in aluminum foil or stored in a sealed glass bottles inside a −20 °C freezer.
11. When the strips are used in traps, a paper clip or safety pin is thread through them to facilitate its use.

Experiments are currently underway to determine the duration of residual attraction to strips stored at ambient conditions. Preliminary results indicate that the nylon strips can remain attractive for a whole year when used only once a week and stored at −20 °C between uses.

2.7 Measuring Biotic and Abiotic Factors

The data collected from mosquito traps are highly dependent on weather conditions and the local environment. It is thus essential to measure these variables during the mosquito-trapping period. A minimum of GPS coordinates, temperature, humidity, and rainfall should be recorded. Temperature and humidity can be measured using data loggers, which automatically registers these variables at set intervals. Manual registration is also possible, although this will result in low measurement frequency. If possible, an anemometer is used to measure the speed of wind. Depending on the sampling method and local environment, moon phase and wind speed (Beaufort scale) can be important additional variables to note. When collections are done inside forested areas, the physical structure of the forest should be measured. Examples include undergrowth density, canopy cover, tree density, tree height, and tree circumference. Here we describe the collection of data on temperature, relative humidity, and rainfall.

1. Rope is used to attach a data logger to a tree or pole close to or at the collection site (<2 m), about 1.50 m above the ground.
2. The rainfall is measured with a rain gauge. A rain gauge is made by placing a funnel in a container with an accurate millimeter scale bar. It is placed outdoors, close to the collection site and away from direct sunlight. The rule of thumb for placement is that all objects (trees, houses, etc.) should be at least twice the height of the object away. So the rain gauge should be placed 10 m away from a 5 m high tree.
3. Ensure both the data logger and rain gauge are placed in a location where neither animals nor people disturb them.
4. The purpose of the data logger and rain gauge is explained to the household members, and any questions are answered fully (*see* **Note 14**).
5. The scale of the rain gauge is read at the same time every day throughout the study period. The height of the liquid surface should be read from the cylinder, not where the water surface meets the cylinder wall. Round up if in doubt between two measurements. During heavy rain, the gauge should be read multiple times a day. Empty the rain gauge after every reading.
6. The data logger data is downloaded onto a computer weekly or monthly.

2.8 Manual Aspiration

This section describes how to perform mouth aspirator collections. This method applies to human landing catches, human-baited net traps, animal landing catches, animal-baited net traps, peripheral net collections, exit/entry traps, and resting shelters.

1. The participants are given a bag containing a clean mouth aspirator, alarm clock, cotton wool, paper/plastic cups (~15 cm high), rubber bands, gauze (15 cm by 15 cm, mesh

size 1.5 mm), torch, spare batteries for torch, plastic sheet, rope, data logger, and water/food (*see* **Note 15**). Dependent on the preference of the participants, the torch can be either a head torch or a handheld torch. Green or blue torch light is preferred, with the light not too intense. Tracing paper or a piece of cloth can be used to change the color and intensity of the torch light.

2. The holding cups are labelled in advance with the time, date, location of collection, and participant number using a permanent marker and masking tape, so that the cups can be reused.
3. The holding cups are covered with a piece of gauze using a rubber band. A small hole is cut in the center of the gauze cover, and the hole is closed with a small piece of cotton wool. The hole should be large enough to insert the tip of the aspirator through.
4. When a mosquito is aspirated, the opening of the aspirator is closed with a finger or piece of cotton wool. Multiple mosquitoes can be collected in one aspirator at one time (maximum of 5).
5. Mosquitoes are carefully transferred into a labelled holding cup. The aspirator is inserted through a hole in the gauze cover, taking care not to allow any already captured mosquitoes to escape. Mosquitoes are blown gently from the aspirator to the cup. The aspirator is then taken out, and the hole is quickly closed using cotton wool.
6. Holding cups with mosquitoes should be placed in a humid and shaded area. Preferably the cups should be placed on top of a small table or chair to temporarily prevent ants from accessing the mosquitoes.
7. After each collection hour/break, new holding cups are used.
8. After the collection period, the empty holding cups are stacked. The cups containing mosquitoes are carefully placed in a cool box. Mosquitoes in the cups have access to 10% sugar water by putting a sugar water-soaked piece of cotton wool on top of the gauze (*see* **Note 16**). A wet towel is placed on the side of the cups to keep the cool box humid (*see* **Note 17**). The mosquitoes and the cool box are kept in the shade at all times (*see* **Note 18**).
9. The cool box is transported back to the field laboratory at the end of the collection period or within 12 h. If mosquitoes are not transported back to the field laboratory immediately, care is taken to protect the samples from ants and other insects and to maintain humidity levels.
10. Aspirators are cleaned using 80% alcohol before the next collection period.

3 Methods

3.1 Human Landing Catches

Human landing catches consist of a human participant collecting mosquitoes off his own exposed lower legs (Fig. 6) [29, 43, 46].

1. The supervisor is contacted a day before the collection period to finalize the exact planning, including the list of participants. The supervisor is asked to check the availability of the participants. If participants are not present, the reserve participants are informed by the supervisor.
2. On the day of collection, the supervisor ensures all participants are present at the collection site about **30** min before the start of the collection period. If necessary, transportation to the collection sites is arranged.
3. Supervisors are provided with a mobile telephone, torch, and umbrella/rain coat.
4. The participants are given a chair and bag containing all equipment necessary for manual aspiration.
5. Participants are placed at the pre-designated sites.
6. Participants are located at least 50 m from each other (*see* **Note 19**). If collections are done outdoors, each participant makes a small makeshift cover (3 m by **3** m) to protect himself from the elements using a plastic sheet and rope. If collections are done indoors, the room description form is filled in (Fig. 7).

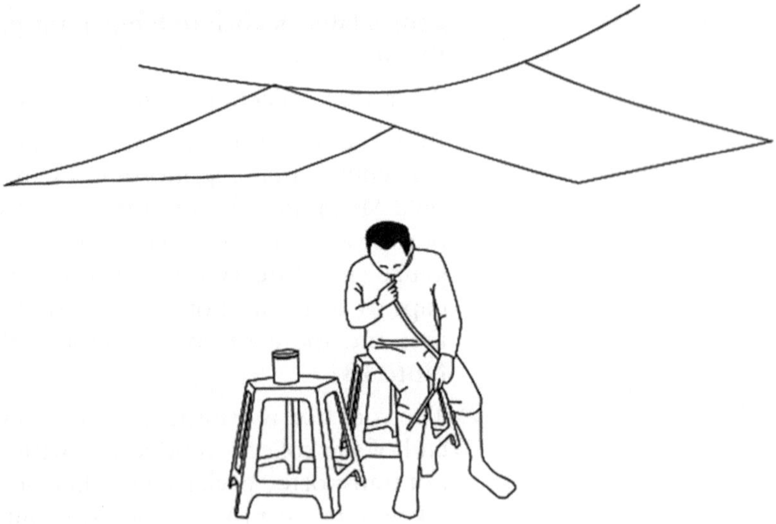

Fig. 6 The human landing catches (reproduced from Tangena et al. [32] with CC BY license [32])

Room description form

<< PROJECT NAME; Title of project >>

Room identification number: ....

Date ....

Name Village ....

Name household head.......................................

Number of houses in household	
Number of beds in household	
Selected house	
House shape	Circular / Line / Corridor/ ....
Roof type	Corrugated/ thatched/................
Number of rooms in house	
Number of bedrooms	
Selected room	
GPS coordinates	
Presence of ceiling	Yes/No
Wall type	Cement/mud/wood/.........
Condition of walls	fully sealed/some holes > 5 cm diameter/many holes >5 cm diameter
Eaves	Closed/open/ screened
Entrance	Door/open/curtain/screened/.....
Windows	Closed/open/ screened/shutters/curtains
Length of room (m)	
Width of room (m)	
Height of room (m)	
Number of beds in the room	
Number of bed nets	Insecticide treated:........................... Non treated:...........................
Use of Indoor Residual Spraying	No/ Yes, date of spraying ....
Use of other insecticides in the room (coil, spray etc.)	No/ Yes, date ....
Number of male sleepers in the room (> 10 years)	
Number of female sleepers in the room (> 10 years)	
Number of children sleepers in the room (< 10 years)	

Number and species of domestic animals within a 10 meter vicinity during day and night

DAY Horses ..../Chickens ..../ Goats ..../Cows ..../Pigs ..../Buffalo

Other, ...

NIGHT Horses ..../Chickens ..../ Goats ..../Cows ..../Pigs ..../Buffalo

Other, ...

Notes

Name and date of fieldworker:..

Fig. 7 Room description form

7. At the start of the collection period, the participants are seated on a chair.
8. The participants expose their legs until the knees. The rest of the body is covered by long-sleeved clothing and closed shoes.
9. The participants calmly sit on a chair with a torch and wait for the mosquitoes to land.
10. The participants collect mosquitoes landing and beginning to probe on their bare legs with an aspirator and torch (*see* **Note 20**).
11. Every hour, collections off the exposed legs are performed for 45 min with a 15 min break. Participants can keep track of the collection time using the provided clock. The supervisor is responsible for the timing of the collection and break periods.
12. Please refer to Subheading 2.8 for a detailed description on collecting and processing the mosquito samples.
13. During the break, participants can eat and drink away from the collection area. Food should preferably be without spices and garlic.
14. The supervisor randomly checks the participants during the collection period to ensure they are adhering to the protocol. Every hour, the holding cups are checked to ensure the correct cup is used.
15. The supervisor is asked to sit at least 20 m from the collection sites when resting, as not to disturb the collections.
16. As human landing collections are laborious, they should last a maximum of 6 h (*see* **Note 21**). If all-night collections are required, then human volunteers should work according to shifts of 3 or 6 h. It is recommended that the order in which the volunteers conduct catches is changed every night, in order to avoid any bias associated with particular individuals always collecting during the first or the second half of the night.
17. For indoor collections, at the end of the collection period, an adjusted room sampling form is filled in (Fig. 8).

3.2 Human-Baited Net Trap

3.2.1 Building a Net Trap Outdoors

1. A foldable bed is placed at the location of collection (*see* **Note 22**).
2. At each corner of the bed, a small hole about 30 cm deep is dug with a shovel. Four poles of 1.2 m are placed into the ground and secured. The sharp edges of the poles are covered with fabric.
3. A small non-insecticide-treated polyester bed net (100 cm high × 200 cm long × 100 cm wide, mesh size 1.5 mm) is hung from the poles. The bed net should cover the bed and reach the ground to prevent mosquitoes from entering.

Room sampling form

<< PROJECT NAME; Title of project >>

Room sampling form: ....

Date ....
Name Village ....
Room identification number: ....
Holding cup number ....
Type of collection: <<CDC light trap/ Suna trap, ...>>
Location of trap: Next to bed net/other..

Name of person in the room at time of collection...............................

Time and date of collection	
Time and date trap is set (24 h Clock)	:
dd/mm/yyyy	- - 201..
Time and date trap is stopped (24h clock)	:
	- - 201..
Time and date trap is removed (24h clock)	:
	- - 201..

Room information previous night (the morning that the traps are collected)	
Number of male sleepers in the room during the night (> 10 years)	
Number of female sleepers in the room during the night (> 10 years)	
Number of children in the room during the night (< 10 years)	
Number of people slept under a net last night?	LLINs, ...
	impregnated, ...
	non-impregnated, ...
Mosquito coils or any other repellent used last night?	Yes / No, ...
Animals outside the room (within 10 m) last night?	
Was trap working when removed? (check this by connecting the trap)	Yes / No

Notes

Name and date of fieldworker: ....

This form can be adjusted for indoor human landing catches, human-baited net traps, pyrethrum collections, exit/entry traps and resting pots.

Fig. 8 Room sampling form

4. A small hole 30 cm deep is dug 30 cm away from each corner of the small bed net. Four poles of 1.5 m are placed into the ground and secured. The tops of the poles are covered with fabric to prevent damage to the bed net.
5. The four poles are covered with the large non-insecticide-treated bed net (100 cm high × 245 cm long × 145 cm wide, mesh size 1.5 mm). The distance between the small and large bed nets should be 30 cm throughout.
6. There should a gap of 30 cm between the outer bed net and the ground for mosquito access. If the gap is too small, the top corners of the bed net are pulled up to increase the distance to the ground. Instead of leaving a gap at the bottom of the large bed net, 28 holes (each 5 cm × 5 cm) can be made for mosquito access.
7. If necessary, a plastic sheet is hung above the construction to protect the participant from the elements.

3.2.2 Building a Net Trap Indoors

1. A piece of rope is attached to the corners of a small non-insecticide-treated polyester bed net (100 cm high × 200 cm long × 100 cm wide, mesh size 1.5 mm).
2. Fabric is sewn onto the corners of the large non-insecticide-treated bed net (100 cm high × 245 cm long × 145 cm wide, mesh size 1.5 mm). These pieces of fabric strengthen the corners, preventing them from tearing when the small bed net is connected.
3. Four small holes (<1 cm) are made in the strengthened corners of the large bed net.
4. The pieces of rope from the corners of the small bed net are threaded through the holes of the larger bed net. The space between the small and large bed nets is 30 cm throughout. Large knots are made in the rope on both sides of the large bed net to secure the net.
5. The remaining rope, which is now attached to both the small and large bed nets, is used to hang the bed net construction inside the house at any convenient place.
6. The bed net construction results in the small bed net touching the floor and the large bed net 30 cm off the floor for mosquito access. If the gap is too small, the top corners of the bed net are pulled up to increase the distance to the ground. Instead of leaving a gap at the bottom of the large bed net, 28 holes (each 5 cm × 5 cm) can be made for mosquito access.
7. A foldable bed is placed inside the small bed net. The bed net should cover the foldable bed completely (Fig. 9).
8. The room description form is filled in (Fig. 7).

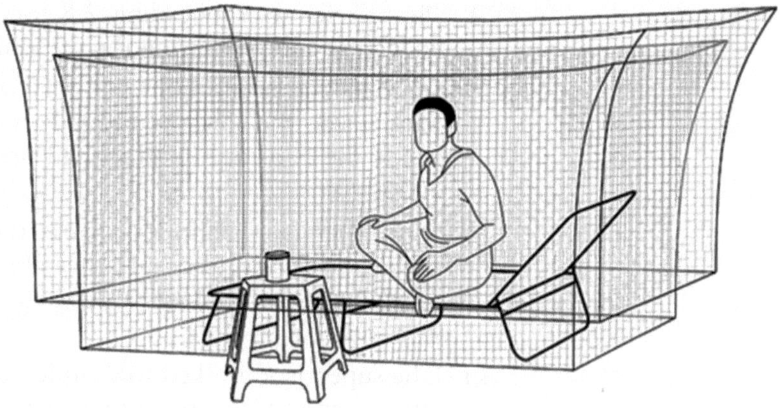

Fig. 9 The human-baited net trap indoors (adjusted from Tangena et al. [32] with CC BY license [32])

3.2.3 Collection Method

The human-baited net trap consists of a participant covered by two untreated bed nets. The participant collects mosquitoes from in between the two nets (Fig. 9).

1. The supervisor is contacted a day before the collection period to finalize the planning, including the list of participants. The supervisor is asked to check the availability of the participants. If participants are not present, the reserve participants are informed by the supervisor.
2. On the day of collection, the supervisor ensures all participants are present at the collection site about 30 min before the start of the collection period. If necessary, transportation to the collection sites is arranged.
3. Supervisors are provided with a mobile telephone, torch, and umbrella/rain coat.
4. The participants are given a bag containing all equipment necessary for manual aspiration.
5. Participants are located at least 50 m from each other (*see* **Note 19**). The human-baited bed net trap is set up and checked for holes and sturdiness. Any unintended holes are closed by the supervisor using a needle and thread.
6. At the start of the collection period, the participant calmly lies down on the foldable bed, completely protected by the smaller inner bed net. They can sleep and relax during this time.
7. Every hour, collections are made for 10 min with a 50 min resting period (*see* **Note 23**). Mosquitoes are collected from in between the two nets using a torch and aspirator. Participants can keep track of the collection time using the provided clock. The supervisor is responsible for the timing of the collection and break period.

8. Please refer to Subheading 2.8 for a detailed description on collecting and processing the mosquito samples.
9. After collecting mosquitoes for 10 min, the participant retires back inside the small bed net. Participants can eat and drink inside the bed net. Food should preferably be without spices and garlic.
10. The supervisor randomly checks the participants during the collection period to ensure they are adhering to the protocol. Every hour the holding cups are checked to ensure the correct cup is used.
11. The supervisor is asked to sit at least 20 m from the collection sites when resting, as not to disturb the collections.
12. As human-baited net trap collections are laborious, collections should last a maximum of 6 h (*see* **Note 21**).
13. For indoor collections, at the end of the collection period, an adjusted room sampling form is filled in (Fig. 8).

3.3 Animal Landing Catches

Animal landing catches consist of a fieldworker collecting mosquitoes off the body of an animal (Fig. 10).

1. A cow or buffalo is generally used as an animal bait, as they are easily obtainable and calm. Depending on the target mosquito species, other animals such as chickens, pigs, and rabbits can also be used (*see* **Note 24**).
2. At the location of collection, the animal is securely tethered to a pole (*see* **Note 25**). The animal is provided with water and food.

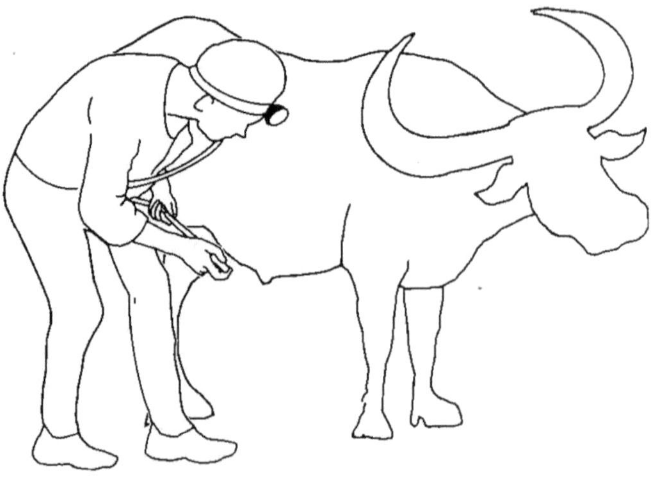

Fig. 10 The animal landing catches

3. If animals are normally protected from the elements, a plastic sheeting can be hung above the animal during the collection period.
4. The participants are given a chair and bag containing all equipment necessary for manual aspiration.
5. If the animal catches are conducted near to houses, the fieldworker can rest in a house. If the animal catches are done outside, the fieldworker prepares his/her own resting place near to the animal, underneath a temporary plastic sheet roof. A non-insecticidal bed net is used to protect the fieldworker from mosquitoes.
6. A fieldworker collects mosquitoes off the animal every 2 or 3 minutes with an aspirator and torch.
7. Please refer to Subheading 2.8 for a detailed description on collecting and processing the mosquito samples.
8. Collections are done for 45 min with a 15 min break. Fieldworkers can keep track of the collection time using the provided clock. During the break, fieldworkers can eat and drink away from the collection area. Food should preferably be without spices and garlic.
9. As animal landing collections are laborious, collections should last a maximum of 6 h (*see* **Note 21**).

3.4 Animal-Baited Net Trap

The animal-baited net trap entails the hourly collection of mosquitoes from inside a bed net that partially covers the animal bait (Fig. 11).

1. A cow or buffalo is generally used as an animal bait, as they are easily obtainable and calm. Depending on the target mosquito

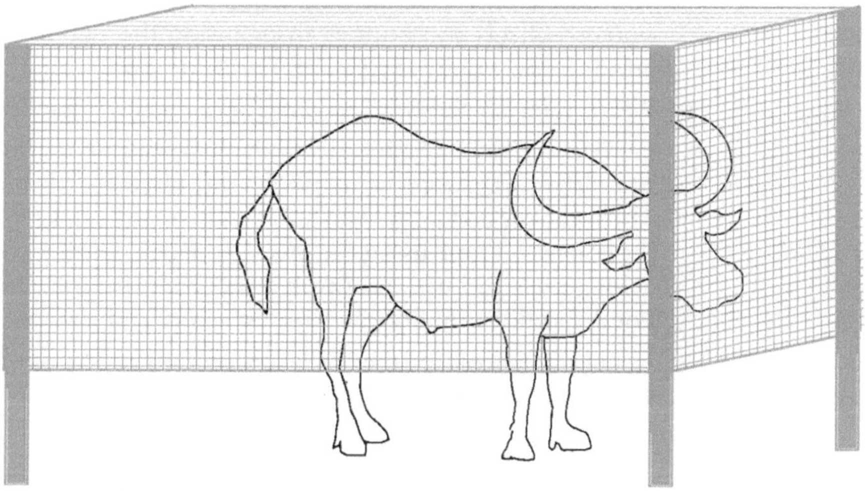

Fig. 11 The animal-baited net trap

species, other animals such as chickens, pigs, and rabbits can also be used (*see* **Note 24**).

2. At the location of collection, the animal is securely tethered to a pole (*see* **Note 25**). The animal is provided with water and food.
3. Fifty to seventy centimeters away from each corner of the animal, a small hole is dug (~ 30 cm deep). Four poles of 2 m length are placed vertically into the holes and secured. The sharp edges of the poles are covered with fabric.
4. The four poles are covered with a bed net (size dependent on the animal), leaving a 30 cm gap between the ground and the bottom of the bed net. The poles ensure that during windy days, the bed net does not move and entangle the animal. Instead of leaving a gap at the bottom of the large bed net, 28 holes (each 5 cm × 5 cm) can be made in the bed nets for mosquito access (*see* **Note 26**).
5. If animals are normally protected from the elements, a plastic sheeting can be hung above the animal during the collection period.
6. The construction is checked for holes and sturdiness. Any unintended holes are closed by the fieldworker using a needle and thread.
7. The fieldworker is given a chair and bag containing all equipment necessary for manual aspiration.
8. If the animal catches are done near houses, the fieldworker can rest in a house. If the animal catches are done outside, the fieldworker prepares his/her own resting place nearby the animal underneath a temporary plastic sheet roof. An untreated bed net is used to protect the fieldworker from mosquitoes.
9. The fieldworker rests at its resting place. After 45 min, the worker collects mosquitoes from inside the net and directly off the animal body for 15 min (*see* **Note 23**).
10. Please refer to Subheading 2.8 for a detailed description on collecting and processing the mosquito samples.
11. The fieldworker returns to his resting place for 45 min, after which the procedure is repeated. Fieldworkers can keep track of the collection time using the provided clock. During the break, fieldworkers can eat and drink away from the collection area. Food should preferably be without spices and garlic.
12. As animal-baited net trap collections are laborious, collections should last a maximum of 8 h (*see* **Note 21**).

3.5 CDC Miniature Light Trap

The CDC light trap is a fan-powered trap with a light source. It is generally placed next to an untreated bed net occupied by a human for overnight indoor malaria vector surveillance (Fig. 12) [43, 70, 71].

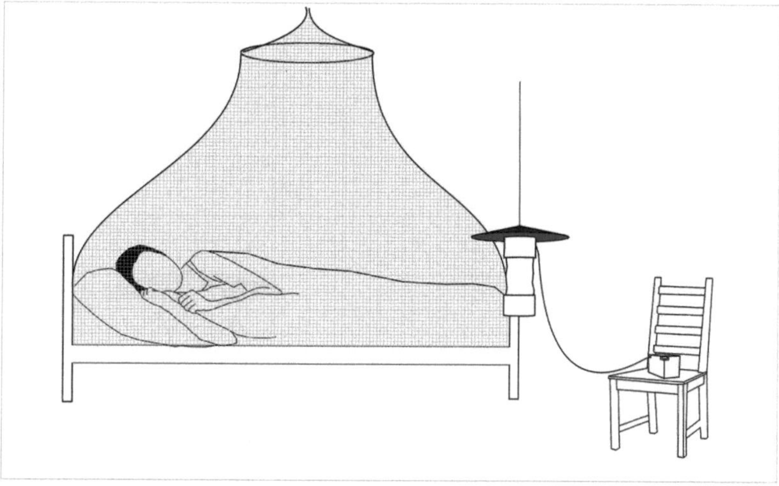

Fig. 12 The CDC miniature light trap next to a human participant sleeping underneath a bed net

1. Households are visited, informed about the project, and asked for permission to use a room for mosquito collection (*see* **Note 27**).
2. The location of the trap is chosen in close collaboration with the community members. The trap is generally place in a shaded and humid area indoors, away from competing light sources [37, 45, 71]. Preferably a room is selected where only one person sleeps every night. More than one person can sleep in the room, as long as this is standardized for all collection rooms. If this variable cannot be standardized, the variability should be taken into account during the data analysis.
3. The room description form is filled in for the selected rooms (Fig. 7).
4. A new untreated bed net is suspended around the bed. The bed net that is routinely used by the residents is properly stored.
5. The trap battery (6 V) is checked, to ensure it is fully charged. It is placed in a battery case, out of the reach of children.
6. To prevent the mosquitoes from desiccating, cotton wool is soaked with water and attached underneath the metal gauze of the collection cup using duct tape.
7. The collection cup is labelled with the date and location of collection using masking tape and permanent marker. Labelling using masking tape allows the label to be easily removed and a new label applied the next time that the trap is used.
8. The CDC miniature light trap with collection container is hung with the fan cylinder about 1.5 m above the ground. The trap is set adjacent to the untreated bed net at the foot end of the bed,

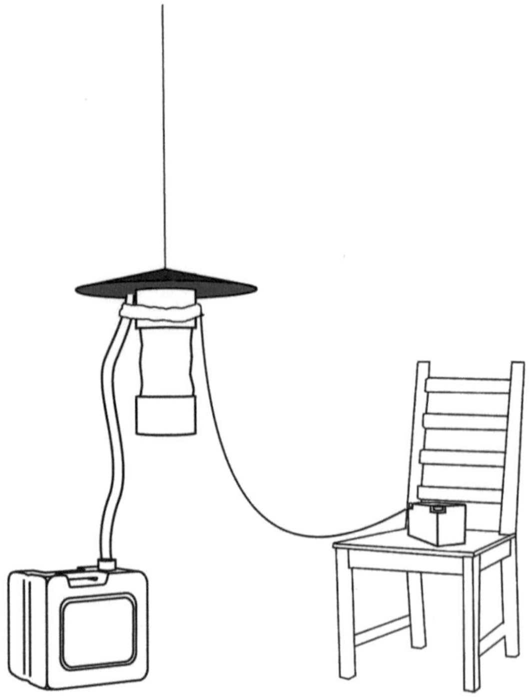

Fig. 13 The location where the attractants should be attached to the CDC miniature light trap (adjusted from Tangena et al. [32] with CC BY license [32])

away from any external light sources. Petroleum jelly is used to oil the rope leading to the trap and the power cable. The petroleum jelly prevents ants and other insects from accessing the collection bag.

9. The battery and CDC miniature light trap are clearly labelled with colored tape, to ease the process of connecting the power cable (red tape for plus, black for minus).
10. Other attractants are added to the trap (*see* **Note 28**). The silicone tube of the CO_2, nylon socks, and/or chemical attractants are attached at the top of the cylinder housing the fan (Fig. 13). The attractants should never be placed above the fan, as the attractant scent will be drawn through the trap attracting mosquitoes to the base of the trap when they are unable to enter.
11. Depending on the project and the involvement of the community members, either the person sleeping in the room or a fieldworker turns the trap on (*see* **Note 29**). The light trap is turned on at dusk by connecting the red-taped area of the light trap power cable to the red-taped area of the battery. The same is done for the black-taped areas.

12. A participant sleeps under the bed net. Mosquitoes are attracted to the odor of the sleeping person, the light source, and the optional additional attractants placed in the trap.
13. At sunrise the community member or fieldworker closes the neck of the collection cup using the attached cord. The battery is then disconnected. The order of first closing the collection cup before turning off the trap is important to prevent mosquitoes from escaping. The trap is left like this until samples are collected (*see* **Note 30**).
14. During collection of the samples, the fieldworker takes off the collection cup and uses a rubber band to close the collection cup more permanently. The collection cups are placed in a cool box for transportation (*see* **Note 18**).
15. The blades of the light trap fan are checked for mosquitoes. Mosquitoes are carefully removed using forceps and stored in a clearly labelled 1.5 mL Eppendorf tubes. A notebook is used to link the Eppendorf tube number to the collection cup number. The Eppendorf tubes are stored in storage boxes in the cool box. The blades of the fan are cleaned using alcohol.
16. Inquiries are made regarding the functioning of the trap during the night and the number of people sleeping in the room. The room sampling form is filled in (Fig. 8).
17. Traps, batteries, and collection cups are transported back to the field laboratory.

3.6 Biogents Suna Trap

The odor-baited counterflow Suna trap is a fan-powered trap that lures mosquitoes with an attractant odor blend and CO_2 (Fig. 14).

1. Households are visited, informed about the project, and asked for permission to use a room or outside area for mosquito collection (*see* **Note 27**).
2. The location of the trap is chosen in close collaboration with the community members. Preferably a room is selected where only one person sleeps every night. More than one person can sleep in the room, as long as this is standardized for all collection rooms. If this variable cannot be standardized, the variability should be taken into account during the data analysis.
3. The room description form is filled in for the selected rooms (Fig. 7).
4. A new untreated bed net is suspended around the bed. The bed net, which is routinely used by the residents, is properly stored.
5. The battery (12 V) is checked, to ensure it is fully charged. It is placed in a battery case, out of reach of children.
6. The collection bag is labelled with the date and collection location using masking tape and permanent marker.

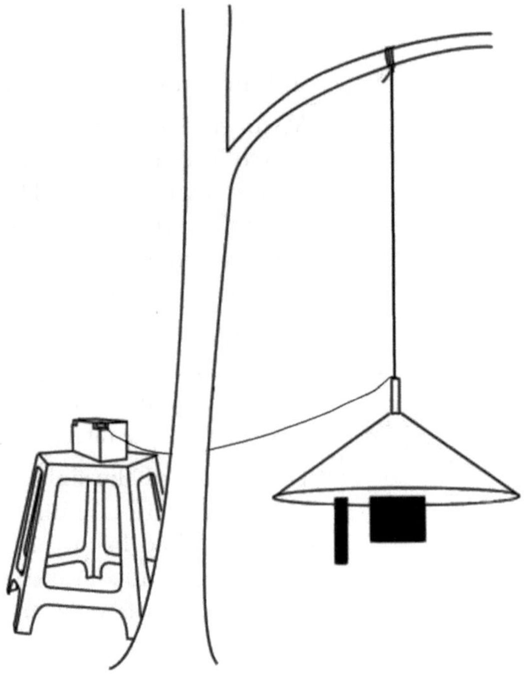

Fig. 14 The Biogents Suna trap. Adjusted from Tangena et al. [32] with CC BY license [32]

7. The trap is hung with the funnel opening **30** cm above ground. Petroleum jelly is used to oil the rope leading to the trap and the power cable. The petroleum jelly prevents ants and other insects from accessing the collection bag.
8. The collection bag is placed inside the trap. The collection bag can be attached before the fan, leading to improved condition of the trapped mosquitoes [72].
9. The attractant (generally nylon strips baited with human or synthetic odor such as MB 5) is hung at the designated area inside the center of the trap at the apex of the gray cover. To maximize the odor distribution, the nylon strips should hang freely.
10. The CO_2 emitting silicone tube (0.5 cm diameter) is attached to the specifically designed CO_2 release pipe.
11. Depending on the project and the involvement of the community members, either the person sleeping in the room or a fieldworker turns the trap on (*see* **Note 29**).
12. The Suna trap is turned on at sunset by connecting the power cable to the battery. The rain-resistant cover is screwed over the connection point.

13. A participant sleeps under the bed net. Mosquitoes are drawn into the trap through a black funnel at the base of the conical trap, where they are collected in a collection bag.
14. At sunrise the trap is turned off by disconnecting the battery. This automatically closes the trap (via a flap in the funnel) and prevents mosquitoes from escaping. The community member or fieldworker makes a visual inspection to check that the flap is closed after disconnecting the power.
15. The collection bags are collected on the same day by the fieldworker (*see* **Note 30**). To collect the collection bags, the trap is left the right way up and turned on. The trap is lightly tapped to encourage the live mosquitoes to fly into the top of the catch bag. The gray cover of the trap is carefully taken off. The collection bag is loosened and closed. The bag is placed in the cool box and the trap is turned off (*see* **Note 18**).
16. The blades of the Suna trap fan are checked for mosquitoes. Mosquitoes are carefully removed using forceps and stored in a clearly labelled 1.5 mL Eppendorf tube. A notebook is used to link the Eppendorf tube number to the collection cup. The Eppendorf tubes are stored in storage boxes in the cool box. The blades are cleaned using alcohol.
17. Inquiries are made regarding the functioning of the trap during the night and the number of people sleeping in the room. The room sampling form is filled in (Fig. 8).
18. Traps, batteries, and collection cups are transported back to the field laboratory.

3.7 Peripheral Net Collection

The peripheral net collection entails placing a large net in the flight path of the mosquitoes. The mosquitoes fly against the net, which encourages them to land long enough to be collected by fieldworkers (Fig. 15) [41].

1. The netting is generally placed between the blood-feeding and resting areas of malaria vector mosquitoes, as the netting does not hinder the visual or olfactory cues. This allows for the collection of both blood-fed mosquitoes and host-seeking mosquitoes on either side of the netting, collecting exophilic and/or exophagic mosquitoes [41, 42].
2. Poles (2.3 m tall) are placed in the ground after using a shovel to dig holes at 2 m intervals along the length of the net (between 20 m and 40 m). The length of the net is dependent on the selected site.
3. The netting (ether polyvinylchloride-coated polyester, 2 m high, and ~20 m to 40 m long) is attached at the top and bottom of the poles using rope or cable ties.

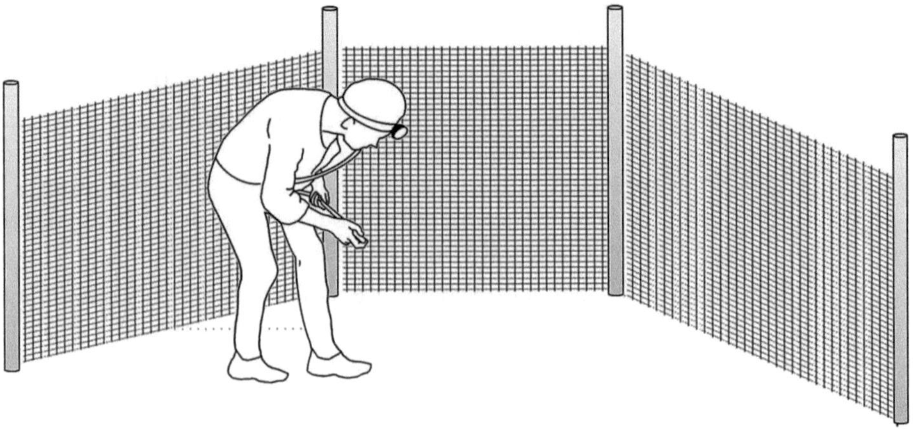

Fig. 15 The peripheral net collections

4. Generally two fieldworkers collect mosquitoes from the peripheral net at the same time. If the net collections are done near houses, the fieldworkers can rest in a house. If the collections are done away from the village, the fieldworkers prepare their own resting place nearby the netting underneath a temporary plastic sheet roof. An untreated bed net is used to protect the fieldworkers from mosquitoes.
5. All possible mosquito blood sources in the collection area (500 m^2) are identified and the locations noted. The locations should preferably be recorded using GPS. If this is not possible, a map of the area should be sketched. Possible hosts include pigs, cows, chicken, and people.
6. The two fieldworkers are provided with a chair and a bag containing all equipment necessary for manual aspiration. If there is interest in gathering data about the resting height, the holding cups can be labelled for different heights (<50 cm, 50–100 cm, 100–150 cm, and > 150 cm).
7. At the start of the collection period, the fieldworkers rest at their resting place for 40 min.
8. The fieldworkers go to the peripheral net and collect all mosquitoes resting on the netting. Each side of the barrier screen is examined for 10 min every hour by the fieldworkers simultaneously, totalling 20 min of collection every hour per fieldworker. Mosquitoes from different sides of the barrier (and at different heights) are stored in different holding cups. The fieldworkers can keep track of the collection time using the provided watch or stopwatch.
9. Please refer to Subheading 2.8 for a detailed description on collecting and processing the mosquito samples.

10. After the 20 min collection period, the fieldworkers return to their resting place for 40 min. During the resting period, fieldworkers can eat and drink away from the collection area. Food should preferably be without spices and garlic.
11. The process is then repeated with new holding cups.
12. As peripheral net collections are labor-intensive, collections should last a maximum of 8 h (*see* **Note 21**).

3.8 Pyrethrum Collection

The pyrethrum collection consists of one or two fieldworkers spraying a room with pyrethrum insecticide, after which all knocked down mosquitoes are collected [29, 43, 44, 73].

1. Households are visited, informed about the project, and asked for permission to use a room for mosquito collection. The owners of the house are asked for their oral approval to spray the room (*see* **Note 31**). A room is selected where only one person sleeps every night. More than one person can sleep in the room, as long as this is standardized for all locations. If this variable cannot be standardized, the variability should be taken into account during the data analysis.
2. The room description form is filled in (Fig. 7).
3. The next morning around 6.30 am, after the participants have left the room, spraying is commenced.
4. All animals, water containers, food items, and small furniture are removed from the room.
5. Windows and doors are closed. The floor and large furniture are covered with large white sheets (Multiple sheets of 2 m × 1 m, 2 m × 2 m, 2 m × 3 m). Sheets are carefully placed underneath the large furniture, such as tables and beds.
6. Fieldworkers wear thick long-sleeved clothing, closed shoes, a mouth mask, gloves, and protective glasses to protect them from the insecticides.
7. Two hand sprayers (double-action type) are filled with a commercial-grade pyrethrin solution (0.2%–0.3%) in kerosene using a funnel.
8. Two fieldworkers, one inside and one outside the room, spray the room simultaneously starting at opposite ends. The field-worker inside the room sprays toward the roof for 45 s, starting from the entrance of the room moving in a clockwise direction. The fieldworker outside the room sprays insecticide into the eaves and windows in an anticlockwise direction (*see* **Note 32**).
9. The fieldworkers close the door and leave the room for 10 min.
10. 1.5 mL Eppendorf tubes are filled with a few silica beads (about ¼ of tube) and topped with cotton wool. Half of the tube is now full. The tubes are labelled with a permanent marker.

11. Information is gathered regarding the presence and use of insecticide-treated nets and coils and insecticide spraying the previous night using an adjusted room sampling form (Fig. 8).
12. Ten minutes after spraying, the doors and windows are opened. The white sheets are checked by two fieldworkers with forceps and a torch. The fieldworkers work from the door in opposite directions. Care is taken not to disturb the sheets (*see* **Note 33**). All knocked down mosquitoes are transferred into clean labelled Eppendorf tubes.
13. Once the sheets are checked, all other possible sites inside the room are surveyed for mosquitoes. Particular attention is paid to areas between the wall and sheets, underneath furniture, between shelves and walls, on bed nets, and under the beds. All mosquitoes are transferred into Eppendorf tubes.
14. In a notebook the Eppendorf tube labels are linked to the collection time, date, room number, and fieldworker names.
15. The tubes containing mosquitoes are placed in a collection box inside a cool box. The mosquitoes and the cool box are kept in the shade at all times (*see* **Note 18**).
16. The cool box is transported back to the field laboratory at the end of the collection period.
17. Due to the residual activity of the insecticide, only a maximum of two surveys a week can be done in any given room.

3.9 Exit/Entry Trap

3.9.1 Building an Exit/Entry Trap

1. Fine untreated netting (UV resistant) is used to cover a wooden frame (45 cm by 55 cm by 55 cm) using a staple gun. All sides are covered with netting, except one 45 cm height by 55 cm length side.
2. Two triangular pieces of netting (45 cm × 28 cm × 28 cm) and two rectangular pieces (55 cm × 26 × 5 cm) are cut from a new piece of netting. The two 28 cm-long sides of the triangular pieces and all three sides of the rectangular-shaped netting (except one 55 cm side) are strengthened with wire (Fig. 16).
3. The two rectangular-shaped pieces of netting are attached to the top and bottom of the open side of the trap (on the non-wired 55 cm edge of the netting). The triangles are

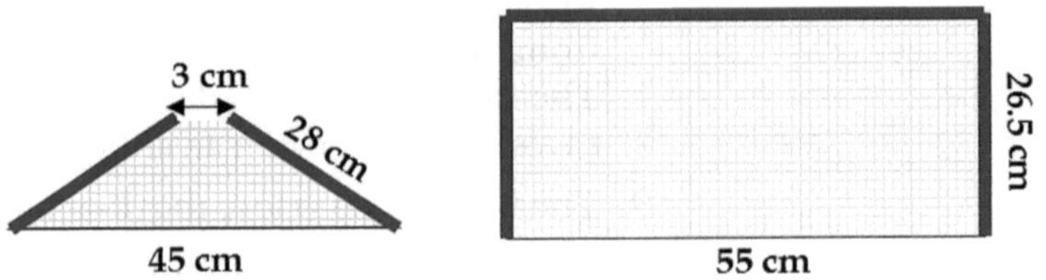

Fig. 16 The triangle- and square-shaped pieces of netting used for the exit/entry trap construction (thick lines represent the places enforced with wire)

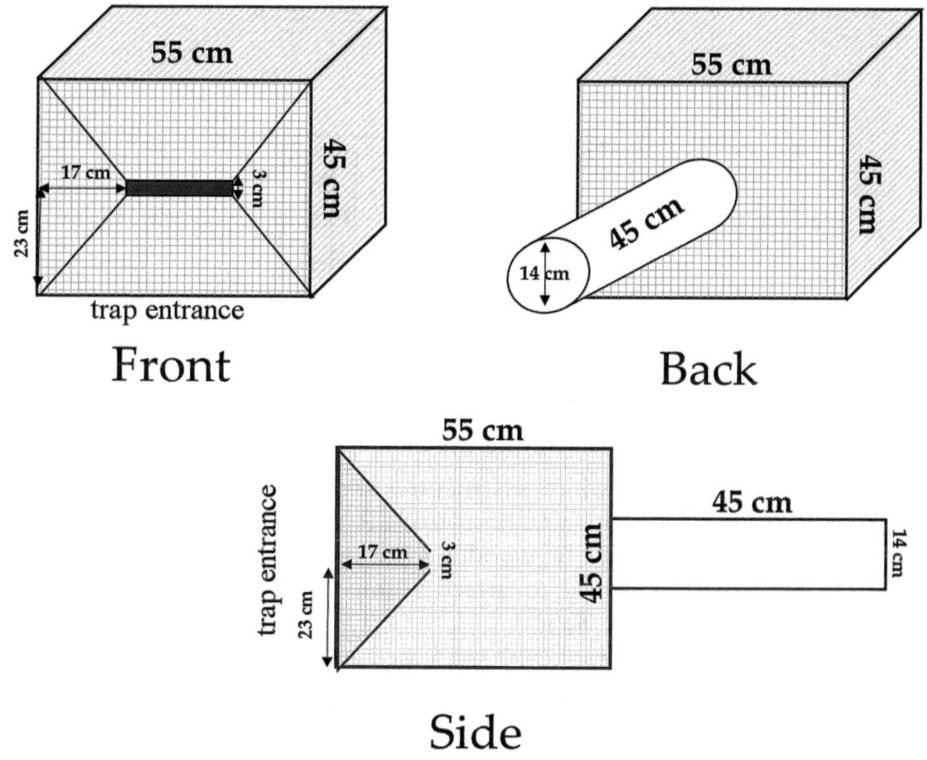

Fig. 17 A schematic representation of the exit/entry trap

attached to the sides (using the non-wired 45 cm edge of the netting; Fig. 17).

4. The strengthened sides are attached to each other to result in a triangular prism using a needle and thread. An opening of 3 cm × 26.5 cm will be present at the top of the triangular prism (Fig. 17). This is the entrance of the trap.
5. A circular hole of 14 cm diameter is cut in the center of the netting on the opposite side of the trap entrance. A sleeve of thick white cotton fabric is attached to the hole (length 54 cm). This is for access inside the trap to collect mosquitoes (Fig. 17).
6. On the trap entrance side, a piece of plywood is placed around the trap using a hammer and nails. Pieces of thick cotton fabric are used to close the gaps between the plywood and trap.

3.9.2 Collection Method

Exit/entry traps are placed in the window or door opening to collect mosquitoes either entering or exiting the rooms (Fig. 18).

1. Households are visited, informed about the project, and asked for permission to use a room for mosquito collection (*see* **Note 34**). A room is selected where only one person sleeps every night. More than one person can sleep in the room, as long as this is standardized for all locations. If this variable

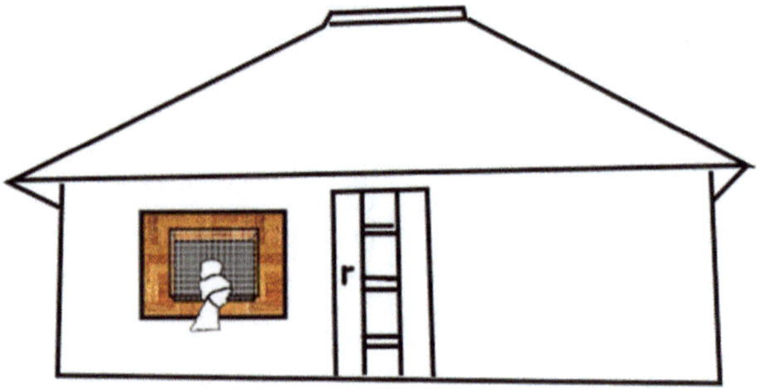

Fig. 18 The exit trap attached to a window

cannot be standardized, the variability should be taken into account during the data analysis.

2. The window structures should be a suitable size and material for the attachment of the traps. Preferably the window frame should be wooden. The owner of the house is asked for oral approval to attach a trap to the window in the room (*see* **Note 31**).
3. The house design impacts the effectiveness of the exit/entry trap [45]. A room description form is therefore filled in (Fig. 7).
4. Before the trap is attached, all possible entry and exit points in the room are closed using banana leaves, bamboo leaves, mud, fabric, or any other locally available products. The eaves are only partially closed (~4 cm gap) to decrease mosquitoes moving through the eaves. If the walls are made from bamboo or other mosquito-permeable material, they are covered with black fabric.
5. The exit/entry trap is attached to the window before sunset (4.00 pm). The sleeve of the trap is closed. The gap between the window frame and trap is closed using banana leaves, bamboo leaves, mud, fabric, or any other locally available product.
6. If the trap is an exit trap, the trap entrance is faced toward the inside of the room. If the trap is an entry trap, the trap entrance is faced toward the outside.
7. The trap is labelled with a number that corresponds to the room description form.
8. The trap is left overnight.
9. The following morning, after the occupants have left the room (8.00 am–9.00 am), the trap entrance is closed using a piece of fabric.
10. The fieldworker is provided with a bag containing all equipment necessary for manual aspiration.

11. The sleeve of the exit trap is opened, and mosquitoes are collected using an aspirator and torch. The exit/entry traps can also be taken off the wall, covered with wet towels and transported back to the field laboratory.
12. Please refer to Subheading 2.8 for a detailed description on collecting and processing the mosquito samples.
13. Information is gathered regarding the presence and use of insecticide-treated nets and coils and insecticide spraying the previous night using an adjusted room sampling form (Fig. 8).

3.10 Resting Shelters

Resting shelters are artificial resting locations developed to attract mosquitoes either before host seeking or when developing their ovaries [30, 46].

3.10.1 Resting Pit

1. In close collaboration with the village leaders, a shaded area close to or inside the village is sought. This area should be shaded throughout the day, either naturally or by a roofing made from locally available products such as banana leaves and bamboo. Areas where digging is challenging are avoided.
2. The owner of the land is asked for oral approval to dig a pit for the collection of mosquitoes. The owner is assured that the pit will be closed after the study.
3. A large rectangular pit measuring 2 m deep, 1.5 m long and 1 m wide is dug using a measuring tape and shovel.
4. The sides of the pit are elevated slightly and sloped to prevent water from flowing into the pit from the surrounding area.
5. Inside the pit ~60 cm from the bottom, several shelters of 30 cm deep, 20 cm high, and 30 cm wide are dug into the sides of the pit (Fig. 19).

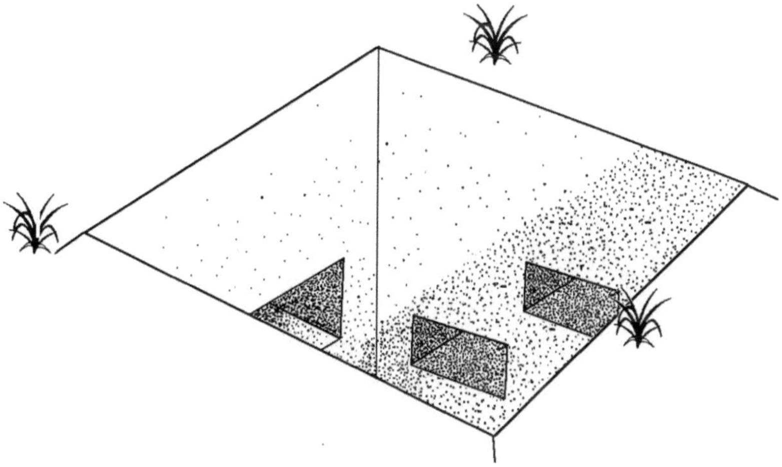

Fig. 19 The resting pit without the outside fencing

6. A fence is placed around the pit to prevent animals and people from accidentally falling into the pit.
7. A schematic image of the pit is drawn and the shelters are numbered.
8. The pit is left for the night.
9. The next morning just before sunrise (5.30 am), the shelters in the resting pit are inspected by a fieldworker. The fieldworker is provided with a bag containing all equipment necessary for manual aspiration.
10. The fieldworker carefully enters the pit with the prepared holding cups and surveys each shelter.
11. All mosquitoes resting in the shelters are collected.
12. Please refer to Subheading 2.8 for a detailed description on collecting and processing the mosquito samples.
13. At the end of the study, in accordance with the preference of the owner of the land, the pit is closed.

3.10.2 Resting Pots

1. In close collaboration with the village leaders, suitable sites for resting ports are selected. For outdoor collections, a shaded area close to or inside the village is sought. This area should be shaded throughout the day. Preferably the collection site is 5 m from a house. For indoor collections, a room is selected where only one person sleeps every night. More than one person can sleep in the room, as long as this is standardized for all locations. If this variable cannot be standardized, the variability should be taken into account during the data analysis.
2. The room description form is filled in (Fig. 7). The owner of the room or plot of land is asked for permission to set the pots (*see* **Note 31**).
3. A hole is drilled in the bottom of the clay pots (~20 L) to decrease the risk of theft and prevent the collection of water (*see* **Note 35**).
4. The pots are placed in groups of three with the opening facing the lateral side (Fig. 20). All pots are placed with the bases together and the openings facing outward.
5. The pots are protected from natural predators where possible, treating the rims of the pots with grease (petroleum jelly) or surrounding them with water. For outdoor collections, a fence is placed around the collection pots to stop animals and people from accidentally moving them.
6. The pots are numbered using masking tape, and their locations are described in detail for later analysis (location of the opening, GPS coordinates, and use of predator preventative methods). If possible, pictures of the pots are made.

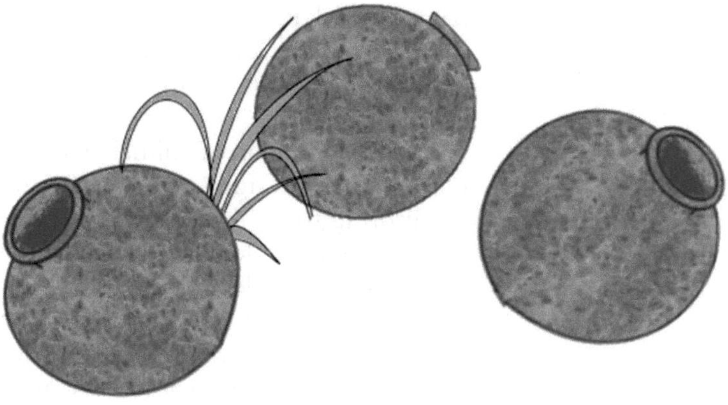

Fig. 20 Three resting pots without the outside fencing

7. The clay pots are left overnight.
8. The next morning just before sunrise (~5.00 am), the collection pots are checked by a fieldworker. The fieldworker is provided with a bag containing all equipment necessary for manual aspiration.
9. All encountered mosquitoes are aspirated from the pots and transferred into the labelled holding cups. If the clay pots are difficult to survey, the entrance of the pot can be covered by a small mosquito cage. The mosquito cage is held toward the light, and the pot is lightly tapped to stir up the mosquitoes. The hole at the bottom of the pot can be used to blow air through the pot, to further stir the mosquitoes. The mosquito cage is taken off the pot and quickly closed. The pot is checked one final time for mosquitoes using an aspirator and torch.
10. Please refer to Subheading 2.8 for a detailed description on collecting and processing the mosquito samples.
11. The inside of the pots are cleaned using a dry piece of cloth. The pots are placed back in the same position as before.
12. For indoor collections, an adjusted room sampling form is filled in after each room is sampled (Fig. 8).

4 Conclusions

Sampling malaria vectors is essential for the proper design and implementation of sustainable malaria control programs. Currently, the human landing catch is the gold standard for sampling mosquitoes biting a human host. The collection of malaria vectors using this method results in a good understanding of vector species composition, the indoor/outdoor biting rate, and man-biting rates. However, human landing catches are becoming more controversial due to its ethical concerns. The human-baited net trap can be a suitable alternative. Animals can substitute human participant altogether if the malaria vector is both anthropophilic and zoophilic.

Where a human or animal host is not available, the fan-powered CDC miniature light trap and Biogents Suna trap are important monitoring tools. These electric traps provide standardized collections and require low labor investment.

Mosquito collection methods that do not use attractants are the peripheral net collection, pyrethrum spray collections, exit/entry traps, and resting shelters. The efficacy of these methods is dependent on the behavior of the mosquitoes and placement of the traps. Peripheral net collections are important to understand the movement of malaria mosquitoes between their blood-feeding and egg-laying areas. Pyrethrum spray collections have been popular in the past, as they give a good indication of indoor-resting rates. However, the intrusion into people's houses and the use of insecticides have made this method less favorable in recent years. Exit/entry traps are key to identifying mosquito house-exiting/entering behavior, with resting shelters important for understanding the behavior of gravid mosquitoes. The description of the different trapping methods in this chapter has hopefully given the reader a better understanding of which sampling methods to use to reach their objective.

The study design related to the sampling method should be written in close collaboration with important stakeholders, using literature and expert advice as guidelines. Activities should be planned ahead of time with the ethics thoroughly evaluated. Throughout the preparatory stages and fieldwork, emphasis should be on good communication and relations with the local community members. They are an integral part of a study.

5 Future Perspectives

Although the use of manual trapping will remain an indispensable part of adult sampling, with funder fatigue and malaria incidence on the rise, it is vital to develop methods which require fewer resources. Independent sampling methods are being developed, which do not need regular involvement of fieldworkers. These traps can, for example, use laser technologies to identify and count mosquitoes entering the traps. The data is then uploaded in real time using cellular networks. This increases the specificity, uniformity, and scale of data. Examples include the Smart counter trap by Biogents and the Project Premonition trap by Microsoft [74, 75]. Resources can further be saved with more involvement of the local communities in the collection of mosquito data [33]. Apart from improving the efficacy of the sampling methods, new technologies are also being used to increase the reach of sampling methods. A great example is the use of solar energy to power traps, making electric traps suitable for resource poor areas.

The development of more efficient traps (with better lure blends) has opened doors for the use of traps as additions to vector control programs using mass removal trapping and push-pull strategies [39, 76]. Mass trapping entails the collection of a significant proportion of the vector population to decrease human exposure to these vectors [77, 78]. Mass trapping is most promising in areas where vector densities are low and when traps are in place early in the transmission season to limit mosquito population growth. The push-pull strategy comprises of repelling vector mosquitoes from areas with human hosts using spatial repellents (push) while attracting them to an area from where they are removed from the environment (pull) [76, 79]. Preliminary results are encouraging. However, the success of these control methods is dependent on the knowledge of the local vector population and, optimization of the luring and repelling methods, for which additional mosquito sampling needs to be done.

6 Notes

1. If human participants are exposed to a higher than normal risk, human landing catches should not be performed. An example is if someone would normally be at risk of *Anopheles* bites during the evening, then conducting human landing catches during that time at that location does not necessarily put the participant at higher risk of infection than other community members.
2. In accordance with the study design, the α can be adjusted for.
3. The responsible governmental bodies should be involved early on in the development of the protocol. The responsible government bodies are generally the Ministry of Health and their ethics committee. However, this can differ between countries.
4. If possible, representatives of the local government office should accompany the field team when the project is presented.
5. The supervisors are recruited to coordinate the fieldwork and act as a liaison between the participants and researchers. They have to meet the same requirements as the participants. They are required to sign the same consent form and receive the same chemoprophylaxis and vaccinations. Generally, the supervisors are well-respected members of the community. The supervisors are responsible for the attendance of the participants at the start of every collection period. They also ensure adherence to the protocol and help the participants with any

issues hindering their fieldwork. Depending on the discussions with village leaders and government officials, the supervisors receive a similar or slightly higher payment than the participants.

6. In some countries it is difficult to find non-smoking participants. In such cases smoking participants can be included in the study. However, participants should be made aware that they cannot smoke during the collection period. Female participants are generally excluded from participation due to concerns over safety at night, different body odors at different stages in the menstrual cycle, and possible pregnancy (which the woman may not be aware of).
7. In some countries it will be challenging to find people who do not eat heavily spiced and garlic-containing food. The protocol can be adjusted to the local situation, as long as it is standardized for all participants.
8. As all participants may not always be available, it is recommended to enrol 10–20% more participants than necessary in the study. These reserve participants sign the consent form and receive the benefits of vaccinations, bed nets, and/or chemoprophylaxis (dependent on the protocol). When insufficient participants are able to participate in the study, the reserve participants are asked to participate. They receive the same compensation on the days when they participate. The role and responsibilities of being a reserve participant should be clearly explained.
9. If participants cannot sign, their fingerprint can be used as an alternative.
10. In some countries it might not be acceptable to provide participants with malaria chemoprophylaxis. Please discuss the local regulations with the authorities and ethics committee before designing your study. If malaria prophylaxis is not allowed in an area with active malaria transmission (drug resistance or religious reasons), it is likely unethical to conduct human landing catches. However, this decision may need to be taken by a local committee.
11. Some participants might be hesitant to take medicine or receive vaccinations. If they are not willing to receive the appropriate medication or vaccinations, they are excluded from the study. Participants claiming to have been previously vaccinated should provide appropriate documentation for this. If this is not possible, they are excluded from the study.
12. The supervisors should have access to a phone. They are provided with sufficient credit to call the study team and organize the participants.

13. It is normal for the nylon strips to retain some oily residue after drying.
14. Some data loggers have a red light that lights up every few minutes during recording. Ensure the community members are aware that they are not being filmed nor any data, except temperature and humidity, is recorded.
15. Discuss with participants whether they will provide their own food and drinks during the collection period or whether the project coordinators should organize this.
16. Ensure the soaked cotton wool does not drip sugar water into the cup.
17. When paper cups are used, the wet towel is separated from the cups using plastic sheeting, to ensure the cups keep their shape.
18. If the collection area is very hot, ice packs covered with towels can be included in the cool box.
19. During collections at night and/or in remote forested areas, the participants can be placed closer together for security reasons. The distance between participants should be standardized throughout.
20. If the density of mosquitoes is too high in the area, more collectors can work together to collect mosquitoes off one human bait (a total of two participants). Alternatively, collection periods can be shortened.
21. The length of a collection period is also dependent on the local regulations and preference of the population.
22. The exact details of the net trap construction are dependent on the timeline of the project. For long-term collections (>1 month), semipermanent bamboo construction is necessary [80], while foldable beds surrounded by netting are sufficient for short-term collections [32].
23. Collections can also be made every 2 h or just once in the morning. These methods are less labor-intensive but will result in a lower number of mosquitoes.
24. Fieldworkers should be properly trained in handling the animals to minimize risk of injury to fieldworkers and animals.
25. Generally, animals placed close to the human houses will collect more anthropophilic mosquitoes, while collections in the forests and animal settlements will collect more zoophilic mosquitoes.
26. If host feeding on the animals needs to be avoided, similar to the human-baited net traps, two bed nets can be used: one inner net protecting the animal and one outer net.

27. Ethical clearance might be necessary to place the trap. The local requirements and regulations need to be checked before conducting the study.
28. Attractants include CO_2 and nylon socks with either human, animal, or a synthetic odor.
29. If the trap has to be turned on and off at specific times, an alarm clock is provided to the community volunteers.
30. For best preservation, the mosquito samples should be collected every day.
31. Written consent may be needed dependent on the ethics requirements for the study.
32. Before spraying the eaves and other openings in the room can be closed completely with banana leaves, fabric, and/or other locally available products. Spraying is then only done inside the room.
33. If it is too dark inside the room, the white sheets can be moved outside for the collection of mosquitoes. This is only possible if there is no wind outside.
34. Completely screened houses are avoided for exit/entry traps. If needed, with written informed consent, the screens can be removed and reinstalled at the end of the study. This should be done at no cost to the owner and in close collaboration with them.
35. The containers can be lined with sticky sheets made with rat glue [81]. The sticky lining decreases the frequency of collections and therefore the labor intensity. However, the mosquitoes stuck to the sheets are difficult to take off the sheets and are more damaged than those which are collected through aspiration.

Acknowledgments

This work was supported by the Yersin project, funded by the Michelin Corporate Foundation. AH was supported by a grant from the Innovative Vector Control Consortium.

References

1. Smith DL, Dushoff J, Snow RW et al (2005) The entomological inoculation rate and *Plasmodium falciparum* infection in African children. Nature 438:492–495
2. Hay SI, Smith DL, Snow RW (2008) Measuring malaria endemicity from intense to interrupted transmission. Lancet Infect Dis 8:369–378
3. Smith T, Killeen G, Lengeler C et al (2004) Relationships between the outcome of *Plasmodium falciparum* infection and the intensity of transmission in Africa. Am J Trop Med Hyg 71:80–86
4. Killeen GF, Ross A, Smith T (2006) Infectiousness of malaria-endemic human populations to vectors. Am J Trop Med Hyg 75:38–45

5. Reddy M, Overgaard H, Abaga S et al (2011) Outdoor host seeking behaviour of *Anopheles gambiae* mosquitoes following initiation of malaria vector control on Bioko Island, Equatorial Guinea. Malar J 10:184
6. Russell TL, Beebe NW, Cooper RD et al (2013) Successful malaria elimination strategies require interventions that target changing vector behaviours. Malar J 12:56
7. Moiroux N, Gomez MB, Pennetier C et al (2012) Changes in *Anopheles funestus* biting behavior following universal coverage of long-lasting insecticidal nets in Benin. J Infect Dis 206:1622–1629
8. Sougoufara S, Diédhiou SM, Doucouré S et al (2014) Biting by *Anopheles funestus* in broad daylight after use of long-lasting insecticidal nets: a new challenge to malaria elimination. Malar J 13:125
9. Dabiré RK, Namountougou M, Sawadogo SP et al (2012) Population dynamics of *Anopheles gambiae* s.L. in Bobo-Dioulasso city: bionomics, infection rate and susceptibility to insecticides. Parasit Vectors 5:127
10. Lwetoijera DW, Harris C, Kiware SS et al (2014) Increasing role of *Anopheles funestus* and *Anopheles arabiensis* in malaria transmission in the Kilombero Valley, Tanzania. Malar J 13:331
11. Githeko A, Adungo N, Karanja D et al (1996) Some observations on the biting behavior of *Anopheles gambiae* s.S., *Anopheles arabiensis*, and *Anopheles funestus* and their implications for malaria control. Exp Parasitol 82:306–315
12. Gryseels C, Durnez L, Gerrets R et al (2015) Re-imagining malaria: heterogeneity of human and mosquito behaviour in relation to residual malaria transmission in Cambodia. Malar J 14:165
13. Killeen G (2014) Characterizing, controlling and eliminating residual malaria transmission. Malar J 13:330
14. Ng'habi KR (2010) Behavioural, ecological and genetic determinants of mating and gene flow in Africa malaria mosquitoes. PhD Thesis, Wageningen University
15. Ndiath MO, Mazenot C, Gaye A et al (2011) Methods to collect *Anopheles* mosquitoes and evaluate malaria transmission: a comparative study in two villages in Senegal. Malar J 10:270
16. Molineaux L, Gramiccia G (1980) The Garki project: research on the epidemiology and control of malaria in the Sudan savanna of West Africa. World Health Organization, Geneva
17. Fontenille D, Lochouarn L, Diagne N et al (1997) High annual and seasonal variations in malaria transmission by anophelines and vector species composition in Dielmo, a holoendemic area in Senegal. Am J Trop Med Hyg 56:247–253
18. Fontenille D, Lochouarn L, Diatta M et al (1997) Four years' entomological study of the transmission of seasonal malaria in Senegal and the bionomics of *Anopheles gambiae* and *A. arabiensis*. Trans R Soc Trop Med Hyg 91:647–652
19. Watson M (1921) The prevention of malaria in the federated Malay states, a record of 20 years progress. E.P. Dutton and company, New York
20. Gater BAR (1935) Aids to the identification of anopheline imagines in Malaya. Goverment of the Straits Settlement and the Malaria Advisory Board, Federated Malay states, Singapore
21. Zwiebel LJ, Takken W (2004) Olfactory regulation of mosquito–host interactions. Insect Biochem Mol Biol 34:645–652
22. Gimnig JE, Walker ED, Otieno P et al (2013) Incidence of malaria among mosquito collectors conducting human landing catches in western Kenya. Am J Trop Med Hyg 88:301–308
23. Chen H-L, Chang J-K, Tang R-B (2015) Current recommendations for the Japanese encephalitis vaccine. J Chin Med Assoc 78:271–275
24. Imwong M, Hien TT, Thuy-Nhien NT et al (2017) Spread of a single multidrug resistant malaria parasite lineage *(PfPailin)* to Vietnam. Lancet Infect Dis 17:1022–1023
25. Ashley EA, Dhorda M, Fairhurst RM et al (2014) Spread of artemisinin resistance in *Plasmodium falciparum* malaria. N Engl J Med 371:411–423
26. Le Goff G, Carnevale P, Fondjo E et al (1997) Comparison of three sampling methods of man-biting anophelines in order to estimate the malaria transmission in a village of South Cameroon. Parasite 4:75–80
27. Seng CM, Matusop A, Sen FK (1999) Differences in *Anopheles* composition and malaria transmission in the village settlements and cultivated farming zone in Sarawak, Malaysia. Southeast Asian J Trop Med Public Health 30:454–459
28. Rubio-Palis Y, Curtis CF (1992) Evaluation of different methods of catching anopheline mosquitoes in western Venezuela. J Am Mosq Control Assoc 8:261–267
29. Service MW (1977) A critical review of procedures for sampling populations of adult mosquitoes. Bull Entomol Res 67:343–382
30. World Health Organization (1975) Methods and techniques. Manual on practical entomology in malaria. WHO, Geneva

31. Hamon J (1964) Observations sur l'emploi des moustiquaires-pieges pour la capture semi-automatique des moustiques. Bull Soc Pathol Exot 57:576–588
32. Tangena J-AA, Thammavong P, Hiscox A et al (2015) The human-baited double net trap: an alternative to human landing catches for collecting outdoor biting mosquitoes in Lao PDR. PLoS One 10:e0138735
33. Chaki PP, Mlacha YP, Msellem D et al (2012) An affordable, quality-assured community-based system for high-resolution entomological surveillance of vector mosquitoes that reflects human malaria infection risk patterns. Malar J 11:172
34. Singh N, Mishra AK (1997) Efficacy of light-traps in sampling malaria vectors in different ecological zones in Central India. Southeast Asian J Trop Med Public Health 28:196–202
35. Kilama M, Smith DL, Hutchinson R et al (2014) Estimating the annual entomological inoculation rate for *Plasmodium falciparum* transmitted by *Anopheles gambiae s.l.* using three sampling methods in three sites in Uganda. Malar J 13:111
36. Lines JD, Curtis CF, Wilkes TJ et al (1991) Monitoring human-biting mosquitoes (Diptera: Culicidae) in Tanzania with light-traps hung beside mosquito nets. Bull Entomol Res 81:77–84
37. McDermott EG, Mullens BA (2017) The dark side of light traps. J Med Entomol 55:251–261
38. Hiscox A, Otieno B, Kibet A et al (2014) Development and optimization of the Suna trap as a tool for mosquito monitoring and control. Malar J 13:257
39. Homan T, Hiscox A, Mweresa CK et al (2016) The effect of mass mosquito trapping on malaria transmission and disease burden (SolarMal): a stepped-wedge cluster-randomised trial. Lancet 388:1193–1201
40. Hiscox A, Maire N, Kiche I et al (2012) The SolarMal project: innovative mosquito trapping technology for malaria control. Malar J 11:O45
41. Burkot TR, Russell TL, Reimer LJ et al (2013) Barrier screens: a method to sample blood-fed and host-seeking exophilic mosquitoes. Malar J 12:49
42. Marcombe S, Bobichon J, Somphong B et al (2017) Insecticide resistance status of malaria vectors in Lao PDR. PLoS One 12:e0175984
43. World Health Organization (2013) Malaria entomology and vector control. Guide for participants. WHO, Geneva
44. Harbison JE, Mathenge EM, Misiani GO et al (2006) A simple method for sampling indoor-resting malaria mosquitoes *Anopheles gambiae* and *Anopheles funestus* (Diptera: Culicidae) in Africa. J Med Entomol 43:473–479
45. Govella NJ, Chaki PP, Mpangile JM et al (2011) Monitoring mosquitoes in urban Dar Es Salaam: evaluation of resting boxes, window exit traps, CDC light traps, Ifakara tent traps and human landing catches. Parasit Vectors 4:40
46. Silver JB (2008) Field sampling methods. Mosquito ecology, 3rd edn. Springer, Dordrecht
47. Muirhead-Thomson RC (1958) A pit shelter for sampling outdoor mosquito populations. Bull World Health Organ 19:1116–1118
48. Kweka EJ, Mwang'onde BJ, Kimaro E et al (2009) A resting box for outdoor sampling of adult *Anopheles arabiensis* in rice irrigation schemes of lower Moshi, northern Tanzania. Malar J 8:82
49. Service MW (1993) Mosquito ecology. Field sampling methods. Elsevier Applied Science, London
50. Odiere M, Bayoh MN, Gimnig J et al (2007) Sampling outdoor, resting *Anopheles gambiae* and other mosquitoes (Diptera: Culicidae) in Western Kenya with clay pots. J Med Entomol 44:14–22
51. Sikaala CH, Killeen GF, Chanda J et al (2013) Evaluation of alternative mosquito sampling methods for malaria vectors in lowland south - East Zambia. Parasit Vectors 6:91
52. Rosner B (2010) Chapter 8 hypothesis testing: two-sample inference. In: Fundamentals for biostatistics. 7th edn
53. Detinova TS (1945) Determination of the physiological age of female *Anopheles* from the changes of the tracheal system of the ovaries. Med Parazitol (Mosk) 14:45–49
54. World Health Organization (2016) Test procedures for insecticide resistance monitoring in malaria vector mosquitoes, 2nd edn. The WHO susceptibility test for adult mosquitoes, Geneva
55. Cooper RD, Frances SP, Popat S et al (2004) The effectiveness of light, 1-octen-3-ol, and carbon dioxide as attractants for anopheline mosquitoes in Madang Province, Papua New Guinea. J Am Mosq Control Assoc 20:239–242
56. Barr AR, Smith TA, Boreham MM et al (1963) Evaluation of some factors affecting the efficiency of light traps in collecting mosquitoes. J Econ Entomol 56:123–127
57. Gillies MT (1970) The role of carbon dioxide in host-finding by mosquitoes (Diptera: Culicidae): a review. Bull Ent Res 70:525–532

58. Smallegange RC, Schmied WH, van Roey KJ et al (2010) Sugar-fermenting yeast as an organic source of carbon dioxide to attract the malaria mosquito *Anopheles gambiae*. Malar J 9:292
59. Mweresa C, Omusula P, Otieno B et al (2014) Molasses as a source of carbon dioxide for attracting the malaria mosquitoes *Anopheles gambiae* and *Anopheles funestus*. Malar J 13:160
60. van Loon JJA, Smallegange RC, Bukovinszkiné-Kiss G et al (2015) Mosquito attraction: crucial role of carbon dioxide in formulation of a five-component blend of human-derived volatiles. J Chem Ecol 41:567–573
61. Mburu MM, Mweresa CK, Omusula P et al (2017) 2-butanone as a carbon dioxide mimic in attractant blends for the Afrotropical malaria mosquitoes *Anopheles gambiae* and *Anopheles funestus*. Malar J 16:351
62. Smallegange RC, Knols BG, Takken W (2010) Effectiveness of synthetic versus natural human volatiles as attractants for *Anopheles gambiae* (Diptera: Culicidae) sensu stricto. J Med Entomol 47:338–344
63. Schmied WH, Takken W, Killeen GF et al (2008) Evaluation of two counterflow traps for testing behaviour-mediating compounds for the malaria vector *Anopheles gambiae* s.S. Under semi-field conditions in Tanzania. Malar J 7:230
64. Njiru BN, Mukabana WR, Takken W et al (2006) Trapping of the malaria vector *Anopheles gambiae* with odour-baited MM-X traps in semi-field conditions in western Kenya. Malar J 5:39
65. Logan JG, Birkett MA (2007) Semiochemicals for biting fly control: their identification and exploitation. Pest Manag Sci 63:647–657
66. Acree F, Turner RB, Gouck HK et al (1968) L-lactic acid: a mosquito attractant isolated from humans. Science 161:1346–1347
67. Braks MAH, Meijerink J, Takken W (2001) The response of the malaria mosquito, *Anopheles gambiae*, to two components of human sweat, ammonia and l-lactic acid, in an olfactometer. Physiol Entomol 26:142–148
68. Okumu FO, Killeen GF, Ogoma S et al (2010) Development and field evaluation of a synthetic mosquito lure that is more attractive than humans. PLoS One 5:e8951
69. Mukabana WR, Mweresa CK, Otieno B et al (2012) A novel synthetic odorant blend for trapping of malaria and other African mosquito species. J Chem Ecol 38:235–244
70. Odetoyinbo JA (1969) Preliminary investigation on the use of a light-trap for sampling malaria vectors in the Gambia. Bull World Health Organ 40:547–560
71. Mboera LE, Kihonda J, Braks MA et al (1998) Influence of centers for disease control light trap position, relative to a human-baited bed net, on catches of *Anopheles gambiae* and *Culex quinquefasciatus* in Tanzania. Am J Trop Med Hyg 59:595–596
72. Verhulst NO, Bakker JW, Hiscox A (2015) Modification of the suna trap for improved survival and quality of mosquitoes in support of epidemiological studies. J Am Mosq Control Assoc 31:223–232
73. Williams J, Pinto J (2012) Training manual on malaria entomology, for entomology and vector control technicians (basic level). United States Agency for International Development, Washington, DC
74. Microsoft (2015) Project premonition https://www.microsoft.com/en-us/research/project/project-premonition/. Accessed 22 Dec 2017
75. Biogents (2016) BG-counter: remote mosquito monitoring. https://www.bg-counter.com/. Accessed 24 Dec 2017
76. Menger D, Otieno B, de Rijk M et al (2014) A push-pull system to reduce house entry of malaria mosquitoes. Malar J 13:119
77. Kydonieus AF, Beroza M (1982) Insect suppression with controlled release pheromone systems, vol 1. Pheromones and their use. RC Press, Boca Raton, FL
78. Poulin B, Lefebvre G, Muranyi-Kovacs C et al (2017) Mosquito traps: an innovative, environmentally friendly technique to control mosquitoes. Int J Environ Res Public Health 14:313
79. Cook SM, Khan ZR, Pickett JA (2007) The use of push-pull strategies in integrated pest management. Annu Rev Entomol 52:375–400
80. Tangena J-AA, Thammavong P, Malaithong N et al (2017) Diversity of mosquitoes (Diptera: Culicidae) attracted to human subjects in rubber plantations, secondary forests, and villages in Luang Prabang province, northern Lao PDR. J Med Entomol 54:1589–1604
81. Pombi M, Guelbeogo WM, Kreppel K et al (2014) The sticky resting box, a new tool for studying resting behaviour of Afrotropical malaria vectors. Parasit Vectors 7:247

Chapter 18

Insecticides and Insecticide Resistance

Mamadou Ousmane Ndiath

Abstract

Vector control has significantly reduced malaria morbidity in many regions of the world where the disease was endemic and is now moving toward malaria elimination. Among the tools available for vector control, the use of long-lasting insecticidal bed nets (LLINs) and indoor residual spraying (IRS) has proved most effective. However, *Anopheles* mosquitoes are becoming increasingly resistant to insecticides. In this chapter, we describe the main aspects of vector control—with a particular focus on insecticidal products commonly used in vector control as well as on mechanisms of insecticide resistance. We also discuss the impact of insecticide resistance on malaria transmission.

Key words *Anopheles*, Insecticide resistance, Vector control, Residual malaria transmission

1 Introduction

Vector control (VC) is the most effective way to prevent malaria and one of the four fundamentals of the Global Malaria Control Strategy (Amsterdam Ministerial Conference) [1]. For malaria transmission to occur, the vector must live long enough to ensure the development of the parasite and the production of sporozoites [2]. The culmination of this long process requires two essential parameters in the vector, namely, vectorial capacity (interaction between vector and environmental factors, such as population, host preference, feeding time, longevity, etc.) and vectorial competence (interaction between vector and pathogen governed by intrinsic, genetic factors that influence the ability of a vector to transmit a pathogen).

The main objective of VC is to act on the pathogen by reducing mosquito life span, eliminating potentially dangerous mosquitoes or simply preventing them from thriving. In the era of genetics, much more advanced VC tools are currently being studied. These act on vectorial competence, which determines the degree of coadaptation between vector and parasite. These new tools are designed to block the development of the parasite in the mosquito

Frédéric Ariey et al. (eds.), *Malaria Control and Elimination*, Methods in Molecular Biology, vol. 2013,
https://doi.org/10.1007/978-1-4939-9550-9_18,

[3]. Examples are the use of the bacterium *Wolbachia* and genetically modified mosquitoes [4].

The end goal of VC is to permanently interrupt transmission or more often to reduce transmission to such an extent that the disease is no longer a public health problem [5]. The methods used are aimed either at reducing human-vector contact, thus preventing mosquito bites through personal protection, or at reducing mosquito infectivity, longevity, and density. The latter is achieved through a decrease in larval production or control of the adult population resulting in collective protection. However, for VC to be effective, the choice of either method must take into account the bioecology of the targeted species, their behavior, and the epidemiological context in which transmission takes place [6].

In addition, VC prevents epidemics, fights outbreaks in malaria-free areas, controls transmission in high-risk areas, and reduces transmission in areas of high resistance to antimalarials [7]. It can be subdivided into two main parts: larval control and fight against adult mosquitoes. For each control method, several tools can be used, which should take into account the following characteristics: (a) the entomological, epidemiological, and ecological characteristics, which will determine the effectiveness of the vector control, and (b) the economic and sociopolitical situation as well as anthropological characteristics that will determine the success of VC. Finally, VC requires some ingenuity and technicality in the choice of methods and the products to be used as well as in the selection and evaluation of the indicators.

1.1 Larvae Control

Larvae control (LC) is achieved by mechanical, chemical, or biological methods. Mechanical methods are based on large-scale environmental changes such as drainage, water flow, hole fillings, destruction of sheltering receptacles, and modification of rivers and lakes in order to reduce breeding sites for *Anopheles* larvae [8]. The use of larvicidal pesticides such as malathion, temephos, methoxychlor, and methyl-dursban is a typical example of chemical control. Biological control often involves the use of larvivorous fish (*Gambusia affinis*), invertebrate predators (*Toxorhynchites*), parasites (nematodes, protozoa, fungi), or pathogenic bacteria (*Bacillus thuringiensis israeliensis*, *Bacillus sphaericus*) [9].

LC is very difficult to implement in the field. Therefore, its implementation should be controlled and should only be considered under certain conditions: appropriate expertise, qualified personnel, easy access to breeding sites, nature and type of breeding sites, and also acceptance by the population. In short, for LC to be effective, it must be inclusive, that is, take into consideration the technical, economic, and sociocultural aspects of the region.

1.2 Adult Mosquito Control

Control of adult mosquitoes relies heavily on indoor residual spraying (IRS) and the use of long-lasting insecticidal nets (LLINs) [6]. In addition, it may be necessary to add innovative methods such as genetically modified mosquitoes.

1.2.1 Indoor Residual Spraying

The effectiveness of IRS depends primarily on the vector biology [10], which includes the vector anthropophily, which determines the choice of the host, and the vector aggressiveness cycle, which determines the location of the bite and the mosquito's resting place. In general, IRS will be effective for anthropophilic, endophageous, and endophilic mosquitoes. On the other hand, they will be much less effective against exophageous and exophilic species [11, 12].

In Africa, the first IRS campaigns after the Second World War (1955) were marked by the massive use of residual insecticides such as dichloro-diphenyl-trichloroethane (DDT), hexachlorocyclohexane (HCH), and the Dièldrine. DDT comes in a liquid form that dries and forms a crystalline deposit with residual effect on the sprayed surfaces. It has proved very effective, but its toxicity to environment, animals, and humans limits its massive use, hence its prohibition in the 1970s. Today, the IRS application has been carefully standardized, and very clear specifications exist on the material and insecticides to be used [13].

IRS is particularly recommended for the prevention of epidemics as a result of potentially alarming events such as heavy rain, the migration of nonimmune subjects, and the increase in minimum temperatures. However, the choice of insecticide and the formulation to be applied is based primarily on the susceptibility to insecticides of local vectors, the characteristics of the various compounds, the value for money, and sustained collaboration of the population. The insecticides recommended by WHO for IRS are listed in Table 1.

The use of insecticides may lead not only to an increase in the zoophilic tendencies of mosquitoes, due to their repellent action, but also to the appearance of insecticide resistance within *Anopheles* populations [14].

1.2.2 Long-Lasting Insecticidal Nets (LLINs)

The use of mosquito nets has a long history. Already in 1911, Ronald Ross, in his book entitled *Prevention of Malaria*, advocated the use of mosquito nets to protect against mosquito bites. The effectiveness of the nets was particularly improved after impregnation with a pyrethroid insecticide. The first impregnation experiments were carried out in 1984 at the experimental station of Soumousso, Burkina Faso [15]. While impregnation was once done by hand, today impregnated nets are manufactured and respect quality control standards that take into account the composition, mesh size, denier, toughness, weight, flammability, resistance to bursting, and tearing rendering them more efficient [16].

Table 1
WHO recommended insecticides for indoor residual spraying (IRS) against malaria vectors

Insecticide compound and formulation[a]	Class group[b]	Dosage (g a.i./m^2)	Mode of action	Duration of effective action (months)
DDT WP	OC	1–2	Contact	>6
Malathion WP	OP	2	Contact	2–3
Fenitrothion WP	OP	2	Contact and airbone	3–6
Pirimiphos-methyl WP & EC	OP	1–2	Contact and airbone	2–3
Pirimiphos-methyl CS	OP	1	Contact and airbone	4–6
Bendiocarb WP	C	0.1–0.4	Contact and airbone	2–6
Propoxur WP	C	1–2	Contact and airbone	3–6
Alpha-cypermethrin WP & SC	PY	0.02–0.03	Contact	4–6
Bifenthrin WP	PY	0.025–0.05	Contact	3–6
Cyfluthrin WP	PY	0.02–0.05	Contact	3–6
Deltamethrin SC-PE	PY	0.02–0.025	Contact	6
Deltamethrin WP, WG	PY	0.02–0.025	Contact	3–6
Etofenprox WP	PY	0.1–0.3	Contact	3–6
Lambda-cyhalothrin WP, CS	PY	0.02–0.03	Contact	3–6

Note: WHO recommendations on the use of pesticides in public health are valid ONLY if linked to WHO specifications for their quality control. WHO specifications for public health pesticides are available on the WHO homepage at http://www.who.int/whopes/quality/en/

[a] *CS* capsule suspension, *EC* emulsifiable concentrate, *SC* suspension concentrate, *SC-PE* polymer enhanced suspension concentrate, *WG* water dispersible granule, *WP* wettable powder

[b] *OC* organochlorines; *OP* organophosphates, *C* carbamates, *PY* pyrethroids

Pyrethroids are the only insecticides recommended for impregnation of mosquito nets because of the rapidity of their actions, their excito-repellent effects, and their low toxicity in humans. The double barrier of nets, i.e., physical and chemical, used in a generalized way, considerably reduces the human-vector contact and thus malaria transmission. It also reduces the *Anopheles* density [17]. Impregnated mosquito nets can have several effects depending on the products used, which can be (a) deterrent, by preventing mosquitoes from entering the living rooms; (b) excito-repellent, by repelling mosquitoes outside the living rooms; (c) knockdown (kdr), in which case the mosquito is stunned; or (d) lethal, when the mosquito dies shortly after contact with the insecticide.

The permanent and large-scale use of LLINs has revolutionized VC by dramatically reducing malaria transmission worldwide [18]. The combined actions of LLINs and IRS, if maintained and associated with new tools, should enable the elimination of the disease in multiple countries by 2030.

However, like in an arms race, *Anopheles* are becoming increasingly resistant to several classes of insecticides, which jeopardizes the hope of malaria eradication [19]. Resistance is a very difficult problem, especially as it has emerged for next-generation insecticides such as pyrethroids [19, 20]. These difficulties account for the new strategies for adult mosquito control. The concept of personal protection is put forward with the use of next-generation LLINs such as Interceptor2, which is a combination of alpha-cypermethrin, a pyrethroid, and chlorfenapyr, a synthetic pyrrole insecticide, which is metabolized after penetrating the insect. Chlorfenapyr is used in agriculture and for urban pest control. There is also PermaNet® 3.0, the first LLIN combining a synergist piperonyl butoxide (PBO) and deltamethrin, a pyrethroid. Other LLINs such as DawaPlus 3 and 4 are based on the same principle [21]. These third-generation mosquito nets are an ideal choice in areas where mosquitoes have developed insecticide resistance. Table 2 summarizes the insecticides recommended by the WHO for the treatment of mosquito nets.

1.2.3 Genetically Modified Mosquitoes

Studies on vector competence have allowed the identification of mosquito genes likely to be involved in the mosquito immune response to the development of the malaria parasite [22]. The aim of the approach is to replace wild *Anopheles* populations with genetically manipulated mosquitoes that have lost the ability to host and/or transmit the parasite. Importantly, these genetically modified vectors refractory to parasite infection will, once released into the wild, have to replace the wild *Anopheles* populations in order to effectively reduce or block malaria transmission [23]. However, the effectiveness of such an approach on the ground is still unclear as several factors must be taken into consideration, specifically, (a) the heterogeneity of the vectors and the potential competition between vectors belonging to different complexes or groups of species, (b) the habitat diversity and *Anopheles* behavior, and (c) the great genetic diversity of the parasite.

Despite these difficulties, studies have provided new insights into mosquito biology and their ability to adapt to the environment (mainly in *An. gambiae*), which in turn should serve to improve malaria control in the near future [24, 25]. In addition, thanks to the development of genetic engineering, significant progress has also been made with the use of the bacterium *Wolbachia* to block the development of the parasite in the mosquito [26].

Table 2
WHO recommended insecticide products for treatment of mosquito nets for malaria vector control

Insecticide	Formulation[a]	Dosage[b]
Conventional treatment		
Alpha-cypermethrin	SC 10%	20–40
Cyfluthrin	EW 5%	50
Deltamethrin	SC 1%; WT 25%; and WT 25% + binder[c]	15–25
Etofenprox	EW 10%	200
Lambda-cyhalothrin	CS 2.5%	10–15
Permethrin	EC 10%	200–500

Product name	Product type	Duration of efficacy
Long-lasting treatment of polyester nets		
ICON®MAXX	Lambda-cyhalothrin 10% CS + binder in twin sachet pack. Target dose 62 mg Al/m^2 for family-size net (130 × 180 × 50 cm); dose range from 50 mg Al/m^2 (for a large family-size net) to 83 mg Al/m^2 (for a single-size net)	30–36 months

[a]*EC* emulsifiable concentrate; *EW* emulsion, oil in water; *CS* capsule suspension; *SC* suspension concentrate; *WT* water dispersible tablet
[b]Milligrams of active ingredient per square meter of netting
[c]K-O TAB 1-2-3®

2 Insecticides Used in Vector Control

An insecticide is an active substance or a preparation that belongs to the group of pesticides and can kill insects, their larvae, or their eggs. It is important to remember that originally insecticides were not intended for vector control but rather for crop pest control. This is the reason why only a very limited number are used in vector control.

The main synthetic insecticides used in VC belong to four main families: organochlorines, organophosphates, carbamates, and pyrethroids. The potential targets for these insecticides are multifold and varied. Nearly 90% of insecticides used are neurotoxic. They act on the voltage-dependent ion channels, at the origin of the nervous activity or on the ionotropic receptors, altering the synaptic transmission (Fig. 1).

2.1 Organochlorines

They represent the oldest group of chemical insecticides, as they have been used since the 1940s, and display a low toxicity to humans. They all include chlorine atoms in their chemical structure and belong to two main groups: (a) DDT and its analogues (e.g.,

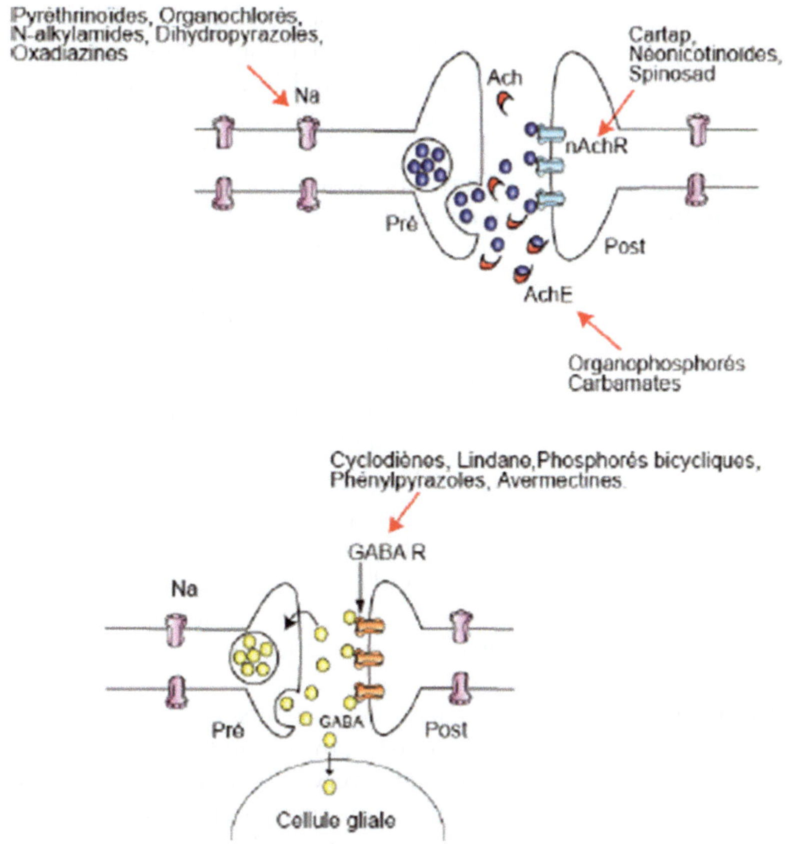

Fig. 1 Schematic representation by (Raymond-Delpech et al. 2005 [27]) of cholinergic (**a**) and GABAergic (**b**) synapses. (**a**) Cholinergic synapse showing the main targets of several classes of insecticides. (**b**) GABAergic synapse also showing sites of action of insecticides. Note that by contrast to acetylcholine, GABA is removed from the synaptic cleft by reuptake into the presynaptic terminal or glial cells. Abbreviations: *GABAR* γ-aminobutyric acid receptor; *n*AChR nicotinic acetylcholine receptor; *Post postsynaptic* element; *Pre presynaptic* element

hexachlorocyclohexane or HCH) and (b) cyclodienes: aldrin, dieldrin, endrin, and endosulfan.

Organochlorines are poorly soluble in water, very stable, and bioaccumulative. Hence, they strongly accumulate in organisms and ecosystems via food chains. Organochlorines may persist for a very long time in soils, plant tissues, and fats. Consequently their use, except DDT for IRS, is now prohibited by the WHO (Convention on Persistent Organic Pollutants). Organochlorines are neurotropic toxins that alter the function of sodium channels essential for the transmission of nerve impulses. DDT, for example, acts on the insect by contact and ingestion, inducing a generalized tremor (motor incoordination) and then a paralysis that sometimes takes 24 h to settle (Fig. 1). DDT has been popular because, like pyrethroids, it has rapid knockdown effect, relative longevity (6–-12 months), and low cost (Table 2). Despite chemical structural differences, DDT and pyrethroids have similar modes of action.

2.2 Organophosphates

They represent a vast group of chemical compounds whose molecules always include a central phosphate radical. Organophosphates are numerous and very heterogeneous with a very low remanence, i.e., the opposite of organochlorines. They are liposoluble and share a mode of action on the nervous system by inhibition of acetylcholinesterase, the enzyme responsible for the hydrolysis of acetylcholine after the transmission of information by this neurotransmitter, resulting in neuromuscular overstimulation and mosquito death (Fig. 1). This mode of action explains their remarkable toxicity toward humans and warm-blooded vertebrates. The most common organophosphates used for IRS are malathion, fenitrothion, and pirimiphos-methyl. They display shorter activity (1–3 months) than pyrethroids and DDT (Table 2). In addition, the organophosphates currently used for vector control are significantly more expensive than other insecticides.

2.3 Carbamates

Carbamates are esters of carbamic acid, which act, like organophosphosphates, by inhibiting acetylcholinesterase (Fig. 1). These products are very effective against mosquitoes, but their use is restricted by their high toxicity and production cost. The best knowns are carbosulfan, propoxur, carbaryl, and bendiocarb. Carbosulfan, effective both as larvicide and adulticide, may be an alternative for impregnating mosquito nets against *An. gambiae* strains resistant to pyrethroids [28]. Carbamates are used for IRS, in the form of bendiocarb. It has short residual activity (2–-6 months) and is more expensive than pyrethroids and DDT (Table 2).

2.4 Pyrethroids

Pyrethroids are synthetic esters of chrysanthemic acid, whose natural compounds, called pyrethrins, are extracted from the *Chrysanthemum cinerariaefolium*. Synthetic pyrethroids are widely used in public health. Depending on the composition of the chemical group that goes into their composition, there are two distinct types of pyrethroids: type I (e.g., bifenthrin, permethrin), which does not have an α-cyano group in their structure, and type II (e.g., permethrin, cyfluthrin, deltamethrin, cyhalothrin), which possesses an α-cyano group.

They are used in the composition of aerosols and smoke coils. Type II pyrethroids are more light stable and have higher insecticidal activity and remanence than type I pyrethroids. Pyrethroids are modulators of voltage-gated sodium channels that are responsible for the depolarization phase of action potentials. Like organochlorines, they kill insects by blocking the functioning of sodium channels essential for the transmission of nerve impulses (Fig. 1). Pyrethroids are used for both IRS and LLINs. They are the only insecticides recommended for impregnation of mosquito nets, because of their fast action at low dose (knockdown effect), their excito-repellent effect, and their safety for humans [13]. Pyrethroids display many modes of action on the mosquito and have relative longevity (3–6 months when used for IRS).

3 Resistance to Insecticides

Resistance of malaria vectors to insecticides is a major concern for public health authorities and especially for national malaria control programs in Africa and beyond, where the prevention of this devastating disease relies heavily on the use of pesticides to control the vector mosquito populations [29]. According to the WHO Expert Committee on Insecticides (1957) [30], resistance is defined as "*the appearance in a strain of insects of the ability to tolerate doses of toxic substances which would exert a lethal effect on the majority of individuals who make up a normal population of the same species.*" Specifically, the insecticide molecule should come into contact with the insect, penetrate its body, and in some cases be transformed into an active metabolite to be transported to its target. Any mechanism capable of modifying one of these steps can therefore lead to resistance [31]. Various mechanisms enable *Anopheles* to resist the action of insecticides, including behavioral, physiological, and biochemical resistance. These mechanisms may allow mosquitoes to resist more than one insecticide (cross-resistance), and *Anopheles* may express more than one resistance mechanism (multiple resistances) [19].

There are generally three types of resistance mechanisms that result in behavioral, physiological, and biochemical changes. Behavioral resistance is observed when a deviant behavior prevents any contact with the insecticide. Physiological resistance is characterized by a reduced penetration, or an increase in the excretion, of insecticides. Finally, biochemical resistance may reflect an increase in the enzymatic activity of the detoxification systems or a decrease in the affinity between the insecticides and its target site. All these resistance mechanisms reduce the toxic action of the insecticide. Very often, there may be cross-resistance between two families (e.g., between DDT and pyrethroids or between OPs and carbamates) (Fig. 2). Finally, resistance may have a cost on the insect biology as it may affect many *Anopheles* life history traits, such as larval development, sexual competition, predation rate, and vector competence [32, 33].

	Biochemical mechanism of resistance				
	Metabolic			Target-site	
	Esterases	Mono-oxygenases	GSH S-transferases	kdr	Altered AChe
Pyrethroids	•	●		●	
DDT		•	●	●	
Carbamates	•	●			●
Organophosphates	●	•			●

Fig. 2 Biochemical mechanisms of insecticide resistance: cross table between insecticides and resistance mechanisms. The circle sizes reflect the relative impact of mechanism of resistance. Abbreviations: *GSH* glutathione, *AChe* acetylcholinesterase, Kdr Knockdown resistance

3.1 Behavioral Resistance

This mechanism of resistance has been demonstrated since the 1950s [34]. However, little research has been done since. Indeed, changes in the behavior of the insect are very difficult to quantify in the laboratory, and their assessment requires extensive field observations. The behavioral resistance mechanism may be stimulus-dependent, implying recognition of the toxic substance by sensory receptors of the insect and creating irritability and repulsion. Irritability will cause the insect to leave the toxic environment, while repulsion will allow the insect to avoid contact with the pesticide [35]. For example, repeated IRS in Thailand habitats has transformed the endophilic and anthropophilic behavior of *An. minimus* mosquito into a more exophilic and zoophilic [36, 37]. It has also been shown that the irritability of DDT leads to absconding or avoidance behavior, so that the mosquito tends to leave treated homes [38]. Much more recent studies have shown that the use of LLINs in Senegal has caused the species *An. funestus* to bite in broad daylight, when people are not under the bed net but outdoors [12].

3.2 Physiological Resistance

To reach their molecular targets, insecticides must penetrate the insect through either the cuticle or the walls of the digestive tract. This penetration takes place at a rate, which, for the same insecticide, varies from one species to another. For example, if the penetration kinetics are slow, then the insecticide will be degraded more quickly by the detoxification systems and will therefore have little effect. Thus, insects will be selected by the pesticide and give birth to a resistant population. Changes in insecticide penetration through the cuticle have been highlighted in several insects, including *Anopheles gambiae* [39] and *Cimex lectularius* [40].

The molecular mechanisms of penetration have been little studied. However, recent studies have attempted to understand these mechanisms, notably by studying the composition of the cuticle in susceptible compared to resistant *Anopheles* strains. The results show significant differences both quantitatively and qualitatively in cuticle composition between susceptible and resistance strains of *An. funestus* [41] and *An. gambiae* populations [42].

3.3 Biochemical Resistance

Once the insecticide enters the insect, it reaches more or less rapidly the cellular level and the target enzymes. This results either in a sharp increase in the activity of the insecticide degradation systems (metabolic resistance) or in a modification of the target of the insecticide (target site modification). The penetration rate of the insecticide is a determinant of biochemical resistance.

3.3.1 Metabolic Resistance

Three types of enzymes participate in insecticide degradation: cytochrome P-450, which introduce an oxygen atom into their substrates; glutathione *S*-transferases, which catalyze the conjugation of molecules having an electrophilic center with the glutathione thiol group; and finally hydrolases, which cleave esters and amides, thus increasing the polarity of metabolites [43, 44].

Cytochrome P-450

They are enzymes involved in the metabolism of juvenile hormones and ecdysones, in the synthesis of pheromones and the protection against toxic substances of plant origin. This enzymatic complex is fixed on the endoplasmic reticulum of cells, more rarely in mitochondria. It is found mainly in the cells of the digestive tract, Malpighian tubules, and fat tissue of insects. They are involved in resistance to pyrethroids, carbamates, DDT, and some organophosphates [45, 46].

Glutathione S-Transferases (GST)

GST play an important role in the detoxification of xenobiotic substances and intervene by catalyzing the conjugation of these substances with endogenous glutathione. There are two forms of GST in insects, GST1 and GST2, each of which plays a role in insecticide resistance. They are mainly localized in the cytoplasm of the cells of fatty substances and wing muscles [47]. GST play a major role in DDT resistance by degrading it into a nontoxic product, DDE [48]. They are also involved in resistance to organophosphorus compounds [45].

Esterases

These enzymes constitute an important group of enzymes that catalyze the introduction of a water molecule at an ester linkage. In insects, esterases are involved in reproduction, hormone metabolism, digestion, and neurotransmission. They are mainly localized in the cytoplasm and on the endoplasmic reticulum of cells of the digestive tract, the Malpighian tubules, the reproductive system, and the fat body. Esterases are of two types depending on whether they preferentially hydrolyze alpha- or beta-naphthyl acetate [48, 49]. Esterases play an important role in organophosphates resistance.

3.3.2 Target Site Modification

More than 90% of the synthetic insecticides are organophosphates, carbamates, and pyrethroids, with sites of action localized in the central nervous system of insects. Among the molecular targets, the three most important ones are acetylcholinesterase (Ache), the voltage-dependent sodium channel (Vdsc), and the gamma-aminobutyric acid receptor (GABAr).

Acetylcholinesterase (Ache)

Ache is the best-known protein acting as a target for organophosphates and carbamates. It is found mainly in the central nervous system and is essential for the proper functioning of cholinergic synapses. In fact, nerve impulses arriving at a synapse result in the release of Ache, which binds to receptors placed on the postsynaptic membrane. This fixation allows the opening of the sodium and potassium channels, which causes the depolarization at the origin of the nerve impulses on the postsynaptic element. The role of Ache is to hydrolyze acetylcholine, which allows the closure of the channels associated with the neurotransmitter receptor. If the action of this enzyme is blocked, the postsynaptic membrane is continually excited, eventually causing the death of the insect [50, 51].

The complete sequence of the genome of *An. gambiae* has shown that there are two genes in the mosquito, *Ace-1* and *Ace-2*, coding for two distinct Aches. The newly identified gene, *Ace-1*, encodes synaptic AChE1, which is the target of organophosphorus and carbamate insecticides in mosquitoes. In *Drosophila melanogaster* and *Musca domestica*, four point mutations located on the *Ace-2* gene render Ache less susceptible to the inhibitory action of insecticides [52]. In *Cx. quinquefasciatus*, *An. albimanus*, and *An. gambiae*, the same Gly/Ser mutation found at position 119 on the *Ace-1* gene confers cross-resistance to OPs and carbamates [53]. Many other point mutations exist on Ache, some of which confer resistance to OPs and carbamates [48, 54].

Voltage-Gated Sodium Channel (CNaVdp)

They are transmembrane proteins composed of 1800 amino acids and 4 homologous domains, each comprising 6 hydrophobic transmembrane segments. They intervene in the transmission of nerve impulses along axons. These channels, once activated (open position), cause a flow of sodium ions from the extracellular medium into the intercellular medium, generating an action potential. This depolarization causes the activation of the nearby CNaVdp and spreads step by step, generating a wave of depolarization that transmits nerve impulses [55].

Pyrethroids and DDT act by modifying the inactivation kinetics of CNaVdp. Exposure of a susceptible *Anopheles* strain to DDT or a pyrethroid leads to uncoordinated movements and then to ataxia, more or less reversible depending on the insecticide and the dose used; we speak of a knockdown (*kd*) effect. The kd effect represents the symptomatological translation of the sensitivity of the insect's nervous system toward the insecticide. From a molecular point of view, data show that the kd effect is due to the binding of pyrethroids or DDT to CNaVdp. A point mutation resulting from the replacement of Leu by Phe at the sixth segment of domain II of CNaVdp (kdr Leu-Phe mutation) confers resistance to pyrethroids and DDT in West Africa [56, 57]. This mutation is found in many mosquito species, including *Aedes aegypti* [58], *Aedes stephensi* [59], *An. gambiae* [20], and *Culex quinquefasciatus* [60]. In East Africa, it is rather the replacement of Leu by Ser in the same position that confers resistance to pyrethroids [61]. Previously, this mutation was observed only in East Africa, whereas it now appears to be invading West Africa, with the direct consequence of the disappearance of the barrier between *kdr-e* and *kdr-w* [62, 63].

Gamma-Aminobutyric Acid Receptors (GABAR)

GABAR are targets of many organohalogen insecticides, including dieldrin and lindane. These insecticides bind to the gamma-aminobutyric acid receptor and inhibit the functioning of the associated chlorine channel [64]. The opening of this channel induces a hyperpolarization of the nerve membrane and its inactivation, which, when prolonged, disrupts the functioning of the nervous system. A single point mutation, namely, the substitution at position 296 of an Ala in Gly on GABA receptors, is responsible for the resistance to cyclodienes and avermectins. As in the case of AChE1, this mutation leads to a structural modification of the active site, thus reducing the binding of inhibitors [65].

4 Impact of Insecticide Resistance on Malaria Transmission

The use of LLINs and IRS has significantly reduced the global malaria burden over the past 15 years. The incidence rate of malaria is estimated to have decreased by 41% globally between 2000 and 2015 [66]. For this progress to translate into the ambitious goal of malaria elimination, many have agreed that VC needs to play a central role [67, 68]. The twenty-first century has witnessed a pronounced increase in the use of insecticides for malaria control. Several major donors have invested heavily in LLIN distributions and IRS activities. Nonetheless, malaria still continues to claim lives, and many questions remain unanswered, particularly with regard to the change in *Anopheles* behavior [12, 69–71].

As much as the impact of vector control (LLINs and IRS) on the transmission of malaria in recent years is known [66], the impact of insecticide resistance on malaria transmission is not yet fully understood. Most of the recent studies focus on alert and projection because in reality, it is very difficult to estimate the precise impact on transmission. However, taking a closer look at this issue, it can be seen from extensive field observations that resistance could jeopardize current and future gains in controlling malaria. It has been shown in West Africa that the use of LLINs has certainly reduced malaria transmission significantly but in the long run has led to a rebound in malaria correlated with an increase in kdr resistance [72, 73]. Other studies have confirmed these observations even though the link between increased resistance and transmission is not as direct as we think, as many other factors such as immunity come into play. However, it is clear that if the efforts made are relaxed, the insecticide resistance will very quickly jeopardize current and future gains in controlling malaria. Therefore, there is an urgent need to manage the resistance phenomenon.

One direct consequence of resistance is described as "residual malaria transmission (RMT)." This term, used in recent years, encompasses the failure of vector control ranging from behavioral resistance to physiological resistance. RMT results from either a behavioral insecticide avoidance or the behavior-related ability of malaria vectors to be unaffected by interventions using insecticides indoors (IRS and LLINs), which is independent of insecticide susceptibility [74]. Two ecological contexts were observed. First, the natural behavioral avoidance occurs when, regardless of the presence of LLINs or IRS, mosquitoes exhibit a behavior that does not bring them in contact with the insecticides, namely, biting outside or early in the evening or morning or mostly biting animals and resting outside. Both IRS and LLINs will mainly affect anthropophilic mosquitoes biting indoors, leaving ample opportunity for more exophilic, exophagic, early-biting, and/or zoophilic vectors to avoid contact with insecticide-treated surfaces and to maintain a certain level of transmission. Second, the protective behavioral avoidance occurs in response to the presence of (indoor) use of insecticides. Insecticide-induced exophily, exophagy, zoophily, or early biting may then occur, e.g., excito-repellent of insecticides (behavioral resistance) [12, 75].

There is also evidence that changes in behavior have apparently been selected as a consequence of vector control and environmental change. *Anopheles* vectors are known to display remarkable adaptative skills that enable their survival in widely varying environmental conditions [76, 77]. Numerous vector species have therefore been implicated in the RMT, and important examples include *An. gambiae* and *An. funestus* (the most common African vectors) [11, 12, 78]. Evidence from a variety of settings over the last half century indicates that RMT occurs even with good access to, and usage of, LLINs or well-implemented IRS, as well as in situations where LLIN use or IRS is not practical [74, 75, 79]. In many malaria-endemic areas, RMT, maintained through a combination of human and vector behaviors, will render malaria elimination extremely difficult.

RMT clearly and unequivocally demonstrates the limits of vector control as designed today. In order to cope with this, a good resistance management policy as defined by the WHO Expert Committee is needed, as well as finding new alternative control methods to reduce or even eliminate the atypical anopheline population responsible for residual transmission of malaria. All this must be supported by regular monitoring of the evolution of resistance in different anopheline populations [80].

5 Conclusion

Insecticides used against arthropod vectors of malaria are a minor group of inputs in modern agriculture. Their intensive use has been the basis of selection of mosquitoes able to survive and reproduce in the presence of pesticides. The consequences of this phenomenon on public health could be catastrophic. Given the worrying state of insecticide resistance, the malaria community must understand its potential impact on the malaria burden. If resistance to currently used insecticides leads to less effective vector control, and no strong action is taken to address resistance, the global malaria burden will increase significantly. However, adequate resistance management can only be achieved if the biotic and abiotic factors influencing the evolution and dispersion of resistance genes in natural populations are well known.

References

1. World Health Organization (1992) Ministerial conference on malaria, Amsterdam, The Netherlands 26–27 October. World Health Organization, Geneva
2. Roberts L (2002) Mosquitoes and disease. Science 298:82–83
3. Esvelt K (2016) Gene editing can drive science to openness. Nature 534:153
4. Baldini F, Segata N, Pompon J et al (2014) Evidence of natural *Wolbachia* infections in field populations of *Anopheles gambiae*. Nat Commun 5:3985
5. World Health Organization (1997) Vector control: methods for use by individuals and communities. World Health Organization, Geneva
6. Mnzava AP, Knox TB, Temu EA (2015) Implementation of the global plan for insecticide resistance management in malaria vectors: progress, challenges and the way forward. Malar J 14:173
7. Chanda E, Mzilahowa T, Chipwanya J et al (2016) Scale-up of integrated malaria vector control: lessons from Malawi. Bull World Health Organ 94:475–480
8. World Health Organization (2013) Larval source management – a supplementary measure for malaria vector control. An operational manual. World Health Organization, Geneva
9. Brownbridge M, Margalit J (1986) New *Bacillus thuringiensis* strains isolated in Israel are highly toxic to mosquito larvae. J Invertebr Pathol 48:216–222
10. World Health Organization (2015) Indoor residual spraying: An operational manual for IRS for malaria transmission, control and elimination, 2nd edn. World Health Organization, Geneva
11. Russell TL, Govella NJ, Azizi S et al (2011) Increased proportions of outdoor feeding among residual malaria vector populations following increased use of insecticide-treated nets in rural Tanzania. Malar J 10:80
12. Sougoufara S, Diedhiou SM, Doucoure S et al (2014) Biting by *Anopheles funestus* in broad daylight after use of long-lasting insecticidal nets: a new challenge to malaria elimination. Malar J 13:125
13. WHO Pesticide Evaluation Scheme (2013) WHO recommended insecticides for indoor

residual spraying against malaria vectors. World Health Organization, Geneva

14. Hamon J, Garrett-Jones C (1963) Resistance to insecticides in the major malaria vectors and its operational importance. Bull World Health Organ 28:1–24
15. Darriet F, Robert V, Vien NT et al (1984) Evaluation de l'efficacité sur les vecteurs du paludisme de la Permethrine en imprégnation sur des moustiquaires intactes et trouées. Organisation mondiale de la Santé, Genève
16. World Health Organization (2001) Spécifications concernant les tulles pour moustiquaires. Rapport de consultation informelle. World Health Organization, Geneva
17. Wilson AL, Dhiman RC, Kitron U et al (2014) Benefit of insecticide-treated nets, curtains and screening on vector borne diseases, excluding malaria: a systematic review and meta-analysis. PLoS Negl Trop Dis 8:e3228
18. World Health Organization (2017) Achieving and maintaining universal coverage with long-lasting insecticidal nets for malaria control. World Health Organization, Geneva
19. Ranson H, Lissenden N (2016) Insecticide resistance in African *Anopheles* mosquitoes: a worsening situation that needs urgent action to maintain malaria control. Trends Parasitol 32:187–196
20. Martinez-Torres D, Chandre F, Williamson MS et al (1998) Molecular characterization of pyrethroid knockdown resistance (kdr) in the major malaria vector *Anopheles gambiae* s.s. Insect Mol Biol 7:179–184
21. WHO Pesticide Evaluation Scheme (2016) Geneva: World Health Organization
22. Beerntsen BT, James AA, Christensen BM (2000) Genetics of mosquito vector competence. Microbiol Mol Biol Rev 64:115–137
23. Curtis CF, Pates HV, Takken W et al (1999) Biological problems with the replacement of a vector population by *Plasmodium*-refractory mosquitoes. Parassitologia 41:479–481
24. Boete C (2005) Malaria parasites in mosquitoes: laboratory models, evolutionary temptation and the real world. Trends Parasitol 21:445–447
25. White BJ, Hahn MW, Pombi M et al (2007) Localization of candidate regions maintaining a common polymorphic inversion (2La) in *Anopheles gambiae*. PLoS Genet 3:e217
26. Walker T, Moreira LA (2011) Can Wolbachia be used to control malaria? Mem Inst Oswaldo Cruz 106:212–217
27. Raymond-Delpech V, Matsuda K, Sattelle BM, Rauh JJ, Sattelle DB (2005) Ion channels: molecular targets of neuroactive insecticides. Invert Neurosci 5(3-4):119–133.
28. Asidi AN, N'Guessan R, Hutchinson RA et al (2004) Experimental hut comparisons of nets treated with carbamate or pyrethroid insecticides, washed or unwashed, against pyrethroid-resistant mosquitoes. Med Vet Entomol 18:134–140
29. Hemingway J, Ranson H, Magill A et al (2016) Averting a malaria disaster: will insecticide resistance derail malaria control? Lancet 387:1785–1788
30. Who expert citation (WHO Expert Committee on Insecticides & World Health Organization. (1957). Expert Committee on Insecticides: seventh report [of a meeting held in Geneva from 10 to 17 July 1956]. World Health Organization. http://www.who.int/iris/handle/10665/40380)
31. Harrison CM (1952) The resistance of insects to insecticides. Trans R Soc Trop Med Hyg 46:255–263
32. Berticat C, Duron O, Heyse D et al (2004) Insecticide resistance genes confer a predation cost on mosquitoes, *Culex pipiens*. Genet Res 83:189–196
33. Ffrench-Constant RH, Bass C (2017) Does resistance really carry a fitness cost? Curr Opin Insect Sci 21:39–46
34. Lockwood JA, Sparks TC, Story RN (1984) Evolution of insect resistance to insecticides: a reevaluation of the roles of physiology and behaviour. Bull Entomol Soc Am 30:41–51
35. Davidson G (1953) Experiments on the effect of residual insecticides in houses against *Anopheles gambiae* and *A. funestus*. Bull Entomol Res 44:231–245
36. Green CA, Gass RF, Munstermann LE et al (1990) Population-genetic evidence for two species in *Anopheles minimus* in Thailand. Med Vet Entomol 4:25–34
37. Chareonviriyaphap T, Bangs MJ, Suwonkerd W et al (2013) Review of insecticide resistance and behavioral avoidance of vectors of human diseases in Thailand. Parasit Vectors 6:280
38. Rostant WG, Bowyer J, Coupland J et al (2017) Pleiotropic effects of DDT resistance on male size and behaviour. Behav Genet 47:449–458
39. Yahouedo GA, Chandre F, Rossignol M et al (2017) Contributions of cuticle permeability and enzyme detoxification to pyrethroid resistance in the major malaria vector *Anopheles gambiae*. Sci Rep 7:1109
40. Koganemaru R, Miller DM, Adelman ZN (2013) Robust cuticular penetration resistance in the common bed bug (*Cimex lectularius* L.)

correlates with increased steady-state transcript levels of CPR-type cuticle protein genes. Pestic Biochem Physiol 106:190–197
41. Wood O, Hanrahan S, Coetzee M et al (2010) Cuticle thickening associated with pyrethroid resistance in the major malaria vector *Anopheles funestus*. Parasit Vectors 3:67
42. Balabanidou V, Kampouraki A, MacLean M et al (2016) Cytochrome P450 associated with insecticide resistance catalyzes cuticular hydrocarbon production in *Anopheles gambiae*. Proc Natl Acad Sci U S A 113:9268–9273
43. Brogdon WG, McAllister JC, Vulule J (1997) Heme peroxidase activity measured in single mosquitoes identifies individuals expressing an elevated oxidase for insecticide resistance. J Am Mosq Control Assoc 13:233–237
44. Hemingway J, Brogdon WG (1998) Techniques to detect insecticide resistance mechanisms (Field and laboratory manual). In: Document WHO/CDS/CPC/MAL/986. World Health Organization, Geneva
45. Ole Sangba ML, Sidick A, Govoetchan R et al (2017) Evidence of multiple insecticide resistance mechanisms in *Anopheles gambiae* populations in Bangui, Central African Republic. Parasit Vectors 10:23
46. Ranson H, N'Guessan R, Lines J et al (2011) Pyrethroid resistance in African anopheline mosquitoes: what are the implications for malaria control? Trends Parasitol 27:91–98
47. Franciosa H, Bergé JB (1995) Glutathione S-transferases in housefly (*Musca domestica*): Location of GST-1 and GST-2 families. Insect Biochem Molec Biol 25:311–317
48. Brogdon WG, McAllister JC (1998) Insecticide resistance and vector control. Emerg Infect Dis 4:605–613
49. Dahan-Moss YL, Koekemoer LL (2016) Analysis of esterase enzyme activity in adults of the major malaria vector *Anopheles funestus*. Parasite Vectors 9:110
50. Kim YH, Lee SH (2013) Which acetylcholinesterase functions as the main catalytic enzyme in the Class Insecta? Insect Biochem Mol Biol 43:47–53
51. Pitman RM (1971) Transmitter substances in insects: A review. Comp Gen Pharmacol 2:347–371
52. Mutero A, Pralavorio M, Bride JM et al (1994) Resistance-associated point mutations in insecticide-insensitive acetylcholinesterase. Proc Natl Acad Sci U S A 91:5922–5926
53. Weill M, Lutfalla G, Mogensen K et al (2003) Comparative genomics: Insecticide resistance in mosquito vectors. Nature 423:136–137
54. Aizoun N, Aikpon R, Gnanguenon V et al (2013) Status of organophosphate and carbamate resistance in *Anopheles gambiae* sensu lato from the south and north Benin, West Africa. Parasit Vectors 6:274
55. Marban E, Yamagishi T, Tomaselli GF (1998) Structure and function of voltage-gated sodium channels. J Physiol 508:647–657
56. Dong K (1997) A single amino acid change in the para sodium channel protein is associated with knockdown-resistance (kdr) to pyrethroid insecticides in German cockroach. Insect Biochem Mol Biol 27:93–100
57. Dong K (2007) Insect sodium channels and insecticide resistance. Invertebr Neurosci 7:17–30
58. Hemingway J, Boddington R, Harris J et al (1989) Mechanisms of insecticide resistance in *Aedes aegypti* (L.) (Diptera: Culicidae) from Puerto Rico. Bulletin of Entomology Research 79:123–130
59. Vatandoost H, Mccaffery AR, Townson H (1996) *Anopheles* electrophysiological investigation of target site insensitivity mechanisms in permethrin-resistant and susceptible strain of *Anopheles stephensi*. Trans R Soc Trop Med Hyg 90:216
60. Chandre F, Darriet F, Darder M et al (1998) Pyrethroid resistance in *Culex quinquefasciatus* from west Africa. Med Vet Entomol 12:359–366
61. Ranson H, Jensen B, Vulule JM et al (2000) Identification of a point mutation in the voltage-gated sodium channel gene of Kenyan *Anopheles gambiae* associated with resistance to DDT and pyrethroids. Insect Mol Biol 9:491–497
62. Djegbe I, Boussari O, Sidick A (2011) Dynamics of insecticide resistance in malaria vectors in Benin: first evidence of the presence of L1014S kdr mutation in *Anopheles gambiae* from West Africa. Malar J 10:261
63. Ndiath MO, Cailleau A, Orlandi-Pradines E et al (2015) Emerging knock-down resistance in *Anopheles arabiensis* populations of Dakar, Senegal: first evidence of a high prevalence of kdr-e mutation in West African urban area. Malar J 14:364
64. Ikeda T, Nagata K, Shono T et al (1998) Dieldrin and picrotoxinin modulation of GABA (A) receptor single channels. Neurorepor 9:3189–3195
65. Zhao X, Salgado VL, Yeh JZ et al (2003) Differential actions of fipronil and dieldrin insecticides on GABA-gated chloride channels in cockroach neurons. J Pharmacol Exp Ther 306:914–924

66. World Health Organization (2016) World Malaria Report 2016. Document WHO/HTM/GMP/2016. World Health Organization, Geneva, p 2
67. Feachem R, Sabot O (2008) A new global malaria eradication strategy. Lancet 371:1633–1635
68. Greenwood BM (2008) Control to elimination: implications for malaria research. Trends Parasitol 24:449–454
69. Roberts R, Enserink M (2007) Malaria. Did they really say ... eradication? Science 318:1544–1545
70. Russell TL, Beebe NW, Cooper RD et al (2013) Successful malaria elimination strategies require interventions that target changing vector behaviours. Malar J 12:56
71. Sokhna C, Ndiath MO, Rogier C (2013) The changes in mosquito vector behaviour and the emerging resistance to insecticides will challenge the decline of malaria. Clin Microbiol Infect 19:902–907
72. Corbel V, Akogbeto M, Damien GB et al (2012) Combination of malaria vector control interventions in pyrethroid resistance area in Benin: a cluster randomised controlled trial. Lancet Infect Dis 12:617–626
73. Trape JF, Tall A, Diagne N et al (2011) Malaria morbidity and pyrethroid resistance after the introduction of insecticide-treated bednets and artemisinin-based combination therapies: a longitudinal study. Lancet Infect Dis 11:925–932
74. Killeen GF (2014) Characterizing, controlling and eliminating residual malaria transmission. Malar J 13:330
75. Russell TL, Lwetoijera DW, Maliti D et al (2010) Impact of promoting longer-lasting insecticide treatment of bed nets upon malaria transmission in a rural Tanzanian setting with pre-existing high coverage of untreated nets. Malar J 9:187
76. Reddy MR, Overgaard HJ, Abaga S et al (2011) Outdoor host seeking behaviour of *Anopheles gambiae* mosquitoes following initiation of malaria vector control on Bioko Island, Equatorial Guinea. Malar J 10:184
77. Trung HD, Bortel WV, Sochantha T et al (2005) Behavioural heterogeneity of *Anopheles* species in ecologically different localities in Southeast Asia: a challenge for vector control. Tropical Med Int Health 10:251–262
78. Moiroux N, Gomez MB, Pennetier C et al (2012) Changes in *Anopheles funestus* biting behavior following universal coverage of long-lasting insecticidal nets in Benin. J Infect Dis 206:1622–1629
79. Durnez L, Coosemans M (2014) Residual transmission of malaria: an old issue for new approaches. In: Manguin SE (ed) Anopheles mosquitoes – new insights into malaria vectors. ISBN: 978-953-51-1188-7 InTech
80. Kelly-Hope L, Ranson H, Hemingway J (2008) Lessons from the past: managing insecticide resistance in malaria control and eradication programmes. Lancet Infect Dis 8:387–389

Part VI

Opinions

Chapter 19

Herbal Remedies to Treat Malaria in Madagascar: Hype and Hope

Arsène Indriambelo, Mamy Arilandy Rakotomamonjy, Rakotondrafara Andriamalala, Harison Rabarison, Michel Ratsimbason, Astrid Knoblauch, and Milijaona Randrianarivelojosia

Abstract

On the island of Madagascar, prior to the arrival of the Europeans, some pathologies including malaria, locally known as *tazo* (fever), were already described. As part of the Malagasy traditional knowledge, traditional medicine mainly based on the use of herbal remedies is part of the malaria treatment still today. Across the country, hundreds of plants are identified as antimalarial, and some compounds from plants show interesting in vitro activities against human *Plasmodium*. However, it has become clear that most of the antimalarial herbal remedies traditionally used are not efficient antimalarials. In order to identify authentic antimalarial herbal remedies, methodical approaches should range from plant selection to biological screening. In this paper, we share our point of view based on our experience on antimalarial plants in Madagascar.

Key words Madagascar, Traditional knowledge and practices, Medicinal plants, Antimalarial remedies

1 Traditional Medicine in Madagascar

Since 2007, traditional medicine has been legalized by a ministerial decree as biomedicine, allowing healers to practice their profession freely in Madagascar. Evidently, traditional medical practices are complex, involving skill and experience based on the beliefs, theories, and indigenous knowledge of different cultures. Traditional medicine, practiced openly as well as secretly, is used in the maintenance of health, as well as in the prevention, diagnosis, and improvement or treatment of physical and mental illness. Traditional healers are found both in rural and urban areas in Madagascar. These can be astrologists, traditional midwives, or herbalists. In many remote and rural areas of Madagascar, traditional healers are respected in the communities, and their advice is followed.

Frédéric Ariey et al. (eds.), *Malaria Control and Elimination*, Methods in Molecular Biology, vol. 2013, https://doi.org/10.1007/978-1-4939-9550-9_19,

1.1 Traditional Healers Have Different Profiles

In Northern Madagascar they are typically elderly people called *dady* (grandmother) or *dadilahy* (grandfather). Elsewhere they are commonly called *ombiasy* or *mpimasy*. This nomenclature is suggestive of a particular power allowing them to be connected to the ancestral spirits, to guess the past and to predict the future. *Ombiasy* refers to medicine men. Women also play an important role as powerful and feared healers, including those who communicate with a queen or king's spirit, for example, through possession.

1.2 Transmission of Traditional Medical Knowledge

Community members learn and continue to administer self-traditional treatment based on what they see and hear around them. Furthermore, children or relatives of traditional healers may inherit the "power" and become accepted as traditional healers themselves. Among the *Sakalava* ethnic group, female twins are believed to have divine gifted hands and are naturally talented massagers for treating trauma. At times people become self-proclaimed healers including those who failed to complete their studies but acquired a rudimentary knowledge in science and medicine. Some healers do not easily reveal the secrets and nuances of their work to strangers. For example, it is not always easy for researchers to access information on medicinal plant use.

1.3 Healers

In subtle ways, traditional healers are considered as "*mpitsabo*" (healers), which is more than just caregivers. They are respected as remedy makers. Yet from a Christian perspective, the Malagasy traditional healers often have a negative connotation, because they may serve as idols and are suspected of practicing witchcraft [1].

Diseases can be perceived as an elementary events resulting from a disorder in the visible or invisible world. The healer's role illustrates the permeability that exists between therapeutic, social, and cultural aspects in Malagasy thought [2]. The therapeutic aspect appeals to empirical practices or to magic, ritual, and symbolic acts that are going to help the healer to restore the harmony, to reinstall his "patient" to the state in which he/she had been before his/her disease. A healer's role is indeed essential in the therapy of more complex diseases attributed to supernatural causes in connection with the Malagasy cosmogony, such as breaking taboos, wizard attacks, or possession by bad spirits, because in that case modern medicine can be perceived as ineffective. The social dimension is represented by the healer's ability to preserve the social cohesion of his community. The cultural dimension is based on beliefs and perceptions that are recognized by both healer and patient. Therefore, these three dimensions do not operate independently of each other but are connected. A traditional healer has the responsibility to take care of the members of his community individually and collectively. However, it is alarming to see traditional healers who are well established in their community and who combine traditional medicine with modern terminology. In the press and on radio, they claim to defeat all pathologies: cancer, leukemia, tuberculosis, and viral diseases.

1.4 Medical Plants

A traditional healer treats diseases using his/her knowledge of the local pharmacopeia. Traditional remedies are mainly developed from plants. They are largely administered orally as tea (decoction or infusion) or by chewing, but they are also used in steam baths or cataplasm. For example, being possessed (including convulsion) can be treated by using a plant, whose unpleasant smell is supposed to chase the evil spirit out of the body of the afflicted individual. Healers can prescribe a single plant or a plant mixture.

1.5 Traditional Medicine in a Legal Context

The practice of the traditional medicine is legal in Madagascar since 2007 and recognized as part of the health-care seeking of Malagasy people. In line with the WHO recommendations, the Malagasy government allows the integration in public health centers of improved traditional remedies produced in Madagascar. The government took the initiative to promote this form of health care in order for it to be used safely and efficiently and for it to complement modern medicine. Key actors take part in this framework, directly or indirectly, such as the Centre National d'Application de Recherche Pharmaceutique (CNARP, a governmental center for pharmaceutical research) or the Institut National de Recherches Appliquées (IMRA, a private research center). Such collaborations have improved traditional remedies including antimalarials.

1.6 Urban Medicinal Plants and the Herbal Tea Vendor

Traditional medicine is practiced both in rural and urban areas, sometimes in parallel with western medicine. In many Malagasy towns, several dozens of medicinal plant vendors are found on market places (Fig. 1). They offer fresh and dry plant materials from the local region or from distant regions. These vendors deliver on demand and advise on plants that can alleviate the symptoms reported by the clients/patients. Interestingly, some vendors look for a particular dry stem of a specific plant among several bits and pieces (Fig. 2). Those who are acquainted with commerce and modern preparations sell remedies in elaborate forms: liquid or pasty, syrups, ointments, and ointments of secret formula bearing only the name of the treated disease on the container. Also, herbal tea vendors are circulating in towns with popular remedies such as the Katrafay, a bitter tea known to combat fatigue, muscle pain, fever, and malaria.

Several plants are prescribed and taken for their antimalarial virtues, but few of them have been examined rigorously. Treating a killer parasitic disease like malaria with ineffective herbal remedies can be a threat from a public health perspective. "We use it and it seems to work" is never a proof of therapeutic efficacy.

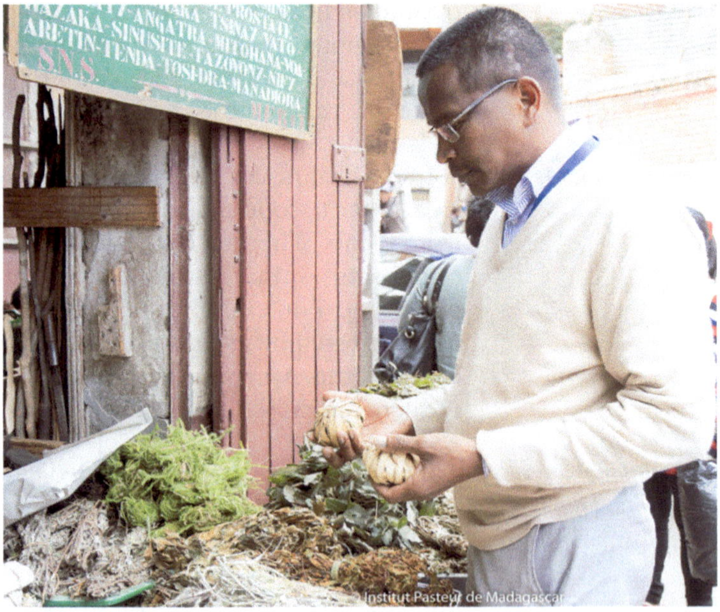

Fig. 1 Medicinal plant vendor providing Katrafay (*Cedrelopsis* sp.) stem bark in Antananarivo (© Institut Pasteur de Madagascar, Juin 2018). Milijaona Randrianarivelojosia (in the photo) asked for plants to treat tazo and fatigue. The vendors suggested a mixture of Asteraceae hidden plants already crushed (2 USD for 15 days treatment: decoction and steam bath) and also Katrafay stem bark (1 USD for 3 days treatment: bath and decoction). The smell of the bark he has in his hands is specific of *Cedrelopsis*. Plant material is from Morondava in the southwestern coastal area of Madagascar

2 Ethnobotanical Survey and Antimalarial Plants

In Madagascar the indication of plants as traditional remedies is widely shared among many ethnic groups. However, some remain tribal, clan, or family secrets. Unfortunately, most of the traditional healers are illiterate and cannot pass on their knowledge in written form. For research purposes and to archive information for future use, there is a need for ethnobotanical surveys.

2.1 Decades of Ethnobotanical Surveys

In the southwestern part of the Indian Ocean, the first written ethnomedical data was published in Mauritius and La Reunion Islands [3–5]. In Madagascar western researchers took the initiative to collect Malagasy ethnomedical information from local populations such as Dandouau [6] and Decary [7]. More specific information on Malagasy antimalarials was published early in the 1900s [8]. Later, other documents on the use of medicinal plants to treat diverse pathologies including fever and malaria were published [9–12]. All of the published data gave valuable information. Some

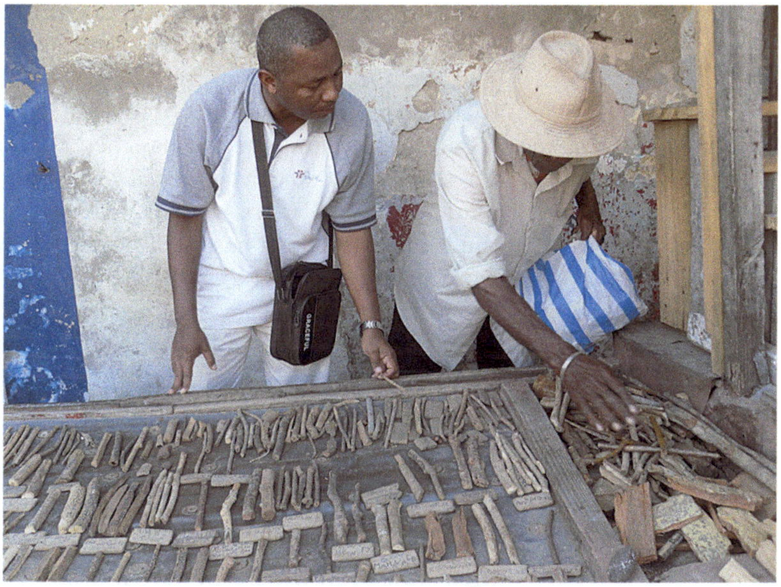

Fig. 2 Medicinal plant vendor on the main marker in the town of Toliara looking for a particular stem (© Indriambelo, Juin 2016). Arsène Indriambelo (on the left) asked for tsivoatolaka (*Gonioma malagasy*, Apocynaceae) to treat malaria. The old man started to search among dry woods already on the table. He said he has got the plant but maybe it is in his stock. Then he poured the content of plastic bag on the table. He searched again. Then, after a couple of minutes, he picked and tended a piece of stem to Arsène. No particular trait confirmed that this was indeed tsivoatolaka

authors attempted to extract data from multiple documents to compile a list of plants used to combat malaria in Madagascar [13]. They found that antimalarial plants represent by far the highest percentage among all listed plants from the documents examined. Two hundred twenty-nine species, of which about 30% are endemic to Madagascar, have been reported as having antimalarial value in Malagasy traditional medicine. They are distributed in 75 families and 176 genera.

2.2 Updating Data Prior to Plant Analysis

Scanning published papers and lay literature is an option for choosing plants to be studied to discover antimalarial drugs. However, it is better to cross-check or to complete the information with fieldwork. From our experience it is worthy going into the forests with traditional healers and interviewing villagers to obtain information. The preparation receipt of herbal remedies, their uses, and plant parts employed are among the key information that must be properly collected. When possible botanical identification is first made by experienced forest keepers and further confirmation made by comparison with specimens deposited at the botanical national park.

The traditional criteria for diagnosing *tazo* are broad, where *tazo* is currently translated as malaria. It is difficult to identify plants that are successfully curing malaria. Consequently, plants used to treat the typical symptoms of malaria, e.g., fever, fatigue, headache, muscle, and joint pain, are classified as antimalarial plants. Now and for the future, surveyors should pay attention to additive remarks made by the villagers. Again, most of the knowledge acquired by the local population has been passed onto them by word of mouth from one generation to another. It is a duty to update ethnobotanical information before they get lost. One-shot transversal surveys do not help establish a link between what is said and what is really done to treat *tazo*. During a survey in August 1993 in and around Andasibe situated at ~130 km east of Antananarivo, the capital of Madagascar [14], a traditional healer told us that "during the colonization period, when foreigners came to the rural village with Madagascan civil servants to ask about the use of plants to cure illness, some local people told lies, indicating plants around their houses to which they attributed imaginary, nonsense uses".

3 Promising Results from Malagasy Antimalarial Plant

Between 1991 and 1995, the Institut Malgache de Recherches Appliquées screened in vitro and in vivo several antimalarial plants against *Plasmodium* mainly selected from the list elaborated by Rasoanaivo et al. [13], as well as from our own prospective ethnobotanical surveys. Most of the plants tested showed weak antimalarial activity. However, there was one exception: the alkaloids isolated from *Strychnos myrtoides* locally called *retendrika* that potentiated chloroquine action against *Plasmodium*.

3.1 Retendrika + Chloroquine Combination to Treat Malaria

A fatal malaria outbreak occurred in Madagascar in the 1980s [15]. The severity of the infection was such that local populations thought it was a new disease. They called it *bemangovitra* (disease of great shivers). The country experienced also economic collapse in that period. Shortage of chloroquine and other modern antimalarial drugs drove the population back to use herbal remedies more often. During ethnobotanical fieldwork conducted between 1990 and 1992 in Andasibe, we sympathized and worked with an experienced ethnobotanist (Abrahama). One day, he kindly revealed to Rasoanaivo (senior researcher) that he was taking the infusions of *retendrika* to prevent malaria. This plant grows in Ankarafantsika, in the western part of Madagascar. Months later the ethnobotanist also mentioned that he and his family use the infusion of *retendrika* stem with one or two chloroquine tablets as a curative treatment against malaria. *Retendrika* was identified later on as *Strychnos myrtoides* Gilg & Buss (Loganiaceae).

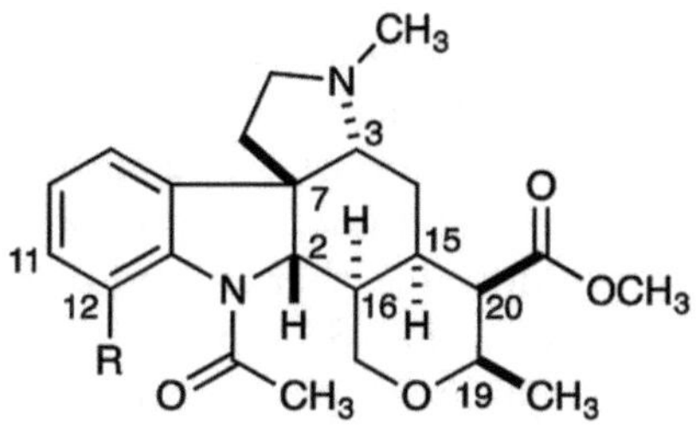

R = H, malagashanine; R = OH, 12-hydroxymalagashanine

Fig. 3 Alkaloids from *Strychnos myrtoides*

3.2 Alkaloids from Strychnos myrtoides Reverse Chloroquine Resistance

We went to Ankarafantsika to identify and collect the stem bark of *Strychnos myrtoides*. We evaluated the intrinsic anti-plasmodial activity of the crude alkaloid extracts in vitro and in vivo, but all had only moderate activity [16]. The insight from Abrahama guided our work toward drug combination assessment, and we isolated a new alkaloid, named malagashanine (Fig. 3) [17].

Malagashanine turned out to be the parent compound of a new subtype of *Strychnos* alkaloid, the C-21, Nb-secocuran indole alkaloid isolated from Malagasy *Strychnos* [18]. It had a weak anti-plasmodial activity, but when combined to chloroquine at concentrations much lower than required for anti-plasmodial effect, it enhanced chloroquine action: (1) in vitro against chloroquine-resistant *P. falciparum* FCM29 and also (2) in vivo against chloroquine-resistant *P. berghei* in mice. This confirmed the validity of the traditional recipe in experimental models [16, 19, 20].

These results were exciting and promising. At that time one of the strategies to combat malaria drug resistance was drug combination. Any reversing agent that overcomes drug resistance is a potential new strategy in malaria chemotherapy [21]. One advantage of this approach in malaria was the possibility of prolonging the chloroquine lifespan, since this antimalarial drug is of good tolerability, limited host toxicity, low cost, and available for both preventive and curative purposes.

3.3 What Does the Clinical Trial Tell Us?

Strychnos myrtoides is among the very few Malagasy medicinal plants that reached the clinical study phase [19]. In 2001, the authors initiated a controlled, double-blind, randomized clinical trial with a standardized alkaloid extract of *Strychnos myrtoides* (as phytomedicine) titrated at 20% malagashanine in Ankazobe to treat uncomplicated malaria. The main objective of the study was to assess the chloroquine resistance reversal activity of the standardized phytomedicine. The 1996 WHO protocol was used to assess therapeutic responses until 14 days of follow-up. Since chloroquine was the recommended first-line treatment in Madagascar and in many African countries at that time, two therapeutic arms were tested: chloroquine + placebo and chloroquine + *Strychnos myrtoides* alkaloid extract. Patients were aged 6–60 years old (mean age was 16 years). The authors did not describe in detail the doses of chloroquine and phytomedicine used. However, the key finding indicated that among patients who completed the 14-day follow-up, 21% (33/157) of the patients were parasitemic in the chloroquine + placebo arm and 18.8% (29/154) in the chloroquine + *Strychnos myrtoides* alkaloid arm. The outcome comparison between the two therapeutic arms demonstrated that there is no statistically significant difference, meaning that *Strychnos myrtoides* alkaloid + chloroquine combination failed to give the expected results.

The *Strychnos myrtoides* story has taught us three lessons: (1) The alkaloids that potentiate antimalarial drugs open new perspectives to understand drug resistance in malaria; (2) the promising in vitro finding was not confirmed in a clinical trial in treating uncomplicated *P. falciparum* malaria; and (3) villagers in Ankarafantsika, to whom our colleague talked, did not mention the use of the combination chloroquine + retendrika to treat malaria. Likely, such practice is not very common. From this perspective, Abrahama, who passed away many years ago, might have added chloroquine to *retendrika* when he noticed that the tazo did not disappear following retendrika intake. Nevertheless, we appreciate that a controlled, double-blind, randomized clinical evaluation of challenging phytomedicine was performed in Madagascar.

4 Crosstalk Between Herbal Remedies and Antimalarial Drugs

For the past decades, antimalarial drugs have been used according to recommendations established and adopted by most of the malaria endemic countries in the tropics. However, traditional remedies mainly made from plants remain extensively used against malaria and fever in general. Thus, in Madagascar traditional medicine has been integrated to primary health-care policies [22]. Since traditional medicine combines long-standing and evolving practices based on indigenous beliefs, their surveillance is particularly challenging, and this compromises practical application of national policies. To tackle this issue, a better surveillance of herbal medications is essential, but this cannot be achieved without thorough plant knowledge. Differences observed in the way local populations make use of them undoubtedly and clearly reflect their wide range of virtues [14, 23, 24]. Unfortunately, although an extensive literature related to conventional drug performance is already available, very little is known about safety and efficacy of plant-based remedies, even the most common ones.

Malaria control strategies in the tropics progressively turned toward the use of artemisinin-containing drugs, called artemisinin-based combination therapies (ACTs). From the peculiar situation of Madagascar, we report herein the main issues encountered when calibrated medications like ACTs are confronted to the use of empiric medicinal plants piloted by traditional practice. First of all, an unavoidable imbalance exists between intake of ACTs and herbal remedies in Madagascar. The competition between these two medicines actually starts as early as their respective accessibility to local communities. Indeed, while medicinal plants are easily available within the village from informal markets, as well as from supermarkets or convenience stores, ACTs remain essentially delivered at health facilities. Herbal drugs are commonly used as self-medication or prescribed by traditional healers to treat a broad range of illness [8, 25]. So-called antimalarial plants are then administrated to treat malaria symptoms, including fever, headache, fatigue, etc. [14, 23, 24], or to enhance the activity of standard antimalarial drugs [26]. Since such intakes cannot easily stay under the control of medical staff prescribing treatments in case of malaria attack, they are susceptible of being taken by patients prior to, during, or after their ACT regimen without any reliable evidence. As mentioned above, the safety and the intrinsic activity of herbal preparations often remain unknown, and in particular no (or few) data are available when they are associated with other active principles. Some observations have reported severe or fatal adverse events following herbal remedy intake in Madagascar. To cite a few, sudden death in a child was reported following the administration of *Crotalaria* sp. (Fabaceae) infusion as "tambavin-jaza" (childhood remedy) [27]; several cases of renal failure have been detected in hospital among children taking "tambavin-jaza" [28]. This suggests that intake of herbal drugs with antimalarials might present risks for the patient to develop adverse reactions, and such events could be excessively attributed to ACT.

Thus, a fundamental constraint emerges. Whether an adverse effect should be attributed to medicinal plants or to ACT itself (when simultaneously taken) is still a matter of debate. In addition, intrinsic activity and clinical efficacy of plants have to be demonstrated if their crosstalk with ACT (or not) has not been investigated yet. Therefore, do we have to consider the intake of herbal drugs as an exclusion criterion during clinical trials? Even though patients would be willing to inform medical staff of any episode of herbal intake, this information is compromised by two major considerations. First, it is impossible to get accurate and reliable plant identifications based on just patient interviews. Second, the secrecy is related to the cultural strength surrounding traditional medicine in general. Since traditions are deeply rooted in Malagasy societies, as they are in most African communities, herbal-based remedies are widespread. Such practices are supported by strong social values and often ruled by secrecy, so that the exact nature of the plant taken and the frequency of intakes, although critical, remain challenging even to estimate. All the aspects related to the use of herbal remedies reported herein converge: In-depth studies of medicinal plants are definitely required to ensure accurate pharmacovigilance of conventional antimalarial drugs. Since national policies in the tropics recommend ACTs as first-line drugs for treating malaria, efforts have to be particularly focused on investigating the effects of herbal intakes in this context. This means that any plant-based intake, even preparations not supposed to act as remedies like (traditional) tea, has to be documented during the follow-up of ACT-treated patients. Moreover, pharmacovigilance programs have to be developed according to an active multi-site form in which the behavior of ACTs in combination with local herbal drugs would be assessed in both rural and urban areas.

To date, concomitant intake of herbal medicines cannot be considered to compromise ACT efficacy and should not constitute an exclusion criterion in clinical studies. Nevertheless, it possibly makes analyses and interpretations more complex for a more accurate final result. For research purposes, volunteers should be discouraged from taking any herbal medicines once enrolled in an ACT study instead of being excluded. The less complex study design, the more accurate the final interpretation. Beyond toxicity risks, there is an obvious crosstalk existing between calibrated modern medicines, like ACTs, and traditional remedies made from plants. Improvement and development of in vitro methods to assess and predict the nature of these interactions are therefore crucial for a better control and a more efficient establishment of new antimalarial treatment strategies [29].

5 Traditional Medicine and Herbal Remedies Used During Malaria Outbreak

The Malagasy national malaria treatment policy was revised in December 2005. The objective was to achieve malaria elimination [29]. Chloroquine has been replaced by the artemisinin-based combination therapy (artesunate + amodiaquine). Mass distribution of insecticide-treated nets was also adopted to control the malaria vector. Malaria diagnostic has been improved with the use of malaria rapid diagnostic test. Nevertheless, multiple fatal malaria outbreaks occurred in various places: in the southeast region in 2012 [30], in Ampandriankilandy in the northwest region in 2012 [31], and in Ankililoaka in the south region in 2015 [32]. The national health system particularly suffered from antimalarial drug stock out.

5.1 Back to Traditional Medicine

We went to Ampandriankilandy to fight the malaria epidemic occurring between May and July 2012 by undertaking malaria case detection and drug administration to outpatients seen at the primary health center. Also, between October and December 2012, we explored local terminology related to malaria, information channels used around malaria, and attitudes toward health-care seeking practices in case of fever [31]. The outbreak was due to *P. falciparum*. In light of the magnitude of the outbreak, local populations perceived other causes of disease. Since mainly children suffered and died from the outbreak, some blamed a recent tetanus vaccination campaign targeting children, which had taken place a few weeks before the outbreak. Others who had received various sensitization messages in the previous months identified dirt and lack of hygiene as a potential cause of the outbreak. Some interviewees puzzled by the immediate consequences of the disease gave a supernatural explanation. The outbreak was then interpreted as a sign coming from above of the ancestors' anger due to the lack of respect for a sacred place.

Following the numerous interpretations regarding the origin of the outbreak, many prevention-related attitudes were revealed such as refusal to participate in vaccination campaigns that followed the outbreak, increased caution of hygiene and food eaten, construction of latrines and wearing amulets, and traditional objects of protection. For a minority of individuals familiar with malaria being transmitted by mosquitoes, a more regular use of bed nets resulted.

Due to the differences between local and biomedical perspectives on malaria, official messages did not have the expected impact on the population in terms of prevention and care seeking. Rather, most information retained about malaria was spread through informal channels. Most interviewees perceived malaria as a disease that is simple to treat. Tazomoka (mosquito-borne fever) is the Malagasy biomedical word for malaria, but populations in the rural commune of Ampandriakilandy do not use it. Tazo (meaning mainly fever) and tazomahery (strong fever) were the terms more commonly used by villagers to refer to malaria-related symptoms. According to local perceptions, tazo and tazomahery are not associated with mosquitoes. Each of these symptoms required specific treatments. The usual fever management strategies consisted of self-medication or recourse to traditional and biomedical caregivers. In the eyes of most Malagasy people, use of bed nets was intermittent and was not directly linked to protection against malaria.

During our mission from May to July 2012, we recorded four cases of death among children with severe malaria. They died 24 h following their arrival at the health center, despite administrated care by our medical team. At admission there were also two other fatal cases among children with uncomplicated malaria. The first case was a 10-year-old boy. When malaria was confirmed, he was treated with artesunate + amodiaquine and paracetamol. We kept him for 30 min following drug administration. His mother was given artesunate + amodiaquine tablets to complete treatment at home for 2 days, in line with the national policy. Surprisingly, she came back to the health center 7 days later with the child severely sick. Malaria was confirmed again. She held in her hand the tablets of artesunate + amodiaquine that she had not given to her son. We asked her why she did not complete the treatment, and she replied: "the other day when we left the health center I met with a friend of mine who said that modern medicine is not enough to combat the fever that kills children, and it is better to go to the traditional healer, so I did. Now, I see that my son gets bad." The child died after 2 h despite quinine administration. We did not ask what the child was given by the traditional healer, but we saw a red mark on his forehead – with a kind of clay and dying mixture.

The second case was a 6-year-old girl. We kept her during 30 min following the artesunate + amodiaquine and paracetamol administration in the morning. Then she went home, and around 5 pm her parents brought her back to the primary health center. She was conscious and able to drink but suffering from epistaxis, urinary incontinence, and agitation. She died in the evening. Her mother reported that the child had been given tambavy (herbal remedies) a couple of days prior to the medical visit.

5.2 Herbal Remedies Used During Malaria Outbreak

Following the malaria outbreak in 2015, malaria recrudescence persisted in Ankililoaka the following year. We were in the village of Andranomanintsy in the commune of Ankililoaka in June 2016 for the malaria index survey. Among 29 randomly selected children aged 6–59 months, 14 (48.3%) had malaria. We went back to Andranomanintsy and spent 2 weeks with the villagers in March 2017. We talked separately to the four traditional healers and collected from them information about the plants used to treat tazo during the malaria outbreak. With the healers we collected 26 plants from 21 plant families used according to traditional recipes. For each plant, samples were sent to the botany department of the Université d'Antananarivo for identification.

5.3 Anti-plasmodial Activities of Herbal Remedies

A selection was made in order to assess the anti-plasmodial activity of the eight most commonly used recipes (Table 1). Herbal remedies were tested against the chloroquine resistance strain of *P. falciparum* FCM29 maintained in culture. The in vitro testing was performed by the use of SYBR Green I-based assay [33]. The *P. falciparum*-infected erythrocytes were plated at 1% parasitemia and 5% hematocrit in 96-well microtiter plates and exposed to different concentrations of the traditional remedies [34] and incubated for 72 h, at 37 °C and in a gas mixture made of 5% CO_2, 5% O_2 and 90% NO_2. We carried out the test with synchronized young parasites. Extraction was performed by boiling 6 g of plant material in 40 ml of distilled water. Controls were performed to assess the background (negative control) and the parasite growth (positive control). Growth curves were obtained, and the concentration of

Table 1
Anti-plasmodial activity of herbal remedies used by traditional healers to treat malaria during the malaria outbreak in Andranomanintsy, Ankililoaka

Species	Family	Local name	Used part	IC50 (μg/ml)	Observation
Artemisia annua	Asteraceae	–	Leaf	1.46 ± 0,1	Active
Acacia sp.	Fabaceae	Tainaondry	Leaf stem	> 325	Inactive
Mascarenhasia sp.	Apocynaceae	Litsaky	Leaf stem	> 275	Inactive
Vernonia sp.	Asteraceae	Maranitratoraka	Leaf stem	> 145	Inactive
Crotalaria sp.	Fabaceae	Voapiky	Leaf stem Flower	> 100	Inactive
Acacia sp.	Fabaceae	Tainaondry	Root	57.2 ± 4,9	Inactive
Terminalia catappa	Combretaceae	Badamera	Leaf	20.8 ± 4,2	Inactive
Annona reticulata	Annonaceae	Baradefo	Leaf stem	17.1 ± 2,6	Inactive
Hypoestes sp.	Acanthaceae	Kidresy foty	Leaf stem	15.0 ± 1,4	Inactive

extract required to inhibit growth by 50% (IC50) was determined graphically by plotting concentration versus percentage inhibition. Tests were made in triplicate. The IC50 calculation was possible, because extracts were finally evaporated and residues weighted. Herbal remedies with IC50 over 10 μg/ml were considered inactive [34]. The in vitro anti-plasmodial activity of the different herbal remedies is listed in Table 1. The anti-plasmodial activity extracted from *Artemisia annua* was confirmed with its IC50 of 1.46 μg/ml. With high IC50s ranging from 15 μg/ml to more than 300 μg/ml, none of the tested herbal remedies displayed anti-plasmodial activity in vitro.

With regret, we witnessed the negative side of the traditional management of fever and malaria in this particular epidemic context in Ampandriankilandy. Even if the traditional treatment is not toxic, the delay in seeking medical care can be fatal.

In Andranomanintsy, among the tested herbal remedies frequently prescribed by traditional healers to treat malaria, none were active in vitro against *P. falciparum*. During the survey the healers were very confident about the effectiveness of their folk medicines. Some villagers emphasized that plants are the nearest pharmacy during the rainy season. But when the chief of village (JC, 53-year-old man) was alone with us as we were leaving the village, he said: "Our plants are fine to treat light tazo. But when the children get the strong tazomoka, plants use is not enough." Also, he asked money (3€) from our colleague, because his daughter was feverish and he planned to take her to the primary health center 2 h walk away from the village. Therefore, the so-called antimalarial herbal remedies prescribed or taken in self-medication to treat tazo and fever are not all antimalarials.

6 Concluding Remarks

It became clear that most of the so-called antimalarial herbal remedies traditionally used are in fact not efficient antimalarials. There is no specific Malagasy word meaning malaria. Malaria is part of *tazo*, while *tazo* is not systematically malaria, and this confusion in the precise definitions of the disease and/or the name of the plant is a major cause of incomprehension between the two partners: the pharmacologist and the traditional practitioner. For a cure to be effective, it is necessary for a given disease to encounter its specific medicinal cure. Plants used empirically to treat the symptoms of malaria such as fever, joint pain, headache (symptoms that are in fact common to other diseases, including viral or bacterial infection, inflammation, etc.) are classified as antimalarial plants. There is a need to decipher the perception of disease (*tazo*) and the reported use of herbal remedies.

South America offered humanity quinine to combat malaria. Asia offered artemisinin that plays a key role in the malaria elimination global program. Madagascar is known for its rich flora that gave rise to the globally used anticancer compound extracted from Malagasy periwinkle. We must persevere in searching for antimalarial plants. In order to identify authentic antimalarial herbal remedies, methodical approaches should range from plant selection to biological screening. Instead of purifying compounds that are extracted from plants by using nonpolar solvents such as chloroform, and screening these compounds on malaria laboratory models, we believe that it is worthwhile testing herbal remedies that are mainly extracts or infusions prepared in water to be closer to their typical uses. However, it must also be accompanied by a careful and scientific study of their possible toxic effects.

References

1. Lefèvre G (2008) Robivelo Adrienne Rodolphe, Le christianisme et l'usage des plantes médicinales à Madagascar: relecture, réconciliation, réhabilitation. Études océan Indien:40–41
2. Pierlovisi C, Pourchez L (2014) Health, culture and society traditional medicine in Madagascar - current situation and the institutional context of promotion. Health Cult Soc 7(1)
3. Bouton L (1857) Medicinal plants growing or cultivated in the Island of Mauritius. R. de Spéville & Co, Mauricee
4. Leclerq J (1864) Des plantes médicinales de l'Iles de la Réunion et de leur application à la thérapeutique. La Malle, Saint-Denis, pp 1–73
5. Daruty C (1886) Plantes Médicinales de l'Ile Maurice et des Pays Intertropicaux. de Spéville et Co, Maurice, pp 3–61
6. Dandouau A (1910) Catalogue alphabétique des Noms Malgaches. Economie de Madagascar X 1910(2 et XI). No. 1
7. Decary R (1946) Plantes et animaux utiles de Madagascar. Annales du Musée Colonial de Marseille 1946. 6ème série vol. 4
8. Ramisiray G (1901) La Médecine des Malgaches. Revue de Madagascar 3:549–555
9. Rakoto-Ratsimamanga A, Boiteau P, Mouton M (1969) Eléments de Pharmacopée Malagasy, Tome I. Imprimerie Nationale, Antananarivo

10. Descheemacker A (1979) Ravimaitso. Imprimerie St Paul, Fianarantsoa
11. Quansah N (1988) Ethnomedicine in Maroantsetra region of Madagascar. Econ Bot 42:370–375
12. Rasoanaivo P, Ratsimamanga-Urverg S, Rakoto-Ratsimamanga A (1989) Résultats d'Enquêtes Ethnobotaniques dans la Région d'Andasibe et de Beza-Mahafafy. Mémoires de l'Institut Malgache de Recherches Appliquées
13. Rasoanaivo P, Petitjean A, Ratsimamanga-Urverg S et al (1992) Medicinal plants used to treat malaria in Madagascar. J Ethnopharmacol 37:117–127
14. Randrianarivelojosia M, Rasidimanana VT, Rabarison H et al (2003) Plants traditionally prescribed to treat tazo (malaria) in the eastern region of Madagascar. Malar J 2:25
15. Randrianarivelojosia M, Raveloson A, Randriamanantena A et al (2009) Lessons learnt from the six decades of chloroquine use (1945-2005) to control malaria in Madagascar. Trans R Soc Trop Med Hyg 103:3–10
16. Randrianarivelojosia M (1994) Mise en évidence de l'action potentialisatrice vis-à-vis de la chloroquine et contribution à l'élucidation de mécanismes d'action d'alcaloïdes de retendrika (*Strychnos myrtoides* Gilg & Busse). Thèse de Doctorat ès sciences, Faculté des sciences, Antananarivo, p. 85.
17. Rasoanaivo P, Ratsimamanga-Urverg S, Milijaona R et al (1994) In vitro and in vivo chloroquine-potentiating action of Strychnos myrtoides alkaloids against chloroquine-resistant strains of Plasmodium malaria. Planta Med 60:13–16
18. Martin MT, Frappier F, Rasoanaivo P et al (1996) ^{1}H and ^{13}C spectral assignment of strychnobrasiline. Magn Reson Chem 34:489–491
19. Ramanitrahasimbola D, Rasoanaivo P, Ratsimamanga S et al (2006) Malagashanine potentiates chloroquine antimalarial activity in drug resistant Plasmodium malaria by modifying both its efflux and influx. Mol Biochem Parasitol 146:58–67
20. Rasoanaivo P, Rakotonandrasana OL, Ramanitrahasimbola D et al (2005) Traditional medicine and resistance modulators. Ethnopharmacologia 35
21. Martin SK, Oduola AMJ, Milhous WK (1987) Reversal of chloroquine resistance in *Plasmodium falciparum* by verapamil. Science 235:899–901
22. World Health Organization (2002) WHO Traditional Medicine Strategy 2002–2005. World Health Organization, Geneva
23. Penali L, Mulholland DA, Tano KD et al (2007) Low antiplasmodial activity of alkaloids and amides from the stem bark of *Zanthoxylum rubescens* (Rutaceae). Parasite 14:161–164
24. Ramisiray G (1901) Pratiques et croyances médicales des malgaches. Faculté de Médecine de Paris, Paris, p 108
25. Novy JW (1997) Medicinal plants of the eastern region of Madagascar. J Ethnopharmacol 55:119–126
26. Ramanitrahasimbola D, Ranaivoravo J, Rafatro H et al (2004) Strychnos myrtoides: a case study of a chemosensitising medicinal plant. In: Willcox M, Bodeker G, Rasoanaivo P (eds) Traditional medicinal plants and malaria. CRC Press, Boca Raton, FL, pp 141–157
27. Boiteau P (1968) De quelques cas d'acculturation concernant les noms vernaculaires de plante: dangers en résultant. Bull Acad Malgache 46:271–272
28. Andriamanjatoarinohatra R (1987) L'insuffisance rénale d'origine toxique (tambavy) chez l'enfant, vol. Doctorat en Médecine. Faculté de Médecine, Antananarivo, p 105
29. Randrianarivelojosia M, Randriasamimanana JR, Martin C (2009) Artemisinin-based combination therapies (ACTs) and herbal drugs crosstalk: facts and perspectives. Parasite 16:243–244
30. Kesteman T, Rafalimanantsoa S, Razafimandimby H et al (2016) Multiple causes of an unexpected malaria outbreak in a high-transmission area in Madagascar. Malar J 15:57
31. Mattern C, Pourette D, Raboanary E et al (2016) "Tazomoka is not a problem". Local perspectives on malaria, fever case management and bed net use in Madagascar. PLoS One 11: e0151068
32. Halm A, Seyler T, Mohamed S et al (2017) Four years into the Indian ocean field epidemiology training programme. Pan Afr Med J 26:195
33. Rason MA, Randriantsoa T, Andrianantenaina H et al (2008) Performance and reliability of the SYBR Green I based assay for the routine monitoring of susceptibility of Plasmodium falciparum clinical isolates. Trans R Soc Trop Med Hyg 102:346–351
34. Bertani S, Bourdy G, Landau I et al (2005) Evaluation of French Guiana traditional antimalarial remedies. J Ethnopharmacol 98:45–54

Chapter 20

Vade Retro Malaria: The Vagaries of Eradication Campaigns

Georges Snounou

Abstract

This paper provides, rather than a systematic review on malaria eradication attempts in history, a personal perspective on the currents that shaped past control strategies and, more briefly, on the prospects of current strategies. This essay is intentionally opinionated.

Key words Malaria, Control, Elimination, Eradication, History

1 The Dawn of Malaria

Pared to its barest bone, malaria is due to a mosquito biting a human twice. The mosquito picks up the parasite during the first bite, necessarily made on parasite carrier, and 10 or more days later, subsequent bites will generally pass it on to another human. There are two ways to break this cycle: (a) prevent the mosquito from biting, and (b) ensure that no carriers are available. Wittingly or not, these approaches are the basis of all efforts to combat malaria from ancient times to the present.

In theory, the ultimate aim of any malaria control program is the disappearance of the disease, and this can only be achieved when the pathogen is also no longer present. Of the four terms used to describe this, the most frequent are eradication and elimination; extirpation is rarely employed, while extermination is mostly used in reference to mosquitoes. All four terms derive from the Latin, either from the word "root" (eradicate, *radix*; extirpate, *stirps*) or from the word "boundary" (exterminate, *terminus*; eliminate, *limes* or *limen* = threshold). In this essay, I will consistently adopt eradication as the term to describe the disappearance of the parasite from a given area; this is indeed the goal that the malaria community is striving to achieve.

Mention of intermittent fevers, whose characteristics clearly mark them as malarious, can be found in the records left by all civilizations, ancient and recent. A common, tough by no means

Frédéric Ariey et al. (eds.), *Malaria Control and Elimination*, Methods in Molecular Biology, vol. 2013, https://doi.org/10.1007/978-1-4939-9550-9_20,

invariant, denominator was the proximity to marshy grounds, justifying the age-old held notion that malaria is due to miasma (noxious or polluted air) released by rotting organic matter. Incidentally, a miasmatic origin was also ascribed to other diseases such as cholera, yellow fever, typhoid, and other epidemics. Indeed, intermittent fevers could be effectively reduced, and in some regions abolished, by draining the surrounding marshes or lands, by moving to higher drier grounds, or by settling away from afflicted communities. Clearly an erroneous conception of malaria epidemiology is not sufficient impediment to successful malaria control.

The discovery and subsequent introduction of cinchona bark in the mid-seventeenth century to the Old World from the Spanish Peruvian possessions provided the first effective and specific drug against malaria. However, the restricted availability and high price of this "Peruvian or Jesuit's Powder/Bark," obtained from ground bark of the cinchona tree bearing the active agent quinine, precluded large-scale use. Moreover, universal trust in this remedy against malaria was gained slowly as the market was rife with bark of low quinine content or from various other plants yielding a powder with characteristic bitter taste but devoid of quinine. Fake drugs are by no means a modern curse of malaria control. The Spanish colony's monopoly was eventually broken in the mid-nineteenth century and taken up by the Dutch who eagerly established plantations of the high quinine-yielding *Cinchona ledgeriana* in Java and became the main producers of the drug, ensuring ample supplies until the invasion of Indonesia by the Japanese in 1942.

The contribution of quinine to the colonial expansions into the tropical regions during the last decades of the 1800s cannot be underestimated. Malaria, a disease among many in the temperate climes, gained preeminence as an existential health and economic threat to the tropical regions. The espousal of the germ theory of disease, formally demonstrated by Louis Pasteur in the 1860s and subsequently expanded and championed by Robert Koch, led to a scramble to find the causative agent of malaria. In 1880, the honor of the discovery of the protozoan organisms responsible went to Alphonse Charles Louis Laveran, a mere provincial French military doctor, thereby vexing the ambition of contemporary eminent medical colleagues whose grudging acceptance took a few years. Laveran named the pathogen *Oscillatoria malariae*, and he long maintained that only a single species existed. The Italian workers begged to disagree, and after careful observations they named three species, and Celli and Marchiafava proposed the genus *Plasmodium* in 1885. Laveran had to wait until 1907 for recognition of the momentous value of his discovery by a Nobel Prize. This fulfilled the first of the two conditions necessary to elaborate a rational malaria control strategy: identification of the pathogen and the ability to detect it accurately, which for malaria requires a simple microscopic examination of blood, a procedure much improved by the introduction of Romanowsky stains in the early 1900s, still used today in the form of Giemsa stain. The second sine qua non condition is knowledge of the mode of transmission. The notion that insects could act as carriers was established with Patrick Manson's demonstration in the late 1870s of the transmission of filarial nematodes by mosquitoes. In 1894 Manson, who had by then retired to London, convinced Ronald Ross of the Indian Medical Service to investigate the role of insects in the transmission of malaria. The observation in 1897 of oocysts in mosquitoes fed on infected human marks a first landmark, the second followed a year later with the mosquito transmission of bird malaria, and the third was made independently (which was vehemently contested by Ross) by Grassi in 1898–1899 in Italy in which he demonstrated the transmission of malaria to humans and established that the parasite was passed specifically by anopheline mosquitoes. For reasons best known to the Nobel committee, Ross alone was awarded the Nobel Prize in 1902, though one should not underestimate the contribution of national pride and ambition of Europe's Great Powers.

2 A Consequential Clash of Two Schools

Thus, at the turn of the nineteenth century, the stage was set for the elaboration of first earnest and rational strategies to eradicate malaria. From 1899 on, two broad schools of thought dominated: extermination of the mosquito principally by reduction of breeding sites and antilarval measures was championed by Ronald Ross [1], while extermination of the parasites in human carriers through systematic quinine treatment of carriers was championed by Robert Koch [2]. Until activities were disrupted by the outbreak of World War I, numerous malaria control schemes targeting the vector or the parasite, and in some both, were deployed in a diversity of endemic localities, to yield equally disparate results. Generally, the factors that contributed to success or failure varied with the localities where the schemes were deployed. More often than not, successes were lauded, while failures were ascribed to faulty implementation, aptly demonstrating that human nature is more predictable than malaria control.

In retrospect, the principal outcome of these valiant efforts was the birth of malariology and its adoption by a broad range of scientists and medical doctors throughout the world (at that time, few countries were free of malaria). Thus, major advances were made in all aspects of the biology of the parasite and its vector, while observations of the course of natural and experimental infections started to shed light on malaria pathology and immunology and helped improve treatment regimen. Carefully conducted field observations across the continents laid the foundations of malaria epidemiology and brought tantalizing glimpses into the intricate interplay between variable social, environmental, entomological, and parasitological factors, such that the malaria picture could differ unpredictably and drastically between two neighboring areas. In the context of eradication, two overarching conclusions could be drawn. First relatively modest efforts are sufficient to alleviate the burden of malaria within a few years or transmission seasons, often dramatically, and should these efforts diminish or stop malaria often quickly reverts to its initial levels. Second, malaria control programs are expensive to implement, to administer, and, especially, to maintain. Thus, adequate finances could only be secured when the funders deemed that the economic benefits were sufficiently offset by the expenditure. Ultimately, the key to the success of any control strategy depends on an appreciation of the importance of local conditions and of the prospects of long-term sustainability, "lessons" gleaned early last century and that are still valid today.

Of all the different experimental malaria control projects undertaken early in the twentieth century, one in my opinion merits special mention, because it sparked a philosophical rift that had a significant long-lasting impact on global strategies for malaria control two decades later. Ross' credo of an "all-out war against mosquitoes" inspired the Colonial Indian administration to attempt such an attack, and two medical officers with a keen interest in entomology and malaria, Samuel Rickard Christophers and Sydney Price James, were selected to undertake it. They were directed by Ross to select a site he considered suitable: Mian Mir, a military cantonment in Lahore, known to be highly malarious, relatively isolated and provided with an ample supply of manpower [3, 4]. Following an initial malaria survey in 1901, diverse extensive antilarval measures were devised and implemented over the next years, with little impact on the number of malaria cases. In 1909 the experiment was declared a failure, prompting in equal measure virulent personal attacks from Ross and a distrust of mosquito control in James; neither position was fully justifiable. Ross who was adept at dismissing or diminishing any failures was comforted by two well-publicized successes. A ruthless and quite expensive anti-mosquito campaign instigated by William Crawford Gorgas led to reduce yellow fever and malaria to the very low levels needed to complete the construction of the Panama Canal (1904–1914). The other was achieved by Malcolm Watson working in the Federated Malay States from 1901 onward, who obtained significant reduction of malaria by specifically targeting those mosquito species that transmit the disease to workers in the rubber plantation close to Kuala Lumpur [5, 6]. This work strongly impressed Nicolaas Hendrik Swellengrebel who was grappling with malaria in Dutch Indonesia. He melded his own careful entomological work with the work of Watson and formulated the important concept of species sanitation [6, 7].

The impact of the Mian Mir failure on the direction of control strategies was only felt when James became an internationally influential malariologist in the early 1920s. Already recognized as a tropical disease expert and an outstanding malariologist, James was chosen to set up the Malaria Therapy Centre at Horton Mental Hospital in England around 1923, in which induced malaria served to treat neurosyphilitic patients, a surprisingly successful approach devised and pioneered by Julius Wagner-Jauregg in Vienna in 1917. The insightful and detailed observations made at Horton, from its earliest day and for the next decades, propelled James's fame and reputation as a malariologist. More importantly it opened the way to unravel many of the biological characteristics of the malaria infection, of the complex relationships between the parasite and its hosts, and further allowed to conduct drug efficacy studies. It was not surprising that James was sought in 1923 to join the other respected malariologists of that time as a member of the newly formed Malaria Commission of the League of Nations. This body exerted considerable influence on the direction of malaria control policies in European nations, most of which were malarious and, by extension to their colonies, which then covered much of Africa, the Middle East, and the sub-Indian continent and most of Southeast Asia [7]. A highly affable and persuasive person, James's distrust of antilarval measures "à la Ross" was transmitted to his colleagues, and members of the Malaria Commission favored the notion that malaria had a social basis and promoted measures aimed at improving general health and socioeconomic conditions. Thus, strategies primarily based on quinine treatment were advocated since alleviating disease was considered of paramount importance [8–10]. In general, the Malaria Commission's elaborated control measures concorded with, and were guided by, the new knowledge on malaria obtained through scientific experimentation.

In the United States, the International Health Board of the Rockefeller Foundation, who had contributed to the success in Panama, opted for larval control as a means to eradicate malaria, a stance they maintained from the 1920s on. Failures of their vector species eradication strategy in various setting over the next 10 years nearly led them to abandon this approach, but the success of Frederick Lowe Soper in eradicating *Aedes aegypti* in 1934, and then the recently introduced *Anopheles gambiae* from northeastern Brazil in 1940 [11–13], rekindled their zeal (discretely extinguished with the failure to rid Sardinia of *Anopheles labranchiae* in 1950 [3, 14]). In 1924 the Rockefeller Foundation dispatched a first emissary, Lewis Wendell Hackett, to set up a malaria research laboratory in Italy. Hackett was keen to test a new larvicide, Paris green. This earned him a cool reception from the Malaria Commission. Paris green, an easily deployed powdered compound substantially more practical and safer to use than the oils previously used to smother larval breeding sites, would have merited a better reception. Consequently, the reticence of Malaria Commission created substantial tension between it and the Rockefeller Foundation, at the time two dominant actors in the field of global malaria control. I further suspect that this generated a soupçon of distrust between US and British malariologists that persisted beyond the 1940s.

3 New Weapons for a Global Eradication Strategy

At the dawn of World War II, the malaria control was a patchwork of successes and failures of a plethora of strategies ideologically aligned to one or other dogmas: vector control or health and socioeconomic improvement. For both, the weapons used, principally larvicides and quinine, were as insufficient as they were inadequate. The ability of anopheline populations to survive extraordinary attacks was often underestimated, while quinine, though a good schizonticidal drug, was inefficient at killing gametocytes and at preventing *P. vivax* relapses, and furthermore its side effects did not endear it to patients. As it has been often the case, wars act as an accelerator of scientific discoveries. The first synthetic antimalarial drugs, plasmochin and Atebrin, were produced by German scientists as a response to the shortage of quinine during World War I, though neither proved better than quinine. Similarly, the occupation of the Indonesian *Cinchona* plantations by the Japanese forces in 1942 led to acute shortages of quinine during World War II, precipitating the second major search for novel synthetic antimalarial drugs by the Allied nations [3]. This led to chloroquine and amodiaquine and a little later to primaquine (United States), as well as pyrimethamine and eventually sulfadoxine (United Kingdom). Primaquine remains the only licensed drug capable of eliminating hypnozoites, though as for all other 8-aminoquinolines including the latest tafenoquine, potential severe hemolysis in persons with glucose-6-phosphate deficiency restricts their widespread use. Chloroquine, sulfadoxine, and pyrimethamine became the preeminent antimalarials for the following decades until the emergence of resistance in *P. falciparum* restricted their use. At present chloroquine is only used to treat vivax and ovale malaria, and the sulfadoxine-pyrimethamine combination is restricted to intermittent preventative treatment in pregnant women.

Efficient as they were, these new antimalarials could not on their own justify any notion of a global strategy to control malaria. The spark that ignited such an ambitious undertaking was provided by the discovery in 1939 of the spectacular insecticidal properties of DDT, a compound first synthesized in 1874, by Paul Hermann

Müller in Switzerland. Initially used to get rid of clothes moths and crops of Colorado beetles, the compound came to the notice of the Allies military authorities who then ran various tests that were so convincing that it was given equal priority with penicillin. Prior to DDT, pyrethrum spray was used to reduce mosquito numbers, but application is needed to be done daily. DDT, on the other hand, remained on the sprayed surfaces for months, during which it fully retained to kill any insect that came in brief contact with it. The potential of DDT to malaria control was provided by its success in eliminating *A. gambiae* from Egypt, introduced to the Nile valley by boats from Soudan. This campaign was devised by Soper, who remains today the only person who can claim success in the eradication of an anopheline twice! Soper called DDT an "almost perfect insecticide." By the close of the 1940s, DDT was found to have been remarkably effective at reducing malaria incidence in Ceylon, Venezuela, and Greece.

After World War II, the League of Nations was dissolved in 1946 to emerge as the United Nations, and its Health Division became the World Health Organization (WHO) in 1948. By then most of the members of the old Malaria Commission had retired or passed away, and a new generation of malariologist emerged to form an Expert Committee on Malaria. They were aware of the potential of chloroquine, and more pertinently many had already personally established the credentials of DDT, rekindling the hope of a total war against malaria. However, in the early 1950s, the first reports of resistance to DDT appeared, but paradoxically, instead of checking such hopes, they accelerated the formulation and then the adoption of the Malaria Eradication Program on the 26th of May 1955 by the Eighth World Health Assembly [3, 15–20]. The rationale was as follows: it was estimated that it would take 6 years for resistance to DDT to emerge and that a concerted attack on mosquitoes over 4 years coupled with treatment of all cases throughout (principally by chloroquine) should lead to the disappearance of malaria *before* any resistance to DDT could emerge. The aim was no longer to eradicate the vector but to deprive it of the pool of carriers that sustain endemicity, until such a time that the parasite has been eradicated from the mosquito; recovery of anopheline populations would thereafter be of no consequence. In effect this represents a combination of the opposite dogmas proposed by Ross and Koch, into one that combines both.

The eradication strategy was straightforward: following an initial year for surveys (preparation), spraying and treatment of malaria cases begin at year 1 (attack) and continue until the infant parasite rate is recorded as negative for 3 consecutive years, followed by years during which residual foci are carefully sought and cleared (consolidation/surveillance). Eradication is officially declared after 3 consecutive years where no autochthonous cases are recorded, and thereafter surveillance continues (maintenance) until such a time malaria is no longer present globally. It was thereby expected that 10 years at most would be needed to achieve malaria eradication, irrespective of initial endemicity. The operative words were "time is of the essence" and "strict, vigilant, and sustained surveillance." An implicit condition for success was that the attack should be initiated simultaneously, not only countrywide but also region-wide, with coordination of activities in bordering regions, and to ensure that spraying will not exceed 6 years.

Over the next 14 years, initial optimism and enthusiastic uptake gave way to a grudging realization that all was not proceeding to plan. This culminated in an official recognition of shortcomings in 1969, followed by the inexorable demise of the Eradication Campaign by the mid-1970s. Malaria had undeniably disappeared from many of the countries that took up the challenge [21, 22], but unfortunately the respite that many tropical endemic regions had been afforded tragically ended with a resurgence of malaria, often as deadly epidemics. Much was written, then and since, about the plethora of factors that have contributed to this [17–20, 23]. These can be broadly grouped as (a) failure of the vectors and parasites to behave as expected, (b) fallibility of human nature extending from honest errors to outright corruption, and (c) waning funding, particularly after initial success. The fact that the timing of the Eradication Campaign coincided with postcolonial upheavals and the Cold War should not be neglected. Discussion of these numerous and varied factors is likely to be more tedious than informative; in fact, one can safely state that *all* the factors influenced progress toward eradication, but their relative contributions as obstacles varied from site to site, region to region, and country to country. Ultimately, the far-reaching consequence was that the notion of malaria eradication became discredited leading the WHO to revert to one of malaria control, whose disadvantages were decried only a few years previously. To some extent, in my opinion, this shift in vision prevented the malaria community from drawing the true lessons inherent to this admittedly embarrassing failure. It is not a little ironic that the drive to conquer malaria by attacking the vector succeeded paradoxically in depleting the ranks of field-experienced malariologists and medical entomologists, bringing the era of classical malariology to an end.

4 Eradication Phoenix

As the euphoria of the Eradication Campaign faded, new knowledge on antibodies in the late 1950s kindled the prospects of an effective vaccine against malaria. This kept the dwindling flame of eradication from being fully extinguished. Indeed, the seminal observations of Cohen, McGregor, and Carrington on the inhibitory antibodies from hyperimmune patients (1961 onward) and of

William HG Richards and then Jerome P Vanderberg and Ruth S Nussenzweig on immunization with inactivated sporozoites (1966 onwards), to name a few, brought forth the possibility of developing an efficient vaccine against malaria. Expectations to achieve this were sharply raised within a few short years in the mid-1970s with the advent of monoclonal antibodies, the development of genetic engineering, and the in vitro cultivation of *P. falciparum*. Thus, the search for an antimalarial vaccine came to dominate the research agenda from the late 1970s and remains a current research priority.

The strategy for the control of malaria during the last decades of the last century rested principally on the pillar of drug treatment. Indications that drug-resistant *Plasmodium* parasites can be readily selected were obtained for chloroquine and antifolates as early as the late 1950s. The history of the emergence and spread of drug resistance is rich in lessons and would merit a chapter. Briefly, through a combination of inadequate monitoring and an overreliance on monotherapy, by the late 1990s, malaria control programs were faced with widespread resistance to nearly all antimalarial drugs. Furthermore, this was much exacerbated by a remarkably meager financial support for research and antimalarial activities. An ambitious program, Roll Back Malaria, was promoted and launched in the early 2000s to counter the fast deteriorating malaria situation and to revive the flow of funding. To some extent, the goals set in this scheme were elevated when in 2007 Bill and Melinda Gates, emboldened by the development of new control tools and the promise of new technologies, called for the global eradication of malaria, rehabilitating in one stroke an aspiration long shunned by the malaria community. This galvanized governments, international agencies, and charitable foundations to increase their pledges for support, and malaria regained a much-valued visibility and weight on the world stage.

The first of these new tools is the insecticide-treated bed net, a highly effective and practical strategy to reduce malaria burden and transmission that was developed in the early 1980s and oft validated thereafter. The second is the rapid diagnostic test (RDTs) making it possible to confirm or establish correct diagnosis within minutes without the need of an army of trained microscopists and the associated expenses for materials and equipment. The rather rudimentary versions that first appeared in the late 1990s have now been supplanted by diverse, relatively cheap, and validated iterations. The third tool was the development of a rational framework, combining pharmacological and biological parameters, for the adoption and deployment of chemotherapeutic strategies that procure a rapid return to health along with protection from drug resistance. This culminated with the adoption toward the middle of the 2000s, after much tribulations and opposition, of artemisinin-based combination therapy (ACT) as the standard first-line treatment for *P. falciparum*.

The renewed hopes for eradication were reenforced by the distant promise inherent to the modern advances in genomics that provided the first complete genomes from a growing number of parasite and vector species and those in gene modification technologies that offered the potential to manipulate vector or parasite populations to benefit mankind. Furthermore, recent progress in whole organism-based vaccines brought some hope to reverse the failure of subunit-based vaccines to achieve full protection against infection. Indeed, vaccines that do not offer sterile protection in a high proportion of recipients are unlikely to offer much in the context of eradication.

5 An Outcome in the Balance

Over the last decade, malaria eradication efforts have yielded a global and welcome decline in malaria, with some countries declared malaria-free and many others expected to attain this status within a short time. The apparent pause in this decline over the last 2 years is worrying. The historian AJP Taylor once acerbically stated that "Napoleon III learned from the mistakes of the past how to make new ones." It seems important for the malaria community to ensure not only that they are not making new ones, but, more pertinently, that they are not repeating the old ones. Given that they share the same goal, eradication, it is not surprising that similarities in overall strategy exist between the old and the recent campaigns. I venture to suggest that of these some should be a cause for immediate concern. The three tools listed above each suffer from potentially serious deficiencies, some biological outside our control and others not. (a) Resistance to current insecticides is emerging and spreading. Furthermore, insecticide-treated bed nets, or for that matter residual spraying, do not protect from mosquitoes that bite and rest outdoors or that bite mainly at dusk or dawn. (b) Failure to respond early and decisively to the first signs of emergence of resistance to artemisinins, or at the very least to agree and adopt a future response strategy, has translated in the dissemination or emergence of such resistant parasites far beyond their initial focus. It is not clear that the new compounds feeding the pipeline to licensing will become available in time to safeguard from a potentially disastrous situation, nor that they will eventually avoid the same fate of a short therapeutic lifespan. (c) Persistence of the parasite at low levels, undetectable by RDTs and microscopy alike, as asymptomatic infections in a significant proportion of the population even in areas of low endemicity, constitutes an insidious obstacle to eradication. Failure to reduce this pool of carriers will ensure continued transmission. (d) These chinks in the eradication armor have in the last few years been accompanied with a global economic downturn that threatens the levels of funding and an increase in political instabilities that have led to global large-scale migrations and population displacements. The parallels with the situation of the Eradication Campaign in the early 1960s are obvious. Hubris, then, shielded that campaign from criticism, which helped deflect and minimize early warning signs of failure. I suggest that success of the current strategies is best served by concentrating on areas of potential or actual failure.

From my point of view, two interrelated conditions are necessary for successful eradication or, for those who still prefer it, for sustainable control. First is the true appreciation of the biological characteristics of the distinct parasite species and their manifold vectors. The near 120 years of research conducted from the time of discovery of the parasite have provided major insights, to which modern technologies are adding many more, but many important gaps remain to be filled. For example, we do not yet understand the fundamental basis of the immune responses to the infection nor the factors that govern the dynamics of the malaria infection and its transmission. In this context, the predictions from worthy mathematical modelling efforts should be treated with caution. The acquiring of this fundamental knowledge of the malaria infection merits and requires the provision of sufficient funding. Second, a recognition that the epidemiology of malaria is defined locally must guide future strategies. Minor environmental differences that occur between neighboring localities could have a substantial influence on endemicity and all its measurable factors. This makes it necessary to tailor any control measures to local conditions. The old adage "you are never as well served as when you serve yourself" is particularly pertinent. In my opinion, trained personnel are an element key to successful eradication. In this context, training must instill a solid grounding in all aspects of practical malariology and must be extended to the myriad staff recruited at the village or district level. Crucially, it is them who implement the malaria control measures, and they should be endowed with the know-how to assess the local epidemiological situation and the authority and latitude to devise and vary these measures accordingly.

Ultimately, success is not measured by the initial impressive and newsworthy reductions in endemicity, but in the ability to bring forth and sustain the much more exacting reductions over the many years that follow. The many species of malaria parasites and their vectors are highly diverse and remarkable to adapt and persist in the face of attack and to resurge should the measures against them weaken. The seemingly increasing yearly gap in the estimated funds needed to implement current malaria control efforts does not bode well for future success. The onus is on the global agencies to ensure that the levels of funding and the commitment to the training and support of those at the coalface of control persist longer than the malaria infection, a pithy statement of intent that is as easy to make as it is difficult to realize.

I do not consider that the outlook for malaria eradication is pessimistic, rather that it is in the balance and that this can be tipped favorably. The long-held belief that malaria recedes before the plow is by no means obsolete. Countries that have attained political stability have seen their malaria problem melt with the consequent increase in wealth and economic maturity that improved living conditions and health alike. As scientists, we can only encourage and applaud those with the political power to bring this about.

References

1. Ross R (1923) Memoirs, with a full account of the great malaria problem and its solution. E. P. Dutton and Company, New York
2. Koch R (1903) Die Bekämpfung der Malaria. Z Hyg Infekt 43:1–4
3. Harrison G (1978) Mosquitoes, malaria and man: a history of the hostilities since 1880. E. P. Dutton, New York
4. Bynum WF (1994) An experiment that failed: malaria control at Mian Mir. Parassitologia 36:107–120
5. Watson M (1921) The prevention of malaria in the federated Malay states. A record of twenty year's progress, 2nd edn. E. P. Dutton and Company, New York
6. Bradley DJ (1994) Watson, Swellengrebel and species sanitation: environmental and ecological aspects. Parassitologia 36:137–147
7. Verhave JP (2011) The moses of malaria. Nicolaas H. Swellengrebel (1885-1970). Abroad and at home. Erasmus Publishing, Rotterdam
8. James SP (1920) Malaria at home and abroad. John Bale, Sons & Danielsson Ltd, London
9. Corbellini G (1998) Acquired immunity against malaria as a tool for the control of the disease: the strategy proposed by the Malaria Commission of the League of nations in 1933. Parassitologia 40:109–115
10. Fantini B (1998) *Unum facere et alterum non omittere*: antimalarial strategies in Italy, 1880–1930. Parassitologia 40:91–101
11. Soper FL, Wilson DB (1943) *Anopheles gambiae* in Brazil. 1930 to 1940. The Rockefeller Foundation, New York
12. Farley JA (1994) Mosquitoes or malaria? Rockefeller campaigns in the American south and Sardinia. Parassitologia 36:165–173
13. Packard RM, Gadelha P (1994) A land filled with mosquitoes: fred L. Soper, the Rockefeller Foundation, and the *Anopheles gambiae* invasion of Brazil. Parassitologia 36:197–213
14. Brown PJ (1998) Failure-as-success: multiple meanings of eradication in the Rockefeller Foundation Sardinia project, 1946–1951. Parassitologia 40:117–130
15. Russell PF (1955) Man's mastery of malaria. Oxford University Press, London
16. Russell PF, West LS, Manwell RD et al (1963) Practical malariology, 2nd edn. Oxford University Press, London
17. Pampana EJ (1969) A textbook of malaria eradication. Oxford University Press, London
18. Litsios S (1997) The tomorrow of malaria, Revised edn. Pacific Press, Ecotrends
19. Bradley DJ (1998) The particular and the general. Issues of specificity and verticality in the history of malaria control. Parassitologia 40:5–10
20. Jackson J (1998) Cognition and the global malaria eradication programme. Parassitologia 40:193–216
21. Bruce-Chwatt LJ, De Zulueta J (1980) The rise and fall of malaria in Europe. A historico-epidemiological study. Oxford University Press, Oxford
22. De Zulueta J (1998) The end of malaria in Europe: an eradication of the disease by control measures. Parassitologia 40:245–246
23. Wilkinson L (1998) Conceptual conflict: malaria control and internecine warfare within a London postgraduate school. Parassitologia 40:239–244

Correction to: The Advanced Development Pathway of the RTS,S/AS01 Vaccine

Lorenz von Seidlein

Correction to:
Chapter 13 in: Frédéric Ariey et al. (eds.), *Malaria Control and Elimination*, Methods in Molecular Biology, vol. 2013,
https://doi.org/10.1007/978-1-4939-9550-9_13

This book was inadvertently published without updating the following corrections:

On p. 178, the word "more" in the sentence "The vaccine was more protective when children were vaccinated between 6 and 12 weeks than between 5 and 17 months of age, and a booster vaccination at 20 months provided added protection" has been replaced with "less". The sentence is updated as "The vaccine was less protective when children were vaccinated between 6 and 12 weeks than between 5 and 17 months of age, and a booster vaccination at 20 months provided added protection" in the revised version of the book.

On p. 179, the numbers 38.5% (7.8 to 59.0) in Table 1 is replaced with 51.3% (47.5 to 54.9)

The updated online version of this chapter can be found at
https://doi.org/10.1007/978-1-4939-9550-9_13

Frédéric Ariey et al. (eds.), *Malaria Control and Elimination*, Methods in Molecular Biology, vol. 2013,
https://doi.org/10.1007/978-1-4939-9550-9_21, © Springer Science+Business Media, LLC, part of Springer Nature 2019

Index

A

Frédéric Ariey et al. (eds.), *Malaria Control and Elimination*, Methods in Molecular Biology, vol. 2013, https://doi.org/10.1007/978-1-4939-9550-9, © Springer Science+Business Media, LLC, part of Springer Nature 2019

B

C

D

K

L

M

O

P

R

S

T

U

V

W

Z

MIX
Papier aus verantwortungsvollen Quellen
Paper from responsible sources
FSC® C105338

If you have any concerns about our products,
you can contact us on
ProductSafety@springernature.com

In case Publisher is established outside the EU,
the EU authorized representative is:
Springer Nature Customer Service Center GmbH
Europaplatz 3, 69115 Heidelberg, Germany

Printed by Libri Plureos GmbH
in Hamburg, Germany